LEPTIN

ENDOCRINE UPDATES
Shlomo Melmed, M.D., Series Editor

J.A. Fagin (ed.): Thyroid Cancer. 1998. ISBN: 0-7923-8326-5
J.S. Adams and B.P. Lukert (eds.): Osteoporosis: Genetics,
Prevention and Treatment. 1998. ISBN: 0-7923-8366-4.
B.-Å. Bengtsson (ed.): Growth Hormone. 1999. ISBN: 0-7923-8478-4
C. Wang (ed.): Male Reproductive Function. 1999. ISBN: 0-7923-8520-9
B. Rapoport and S.M. McLachlan (eds.): Graves' Disease:
Pathogenesis and Treatment. 2000. ISBN: 0-7923-7790-7.
W. W. de Herder (ed.): Functional and Morphological Imaging
of the Endocrine System. 2000. ISBN 0-7923-7923-9
H.G. Burger (ed.): Sex Hormone Replacement Therapy. 2001.
ISBN 0-7923-7965-9
A. Giustina (ed.): Growth Hormone and the Heart. 2001.
ISBN 0-7923-7212-3
W.L. Lowe, Jr. (ed.): Genetics of Diabetes Mellitus. 2001.
ISBN 0-7923-7252-2
J.F. Habener and M.A. Hussain (eds.): Molecular Basis of Pancreas
Development and Function. 2001. ISBN 0-7923-7271-9
N. Horseman (ed.): Prolactin. 2001. ISBN 0-7923-7290-5
M. Castro (ed.): Transgenic Models in Endocrinology. 2001
ISBN 0-7923-7344-8
R. Bahn (ed.): Thyroid Eye Disease. 2001. ISBN 0-7923-7380-4
M.D. Bronstein (ed.): Pituitary Tumors in Pregnancy
ISBN 0-7923-7442-8
K. Sandberg and S.E. Mulroney (eds.): RNA Binding Proteins:
New Concepts in Gene Regulation. 2001. ISBN 0-7923-7612-9
V. Goffin and P. A. Kelly (eds.): Hormone Signaling. 2002
ISBN 0-7923-7660-9
M. C. Sheppard and P. M. Stewart (eds.): Pituitary Disease. 2002
ISBN 1-4020-7122-1
N. Chattopadhyay and E.M. Brown (eds.): Calcium-Sensing Receptor.
2002. ISBN 1-4020-7314-3
H. Vaudry and A. Arimura (eds.): Pituitary Adenylate Cyclase-
Activating Polypeptide. 2002. ISBN 1-4020-7306-2
R.C. Gaillard (ed.): The ACTH AXIS: Pathogenesis, Diagnosis
and Treatment. 2003. ISBN 1-4020-7563-4
P. Beck-Peccoz (ed.): Syndromes of Hormone Resistance on the Hypothalamic-
Pituitary-Thyroid Axis. 2004. ISBN 1-4020-7807-2
E. Ghigo (ed.): Ghrelin. 2004. ISBN 1-4020-7770-X
C.B. Srikant (ed.): Somatostatin. 2004. ISBN 1-4020-7799-8
V.D. Castracane and M.C. Henson (eds.): Leptin. 2006. ISBN 0-387-31415-6
G. Bray and D. Ryan (eds.): Obesity and the Metabolic Syndrome. 2006.
ISBN 0-387-32163-2

LEPTIN

edited by

V. Daniel Castracane, Ph.D.
Professor Emeritus
Texas Tech University School of Medicine
Lubbock, Texas, USA

Michael C. Henson, Ph.D.
Professor and Head
Department of Biological Sciences
Purdue University Calumet
Hammond, Indiana, USA

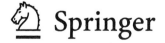

V. Daniel Castracane, PhD
Director of Laboratory Operations
Foundation for Blood Research
P. O. Box 190
Scarborough, ME, USA

Michael C. Henson, PhD
Dept. of Obstetrics and Gynecology
School of Medicine
Tulane University Health Sciences Center
New Orleans, LA, USA

LEPTIN

Library of Congress Control Number: 2005938989

ISBN-10: 0-387-31415-6
ISBN-13: 978-0387-31415-0

e-ISBN-10: 0-387-31416-4
e-ISBN-13: 978-0387-31416-7

Printed on acid-free paper.

© 2006 Springer Science+Business Media, LLC
All rights reserved. This work may not be translated or copied in whole or in part without the written permission of the publisher (Springer Science+Business Media, LLC, 233 Spring Street, New York, NY 10013, USA), except for brief excerpts in connection with reviews or scholarly analysis. Use in connection with any form of information storage and retrieval, electronic adaptation, computer software, or by similar or dissimilar methodology now known or hereafter developed is forbidden.

The use in this publication of trade names, trademarks, service marks and similar terms, even if they are not identified as such, is not to be taken as an expression of opinion as to whether or not they are subject to proprietary rights.

While the advice and information in this book are believed to be true and accurate at the date of going to press, neither the authors nor the editors nor the publisher can accept any legal responsibility for any errors or omissions that may be made. The publisher makes no warranty, express or implied, with respect to the material contained herein.

Printed in the United States of America.

9 8 7 6 5 4 3 2 1

springer.com

Dedication

This volume is dedicated to my parents, who fostered the desire for education, and to a long list of mentors and colleagues who have contributed to my scientific development; but especially to Catherine, Teresa and Jennifer who serve as the continuing inspiration of my life.

VDC

This volume is dedicated to my parents, mentors, trainees and collaborators, and to my colleagues of the Gulf coast, many of whom lost so much in the hurricanes of 2005; but especially to Libby, Kate, Rachel and Chris, who continue to make everything worthwhile.

MCH

CONTENTS

	Dedication	v
	List of Contributors	ix
	Preface	xv
1.	**The obese (*ob/ob*) mouse and the discovery of leptin** V. Daniel Castracane and Michael C. Henson	1
2.	**Leptin receptors** Laura C. Schulz and Eric P. Widmaier	11
3.	**Leptin and obesity** Lauren N. Bell and Robert V. Considine	33
4.	**Leptin and neuroendocrinology** Abhiram Sahu	53
5.	**Leptin-insulin interrelationships** Asha Thomas-Geevarghese and Robert Ratner	79
6.	**Leptin and other endocrine systems** Robert V. Considine	103
7.	**Leptin and immune function, inflammation and angiogenesis** Giuseppe Matarese, Claudio Procaccini and Veronica De Rosa	125

8.	Leptin and bone: central control of bone metabolism by leptin Shu Takeda	139
9.	Roles and regulation of leptin in reproduction Michael C. Henson and V. Daniel Castracane	149
10.	Leptin and cardiovascular disease Kamal Rahmouni, Marcelo L. Correia and William G. Haynes	183
11.	Leptin and cancer Delia-Marina Alexe and Eleni Petridou	201
12.	Lipodystrophy: the experiment of nature to study leptin Rexford S. Ahima and Malaka B. Jackson	225
13.	Pulsatile and diurnal leptin rhythms Luciana Ribeiro, João Vicente Busnello, Ma-Li Wong and Julio Licínio	247
14.	Leptin in farm animals C. Richard Barb, Gary J. Hausman and Timothy G. Ramsay	263
15.	Genetic disorders involving leptin and the leptin receptor I. S. Farooqi	309
16.	Immunoassays for leptin and leptin receptors Jehangir Mistry	319
17.	Clinical applications of leptin Elif Arioglu Oral and Alex M. DePaoli	327
	Index	359

CONTRIBUTORS

Rexford S. Ahima, MD, PhD
    Associate Professor
    University of Pennsylvania School of Medicine
    Department of Medicine, Division of Endocrinology,
      Diabetes and Metabolism
    Philadelphia, PA 19104

Delia-Marina Alexe, MD
    Research Associate
    Department of Hygiene and Epidemiology
    Athens University Medical School
    Athens, Greece

C. Richard Barb, PhD
    Research Leader
    USDA-ARS
    Animal Physiology Research Unit
    Russell Research Center
    Athens, GA 30604-5677

Lauren N. Bell, BS
    Department of Integrative and Cellular Physiology
    Department of Medicine
    Indiana University School of Medicine
    Indianapolis, IN 46202

João Vicente Busnello, MD
    Neuropsychiatric Institute
    David Geffen School of Medicine
    University of California, Los Angeles
    Los Angeles, CA

V. Daniel Castracane, PhD
 Professor Emeritus
 Department of Obstetrics and Gynecology
 Texas Tech University School of Medicine
 Lubbock, TX 79430

Robert V. Considine, PhD
 Department of Cellular and Integrative Physiology
 Department of Medicine
 Indiana University School of Medicine
 Indianapolis, IN 46202

Marcelo L. Correia, MD
 Post –doctoral Research Fellow
 Specialized Center for Research in Hypertension Genetics
 Department of Internal Medicine
 University of Iowa
 Iowa City, IA 52242

Alex M. DePaoli, MD
 Director of Global Development
 Amgen Pharmaceuticals
 Thousand Oaks, CA 91320

Veronica De Rosa, PhD
 Research Associate
 Gruppo di ImmunoEndocrinologia
 Istituto di Endocrinologia e Oncologia Sperimentale
 Consiglio Nazionale delle Ricerche
 c/o Dipartimento di Biologia e Patologia Cellulare e Molecolare
 Università di Napoli "Federico II"
 Via S. Pansini, 5
 80131 Napoli, Italy

I. Sadaf Farooqi, MD, PhD
Department of Clinical Biochemistry
University of Cambridge
Addenbrooke's Hospital
Cambridge CB2 2QQ, UK

Gary J. Hausman, PhD
Research Physiologist
USDA, ARS
Animal Physiology Research Unit
Russell Research Center
Athens, GA 30605

William G. Haynes, MD
Professor of Internal Medicine
Specialized Center for Research in Hypertension Genetics
Department of Internal Medicine
University of Iowa
Iowa City, IA 52242

Michael C. Henson, PhD
Professor and Head
Department of Biological Sciences
Purdue University Calumet
Hammond, IN 46323-2094

Affiliate Scientist
Tulane National Primate Research Center
Covington, LA 70433

Malaka B. Jackson, MD
Endocrinology Fellow
University of Pennsylvania School of Medicine
Children's Hospital of Philadelphia
Philadelphia, PA 19104

Julio Licínio, MD
    Professor of Psychiatry and Biobehavioral Sciences and Medicine/Endocrinology
    Director, Center for Pharmacogenomics and Clinical Pharmacology
    Semel Institute of Neuroscience and Human Behavior
    David Geffen School of Medicine at UCLA
    Los Angeles, CA 90095-1761

Giuseppe Matarese, MD, PhD
    Gruppo di ImmunoEndocrinologia
    Istituto di Endocrinologia e Oncologia Sperimentale
    Consiglio Nazionale delle Ricerche
    c/o Dipartimento di Biologia e Patologia Cellulare e Molecolare
    Università di Napoli "Federico II"
    Via S. Pansini, 5 80131 Napoli, Italy

Jehangir Mistry, PhD
    Vice President, Research and Development
    Linco Research, Inc
    St Charles, MO 63304

Elif A. Oral, MD
    Division of Metabolism, Endocrinology and Diabetes
    Department of Internal Medicine
    University of Michigan
    School of Medicine
    Ann Arbor, MI 48109

Eleni Petridou, MD, MPH
    Professor of Preventive Medicine and Epidemiology
    Department of Hygiene and Epidemiology
    Athens University Medical School
    Athens, Greece

Claudio Procaccini, PhD
   Research Associate
   Gruppo di ImmunoEndocrinologia
   Istituto di Endocrinologia e Oncologia Sperimentale
   Consiglio Nazionale delle Ricerche
   c/o Dipartimento di Biologia e Patologia Cellulare e Molecolare
   Università di Napoli "Federico II"
   Via S. Pansini, 5
   80131 Napoli, Italy

Kamal Rahmouni, PhD
   Assistant Professor
   Specialized Center for Research in Hypertension Genetics
   Department of Internal Medicine
   University of Iowa
   Iowa City, IA 52242

Timothy G. Ramsay, PhD
   Research Physiologist
   USDA, ARS, ANRI
   Growth Biology Laboratory
   Beltsville, MD 20705-2350

Robert E. Ratner, MD
   Vice President for Scientific Affairs
   MedStar Research Institute
   Hyattsville, MD 20783

Luciana Ribeiro, MD, PhD
   Neuropsychiatric Institute
   David Geffen School of Medicine
   University of California, Los Angeles
   Los Angeles, California, USA

Abhiram Sahu, PhD
   Department of Cell Biology and Physiology
   University of Pittsburgh School of Medicine
   Pittsburgh, PA 15261-0001

Laura C. Schulz, PhD
    Postdoctoral Fellow
    Biology Department
    Boston University
    Boston, MA 02215-2406

Shu Takeda, MD
    Department of Orthopedics
    Tokyo Medical and Dental University
    Tokyo, Japan

Asha M. Thomas-Geevarghese, MD
    MedStar Research Institute
    Hyattsville, MD 20783

Eric P. Widmaier, PhD
    Professor
    Biology Department
    Boston University
    Boston, MA 02215-2406

Ma-Li Wong, MD
    Neuropsychiatric Institute
    David Geffen School of Medicine
    University of California, Los Angeles
    Los Angeles, California, USA

PREFACE

The discovery of leptin by Friedman and his colleagues in 1994 was a seminal discovery in the study of metabolism, providing a new tool to study energy expenditure and appetite regulation. Early studies actively investigated many aspects of metabolism, obesity, and diabetes but it was soon evident that leptin was much more than a metabolic hormone. Today leptin, with almost 11,000 reports in the world's literature, is recognized to be important in many areas of physiology with strong suggestions for involvement in clinical conditions as well. Leptin, of course, remains of great interest in obesity and diabetes but other, previously unimagined, areas are now in the realm of leptin physiology. Perhaps leptin and its involvement in many areas of reproductive physiology may be of greatest interest outside of obesity, but other physiological arenas are becoming increasingly involved in the broader understanding of leptin and its pleiotropic functions. These areas include cardiovascular disease, bone physiology, immune regulation, and even cancer and genetics. Clinical trials have suggested other areas of leptin pharmaceutical potential beyond the original promise of obesity management. These topics and others, for the first time, have been collected in one volume as the first comprehensive review of leptin and its many actions. This area will continue to increase and is now compounded by new endocrine factors that have been elucidated in the wake of leptin's explosion onto the physiological scene. The future seems promising for an increased physiological understanding and the development of clinical applications. This volume will serve as the basis for understanding the past and present of leptin, and to indicate where the future direction of leptin may lead.

V. Daniel Castracane, PhD
Michael C. Henson, PhD

Chapter 1

THE OBESE (*ob/ob*) MOUSE AND THE DISCOVERY OF LEPTIN

V. Daniel Castracane[1] and Michael C. Henson[2]

[1]*Texas Tech University School of Medicine, Lubbock, TX and* [2]*Department of Biological Sciences, Purdue University Calumet, Hammond, IN*

Abstract: Early theories describing appetite regulation and energy expenditure suggested the lipostatic theory, which hypothesized that some peripheral signal, probably from adipose tissue, would feedback to central satiety centers to modulate food intake and body weight. However, the experimental techniques needed to validate this hypothesis were lacking at that time. Subsequently, two strains of obese mutants, the *ob/ob* mouse and later the *db/db* mouse, were discovered 50 and 40 years ago, respectively, and proved invaluable to studying the regulation of food intake, energy expenditure, and obesity. Prior to the development of today's more sophisticated techniques for studying biological and biochemical processes, the use of parabiosis, the surgical attachment of two animals with a shared blood supply, provided valuable insights into the obesity. Information gained from studies of these strains of mice, especially in parabiotic studies with normal counterparts, provided evidence for a humoral factor involved in appetite regulation and initiated the search for its identity. Friedman et al discovered leptin in 1994, and demonstrated that this hormone, the product of the *obese* (*ob*) gene, was produced in white adipose tissue and served as the peripheral signal to the central nervous system of nutritional status. After leptin's discovery, the obese mouse model continued to play an invaluable role in the validation of leptin as the missing factor in the *ob/ob* mouse and served as a principal model to delineate the many facets of leptin physiology.

Key words: obesity, *ob/ob* mouse, *db/db* mouse, genetics, mice, leptin

"Corpulence is not only a disease itself, but a harbinger of others."
                                                                                Hippocrates

1. INTRODUCTION

The multiple health risks of obesity have been recognized for centuries, but the last few decades have seen an explosion in its incidence, most particularly in developed countries such as the United States and those in Western Europe. Perhaps the most important findings related to obesity in the last decade are linked to our greater understanding of appetite regulation and energy expenditure that began with the discovery and characterization of leptin in 1994[1], followed by the identification of other associated endocrine factors. The breakthrough which led to this discovery was the finding of a genetic mutation in the mouse that resulted in obesity.[2] This obese mouse (*ob/ob*) provided insights into obesity that led to expectations that some unknown humoral substance was related to the development of obesity in this model. This chapter will describe the initial contributions of the *ob/ob* mouse (and other mouse models) that led to the discovery of leptin and the invaluable role of this model in proving that the newly discovered adipokine was indeed responsible for controlling adiposity in mice.

2. THE OBESE (*ob/ob*) MOUSE

The obese mouse was a fortuitous observation in the summer of 1949 at the Jackson Laboratories in Bar Harbor. Obese mice were first distinguished from littermates at 4-6 weeks of age. Thereafter, they continued to increase in weight and generally weighed four times more than wild type littermates. In the original report, no effect on lifespan through 12 months had been observed. The obese animals were sterile and offspring of heterozygote matings demonstrated the 3:1 ratio characteristic of a recessive gene. The gene responsible was designated *ob (2)* (now *Lep*).

In subsequent reports, the *ob/ob* mouse was reported to come from a noninbred stock where the mutant presented with massive obesity and marked hyperglycemia and was originally considered to be a model of diabetes. The syndrome is inherited as a single autosomal recessive gene located on chromosome 6. The original mutation was transferred to a standard inbred strain (C57BL/6J) by a series of cross-intercross matings. This resultant BL/6 obese mouse was characterized by obesity, hyperphagia, transient hyperglycemia, and elevated plasma insulin concentrations (10-50 times normal) that were associated with a huge increase in the number and size of the beta cells of the pancreas. Mutants of both sexes are infertile.[3] When the obese mutation is expressed on a different genetic background, markedly different diabetic syndromes can result, emphasizing the role of other genetic interactions with the obese mutation.[4]

3. THE DIABETIC (*db/db*) MOUSE

Another mutant strain of obese mouse called diabetes (*db/db*) was discovered, also at the Jackson Laboratory, in 1966.[5] This mutation occurred in an inbred mouse strain (C57BL/Ks) and is characterized by a metabolic disturbance resembling diabetes mellitus. The diabetic mutant is phenotypically similar to the obese mutant but demonstrates symptoms at an earlier age and has a shortened life span. Blood sugar concentrations were 200 mg/dl or greater by 8 weeks of age and reached or exceeded 300 mg/dl by 10 weeks of age. Both *diabetes* (*db*) and *obese* (*ob*) genes are inherited as autosomal recessives with complete penetrance. Diabetic homozygotes are fat, hyperglycemic, and nonfertile, and heterozygotes cannot be visually distinguished from normals. Attempts to control weight by food restriction, as has been successful with the obese mouse, failed in the *db/db* mouse. The *db/db* mouse did not survive on reduced food intake.[5]

The *db* mutation is located on chromosome 4. Homozygous mutants are infertile, obese, hyperphagic, and consistently develop severe diabetes with marked hyperglycemia. Increased plasma insulin concentrations are observed as early as 10 days of age. The concentration of plasma insulin peaks at 6-10 times normal by 2-3 months, then drops precipitously to near normal levels. During the time of elevated insulin, there is a hyperplasia and hypertrophy of the beta cells of the Islets of Langerhans. The decline in plasma insulin is concomitant with islet atrophy and rising blood glucose, which remains above 400 mg/dl until death at 5-8 months.[3]

4. PARABIOSIS

It is important to remember that in 1950 many of the experimental techniques so readily available today had not yet been developed. One of the available techniques that was important in determining the nature of this new obese mutant was parabiosis. Parabiosis is the union of two living organisms, which may occur spontaneously as in the example of conjoined twins or, most often as used in experimental research, following a surgical procedure in laboratory animals such as the mouse or rat.[6,7] This technique allows animals with different physiologies or genetics to be conjoined and to share their blood supplies. Any humoral (endocrine) substances would readily communicate from one parabiont to the other. This technique was most useful in establishing the fact that a humoral substance was involved in the regulation of satiety and adiposity.[8]

Early studies demonstrated the existence of a satiety center within the hypothalamus and that hypothalamic lesions would result in obesity.[9,10] Hervey parabiosed a pair of rats, one being normal and the other bearing hypothalamic lesions that resulted in obesity. This union resulted in severe weight loss and the suppression of appetite in the normal partner. We now appreciate that the increased adipose tissue of the hypothalamic lesioned rat produced excess leptin and affected the normal partner, but not the lesioned rat, since the satiety center had been destroyed.[8]

In a series of important studies, Coleman used the parabiotic technique to great advantage to define the nature of the genetic obese mouse models which had become recognized at his institution. When a normal mouse is parabiosed with an *ob/ob* obese mouse, the obese animal gains weight at a slower rate and approaches the normal body weight, demonstrating that some factor from the normal control mouse crosses to the obese mouse to induce satiety. These results demonstrate that the obese mouse has a deficiency of a satiety factor, but also does not produce any substance which adversely affects the normal partner. The *ob/ob* mouse exhibits an improvement in plasma insulin and blood glucose concentration. In sharp contrast, when the *db/db* obese mouse was parabiosed with a normal mouse, the normal mouse rapidly lost weight, became hypoglycemic and died of apparent starvation within 50 days of surgery.[3,8,11] The *db/db* mouse in this parabiosis pair was resistant to the endogenous factor produced by the normal partner.

Later studies would confirm that leptin was produced in the normal mouse and decreased many aspects of obesity in the *ob/ob* partner. In the *db/db* mouse, the mutation caused a loss of the leptin receptor and therefore was resistant to any leptin effect. Moreover, this mutant produced excess leptin (due to increased adipose tissue), which suppressed appetite severely in the normal partner and resulted in death. Parabiotic studies using rat models have also been valuable in identifying the humoral nature of appetite regulation. As an example, parabiosis of normal pairs of rats, in which one member of the pair was tube fed twice its normal amount, would result in obesity, but the partner had a slight decrease in food consumption from that seen in individuals in normal parabiotic pairs. These studies indicated that some humoral factor from the obese partner would cross the parabiotic union to suppress food intake in the normal partner.[12]

5. EARLY THEORIES OF APPETITE REGULATION

Early hypotheses of the feedback regulation of satiety have been reviewed by Hervey.[12] Three hypotheses were presented to identify the substance responsible for this closed loop regulatory system for energy balance. The first was that the maintenance of body temperature indicated the state of energy balance. The second, the "glucostatic theory" suggested that glucose was the peripheral signaling factor. It was considered unlikely that either of these theories could account for the quantitative accuracy needed for the regulation of energy balance or for its time properties. Variation in body temperature or of blood glucose are short lived and rapidly corrected by intrinsic regulatory mechanisms. It seemed unlikely that these short lived signals could regulate appetite over the 24 hour period.

Early studies by Kennedy[9] and Hervey[10] presented the theory of the "lipostat" model, which proposed that adipose tissue produces some substance that serves as a feedback regulator for appetite suppression. Total fat mass is the variable that was sensed and ultimately regulated. Eventually, leptin was confirmed to be that adipose tissue-derived substance that performed this function. This theory seemed better able to account for the longterm accuracy of energy balance and for the time course of response. Future studies, using the *ob/ob* and *db/db* obese mouse models in different parabiotic unions, would provide evidence to support the lipostatic theory, although still not identifying the responsible signaling molecule.

6. THE STAGE IS SET

Numerous studies, particularly the parabiosis studies by Coleman,[4, 8, 11] had clearly demonstrated that a circulating satiety factor existed, which was absent in the *ob/ob* mouse. The *db/db* mouse was resistant to this satiety factor. Earlier studies had strongly suggested that adipose tissue might be the source of this lipostatic feedback signaling molecule. With this background, Jeffrey Friedman and colleagues at the Rockefeller University began a search to identify this satiety signal. In 1994, Friedman's group[1] was able to isolate and characterize this "obesity hormone" using molecular biology techniques. Following an elegant sequence of experiments, they reported the cloning and sequencing of the mouse *ob* gene and its human homologue. They determined that, in adipose tissue, *ob* encodes a 4.5 kilobase mRNA that features a highly conserved 167 amino acid open reading frame. The predicted amino acid sequence has 84% homology in humans and mice and could be identified as a secreted protein. In codon 105, a nonsense mutation was identified in the original congenic C57BL/6J *ob/ob* mouse strain that expressed a 20-fold quantitative enhancement in *ob* mRNA, while another *ob* mutant, the co-isogenic SM/Ckc-+ $^{Dac}ob^{2J}/ob^{2J}$ strain, did not synthesize *ob* mRNA. Clearly, a collective appraisal of these data indicated that the protein product of the *ob* gene (leptin) functioned as a signaling adipokine that helped to modulate adipose mass. To this end, the authors were intuitive in pointing out that the extensive homology of the described gene product among vertebrate species suggested that its function was highly conserved and that it would now be possible to test for mutations in the human gene. These experiments would mark significant progress toward a better understanding of the alterations to normal metabolic pathways that result in obesity.

7. STUDIES FOLLOWING THE DISCOVERY OF LEPTIN

When the product of the *ob* gene was cloned, it was then possible to test this protein for its presumed role in the regulation of adiposity and the *ob/ob* mouse presented the ideal animal model for such a validation. Pellymounter et al[13] administered daily intraperitoneal injections of recombinant Ob protein at different doses and observed a dose- and time-dependent lowering of body weight, percentage body fat, food intake and serum concentrations of glucose and insulin. In addition, metabolic rate, body temperature, and activity levels were increased by this treatment. These parameters were not changed beyond the levels observed in lean controls, suggesting that the Ob protein normalized the metabolic state of the *ob/ob* mouse. Normal mice treated with Ob protein exhibited a nonsignificant decline in body weight and indicated that the *ob/ob* mouse was more sensitive to the Ob protein than were lean controls. Similar results, using the *ob/ob* mouse, were reported by Weigle et al.[14] Taken together, these studies successfully demonstrated that the Ob protein had a significant role in the regulation of adiposity and metabolism.

Halaas et al[15] also demonstrated the endocrine action of the Ob protein in the *ob/ob* mouse with a reduced food intake and increased energy expenditure, but also found it to be ineffective in the *db/db* mouse. They also found the obese mouse to be more sensitive to treatment with the protein than the wild type mice. They proposed that this 16 kilodalton protein be called leptin, derived from the Greek root *leptos*, meaning thin. Campfield et al[16] demonstrated similar aspects of the Ob protein in the *ob/ob* mouse and its ineffectiveness in the *db/db* mouse. Perhaps most importantly, they compared injection of Ob protein into the cerebral ventricle and found this route to be more effective than the intraperitoneal route of administration, demonstrating the primary action on central neuronal networks that play an important role in feeding behavior and energy balance.

Lipodystrophic mice, lacking white adipose tissue and therefore having very low leptin levels, have a similar phenotype to the *ob/ob* mouse. They are hyperphagic, insulin resistant, and diabetic. Metabolic abnormalities of the *ob/ob* mouse, as well as those of lipodystrophic mice can be normalized with leptin treatment.[17] Similarly, transplantation of white adipose tissue from normal mice to lipodystrophic mice would successfully ameliorate metabolic disturbances.[18] However, adipose tissue transplanted from leptin deficient mice was ineffective[19], indicating the importance of leptin in this corrective action. The transplantation of white adipose tissue to the *ob/ob* mouse had similar results to those reported for the lipodystrophic mice. Specifically, white adipose tissue from normal congenic mice could prevent any further increase in adiposity in young animals, and in both young (40 days) and older (13 months) mice was able to reduce body weight and normalize insulin. White adipose tissue from *ob/ob* mice had no effect.

In addition to the original mutant mouse strains, *ob/ob* and *db/db*, there are other natural mutations and a large number of transgenic mouse models for different forms of obesity, each designed to investigate specific biochemical aspects of the many pathways related to energy and appetite regulation. It is estimated that more than 50 of these genetic models, including both natural and transgenic mutations, exist to study the etiology of obesity[20], with an emphasis on potential pharmaceutical preparations that would serve to suppress appetite via these newly discovered pathways. Virtually every major pharmaceutical company has an interest in developing some medical approach to this exploding clinical obesity epidemic. Studies continue into the roles and mechanisms of leptin action and *ob/ob* and *db/db* mice continue to serve as important tools for these investigations.[21-24] We owe much to those observant individuals who recognized the first mutants and developed those strains that were so useful in understanding leptin before it had a name. They served then as vital investigatory tools to characterize the newly isolated protein and they continue to serve as useful models for better understanding this exciting new hormone.

REFERENCES

1. Y. Zhang, R. Proenca, M. Maffei, M. Barone, L. Leopold and J.M. Friedman, Positional cloning of the mouse *obese* gene and its human homolog. *Nature* **372**:425-432 (1994).
2. M. Ingalls, M.M. Dickie and G.D. Snell, Obese, a new mutation in the house mouse. *J. Heredity* **41**: 317-318 (1950).
3. D.L. Coleman, Diabetes-obesity syndromes in mice, *Diabetes* **32**, Suppl. 1:1-6 (1982).
4. D.L. Coleman, and K.P. Hummel, The influence of genetic background on the expression of the *obese* (*Ob*) gene in the mouse. *Diabetologia* **9**, 287-293 (1973).
5. K.P. Hummel, M.M. Dickie, and D.L. Coleman, Diabetes, a new mutation in the mouse. *Science* **153**, 1127-1128 (1966).
6. M.X. Zarrow, J.M. Yochim, and J.L. McCarthy, Experimental Endocrinology. A sourcebook of basic techniques. Academic Press, New York (1964).
7. J.C. Finerty, Parabiosis in physiologic studies, *Physiol Rev* **32**:277-302 (1952).
8. D.L. Coleman, Effects of parabiosis of obese with diabetic and normal mice. *Diabetologia* **9**, 294-298 (1973).
9. G. C. Kennedy, The role of depot fat in the hypothalamic control of food intake in the rat. *Proc. R. Soc. Lond. B. Biol. Sci.* **140**, 578-596 (1953).
10. G. R. Hervey, The effects of lesions in the hypothalamus in parabiotic rats. *J. Physiol.* **145**, 336-352 (1959).
11. D.L. Coleman, Lessons from studies with genetic forms of diabetes in the mouse. *Metabolism* **32**, 162-164 (1983)
12. G. R. Hervey, Regulation of energy balance. *Nature* **222**, 629-631 (1969).
13. M. A. Pelleymounter, M.J. Cullen, M.B. Baker, R. Hecht, D. Winters, T. Boone, and F. Collins, Effects of the *obese* gene product on body weight regulation in *ob/ob* mice *Science* **269**, 540-543 (1995).
14. D. S. Weigle, T.R. Bukowski, D.C. Foster, S. Holderman, J. M. Kramer, G. Lasser, C.E. Lofton-Day, D.E. Prunkard, C. Raymond and J.L. Kuijper, Recombinant ob protein reduces feeding and body weights in the *ob/ob* mouse. *J. Clin. Invest.* **96**, 2065-2070 (1995).
15. J.L. Halaas, K.S. Gajiwala, M. Maffei, S.L. Cohen, B.T. Chait, D. Rabinowitz, R.L. Lallone, S.K. Burley, and J.M. Friedman, Weight-reducing effects of the plasma protein encoded by the *obese* gene. *Science* **269**, 543-546 (1995).
16. L.A. Campfield, F.J. Smith, Y. Guisez, R. Devos, and P. Burn, Recombinant mouse OB protein: Evidence for a peripheral signal linking adiposity and central neural networks. *Science* **269**, 546-549 (1995).
17. S. Kebanov, C.M. Astle, O. DeSimone, V. Ablamunits, and D.E. Harrison, Adipos tissue transplantation protects *ob/ob* mice from obesity, normalizes insulin sensitivity and restores fertility. *J. Endocrinol.* **186**, 203-211 (2005).
18. O. Gavrilova, B. Marcus-Samuels, D. Graham, J.K. Kim, G.I. Shulman, A.L. Castle, C. Vinson, M. Ekhaus, and M.L. Reitman, Surgical implantation of adipose tissue reverses diabetes in lipoatrophic mice. *J. Clin. Invest.* **105**, 271-278 (2000).
19. C. Colombo, J.J. Cutson, T.Yamauchi, C. Vinson, T. Kadowaki, O. Gavrilova, and M.L. Reitman, Transplantation of adipose tissue lacking leptin is unable to reverse the metabolic abnormalities associated with lipoatrophy. *Diabetes* **51**, 2727-2733 (2002).
20. D.J. Good, Using obese models in research: Special considerations for IACUC members, animal care technicians and researchers. *Lab Animal* **34**, 30-37 (2005).

21. S.M. Turner, P.A. Linfoot, R.A. Neese, and M.K. Hellerstein, Sources of plasma glucose and liver glycogen in fasted *ob/ob* mice. *Acta. Diabetol.* **42**, 187-193 (2005).
22. M. O. Olatinwo, G.K. Bhat, C.D. Stah, and D.R. Mann, Impact of gonadotropin administration on folliculogenesis in prepubertal ob/ob mouse. *Mol. Cell. Endocrinol.* **245**, 121-127 (2005).
23. F. Dong, X. Zhang, X. Yang, L.B. Esberg, H. Yang, Z. Zhang, B. Culver, and J. Ren, Impaired cardiac contractile function in ventricular myocytes from leptin-deficient *ob/ob* obese mice, *J. Endocrinol.* **188**, 25-36 (2006).
24. R. Anzawa, M. Bernard, S. Tamareille, D. Baetz, S. Confort-Gouny, J.P. Gascard, P. Cozzone and D. Feuvray, Intracellular sodium increase and susceptibility to ischaemia in hearts from type 2 diabetic *db/db* mice. *Diabetologia* **20**, 1-9 (2006).

Chapter 2

LEPTIN RECEPTORS

Laura C. Schulz and Eric P. Widmaier
Department of Biology, Boston University, Boston, MA

Abstract: Leptin receptors belong to the class I cytokine receptor family. Although six isoforms of receptor have been identified, only two are thus far known to be linked with intracellular signaling, and only the longest isoform (ObRb) has full signaling capability. Structure/function analyses of the receptor suggest that it exists constitutively as a dimer in the plasma membrane; each receptor of the dimer pair reversibly binds a single leptin molecule. Upon binding, signaling cascades are initiated beginning with activation of receptor-associated janus kinase 2 (JAK2) and phosphorylation of two key tyrosine residues on the intracellular portion of the receptor. Of particular importance for the growing list of leptin actions is that binding of leptin to its longest receptor isoform activates numerous intracellular signals following JAK2 activation, which have been associated with a wide variety of biological actions in different tissues. Expression of the two longest forms of leptin receptor (ObRa and ObRb) appears to be nearly ubiquitous in mammalian tissues, although ObRb is abundantly expressed only in hypothalamus. Total loss of function mutations in ObRb appear to be rare in the human population, but polymorphisms in the regions of the gene that code for extracellular domains of the receptor are not uncommon, and are associated with weight gain and adiposity. An important area of future research will be the identification of the physiological functions of shorter isoforms of the leptin receptor, and continuing characterization of the types and frequencies of receptor polymorphisms in the human population.

Key words: Leptin receptor; domains; signaling mechanisms; localization; receptor structure and function; mouse; human; mammals

1. INTRODUCTION

The *ob/ob* and *db/db* mice display a similar phenotype, which includes obesity, hyperphagia, and infertility. Parabiosis experiments in the 1970s suggested that the *ob* gene encodes a soluble factor that circulates in blood, whereas the *db* gene encodes its receptor[1]. Shortly after *ob* was sequenced, and its product was named leptin[2], the leptin receptor gene was identified using an expression library, and then mapped to the *db* locus[3]. The *db* gene is located on chromosome 4 in mice and 1p in humans[4]. It was the identification of a receptor and the functional link between receptor activation and cell function that defined leptin as a hormone. This review will focus on the structure and function of the mammalian receptor, using the murine and human receptors as well-characterized models. However, it should be noted that partial or complete sequences of leptin receptors have been obtained for many different mammalian species, including *S. scrofa*[5], *B. taurus*[6], *R. norvegicus*[7], *M. lucifugus*[8], and in other vertebrates, and in all cases the structural domains of the receptor are highly conserved (Table 1).

SPECIES	ObRb % nucleotide homology to human
Macaca mulatto (macaque)	97%
Bos taurus (cow)	88%
Canis familiaris (dog)	88%
Sus scrofa (pig)	88%
Ovis aries (sheep)	88%
Myotis lucifugus (little brown bat)	87%
Rattus norvegicus (rat)	83%
Mus musculus (mouse)	81%
Gallus gallus (chicken)	62%

Table 1: Relative similarity of leptin receptor isoform B cDNA sequences of representative species to the human sequence. Mammalian sequences were compared using BLAST. The *G. gallus* comparison is from reference 144.

2. DOMAIN STRUCTURE OF THE LEPTIN RECEPTOR

The leptin receptor is a member of the class I cytokine receptor family, also known as the gp130 receptor family, although unlike many other family members, the leptin receptor does not form oligomers with gp130[9]. Six different isoforms of the leptin receptor, ObRa-f, have been identified, also sometimes referred to as LepRa-f or LRa-f in the literature[10] (Figure 1).

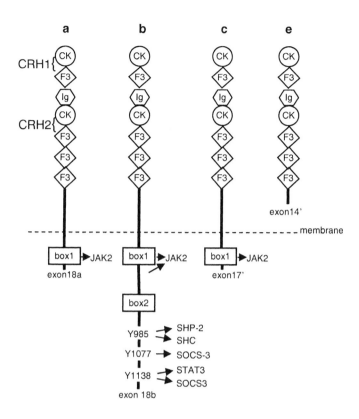

Figure 1: Domain structures of leptin receptor isoforms. Only those isoforms present in multiple mammalian species are shown. CK=cytokine receptor domain; F3 = fibronectin type 3 domain; Ig = immunoglobulin C2 domain; CRH = cytokine receptor homology domain. Y = tyrosines thought to be involved in signaling. Box 1 and 2 are cytokine boxes. The names of the unique terminal exon of each isoform are shown. Arrows symbolize receptor domains or residues that are involved in binding and activation of the signaling proteins indicated (see text for further description of signaling mechanisms).

All six receptor isoforms are products of the *db* gene and share the first 805 amino acids, comprising exons 1-14 in the mouse[11]. The smallest isoform -ObRe- is not a receptor but rather is a soluble binding-protein, as it contains no transmembrane or cytoplasmic domains and is present in the circulation of some species. In rodents, to create ObRe, the splice site at the 3'-end of exon 14 is skipped, and a contiguous sequence, exon 14', which contains a stop codon and a polyadenylation signal, is transcribed. In humans, the sequence 5' of exon 14 does not have a polyadenylation signal, and this may be why no ObRe transcript has been found to exist in humans.

Instead, in humans the ObRe protein is generated by proteolytic cleavage[12,13].

The remaining larger isoforms share exons 1-15, exon 16, which contains the transmembrane domain, and exon 17, which contains the first 29 amino acids of the cytoplasmic domain[11,14]. After this, amino acid 889 in the mouse, ObRa, c, and d have different terminal exons, encoding just 3, 5, and 11 amino acids respectively, whereas the terminal exon of ObRb, also called ObR long or ObRl, has an additional 273 amino acids. Although ObRa-c have been identified in multiple species, ObRd has thus far only been found in the mouse[11], and ObRf has only been found in the rat[14].

All six receptor isoforms possess the extracellular domains of the leptin receptor, which are the only portions of the receptor required for ligand binding[2,15,16]. This part of the receptor is heavily N-glycosylated, with sugars accounting for 36% of its total mass[17]. There are nine disulfide bonds, which contribute to the three dimensional structure of the receptor[17,18]. Near the N-terminus are adjacent conserved cytokine receptor and fibronectin type 3 (FN3) domains, together referred to as a CRH, or *c*ytokine *r*eceptor *h*omologous domain[2]. This CRH is separated from a second CRH by a conserved immunoglobulin C2 domain. There are two additional FN3 domains in the extracellular portion of the receptor, distal to the second CRH. Only the CRH domain closest to the membrane is involved in ligand binding[16,19], possibly via hydrophobic interaction with the a and c helices of leptin[20]. Two amino acids, F-500 and Y-441 are particularly important for leptin binding[21]. The conserved WSXWS motif in the second, but not the first, CRH domain is glycosylated, suggesting that the first CRH domain may be buried within the tertiary structure of the receptor[17].

Each leptin receptor can bind one leptin molecule[21-23]. However, intracellular signaling requires a dimerized receptor in which each receptor in the pair is bound to a leptin molecule. It is the extracellular portion of the leptin receptor that is sufficient for dimerization to occur[22]. Unlike other cytokine receptors, unoccupied leptin receptors exist constitutively as dimers in the cell membrane[22,24,25]. Disulfide bonds within the second CRH domains of each receptor are involved in assembling these pre-formed dimers[20,21]. The binding of two leptin molecules, one to each receptor, does not enhance dimerization, which requires ligand binding in most other cytokine receptors[23-25]. There is evidence, however, that leptin binding induces a conformational change in the dimers[24], and that this in turn may result in clustering of the homodimers[19]. Once activated, the receptors induce intracellular signaling by the Janus kinase/signal transducer and activator of transcription (JAK/STAT) pathway. Two critical cysteine residues in the FN3 domains proximal to the membrane are required for clustering-induced signaling[16,20]. In cells which co-express ObRa and b, heterodimerization does not occur in the absence of leptin[22,24,25], but may occur to a small degree in

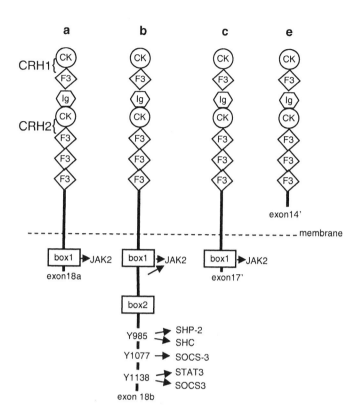

the presence of leptin[26]. Thus, coexpression of ObRa likely does not have any significant affect on signaling by pre-formed dimers of ObRb[26,27]. The extracellular domain is followed by a single, short, hydrophobic domain which spans the membrane, and is contained by exon 16 in the mouse[11].

3. SIGNALING PATHWAYS INITIATED BY INTRACELLULAR DOMAINS OF THE ACTIVATED LEPTIN RECEPTOR

Activation of leptin receptors directly or indirectly activates multiple signaling pathways that involve kinase-induced phosphorylation of proteins, including JAK2/STAT3, erbB2, ERK, IRS1 and rho/rac[15,28-31]. Signaling requires the presence of intact intracellular domains of the receptor. The leptin receptor is an external tyrosine kinase receptor; upon ligand binding each receptor can bind and activate the tyrosine kinase JAK2, which then cross-phosphorylates tyrosine residues in the other receptor in the dimer[32] (Fig. 1). There is an absolute requirement of the intracellular cytokine box 1 motif of the receptor for activation of JAK2. This sequence is present in all the transmembrane isoforms. Most studies, however, have focused on signaling mediated by ObRb, the only isoform which has conserved intracellular tyrosine residues and which is capable of activating the transcription factor STAT3[2,15]. In addition, only ObRb has a cytokine box 2, which does not seem to be required for JAK2 activation, and a sequence of 15 amino acids downstream of box 1 that are required for optimal JAK2 activation[32,33].

The numbering of the crucial tyrosine residues that can be phosphorylated by JAK2 follows the mouse sequence. Phosphorylation of Y1138 is required for binding of the SH2 domains of STATs and of SOCS3, a *suppressor of cytokine signaling* that reduces ObRb signaling partly by inhibiting JAK2 phosphorylation[34-37]. SOCS3 also is activated by binding to Y985 and to a lesser extent to Y1077[38]. Binding of STAT3 or SOCS3 to the phosphorylated leptin receptor enables their phosphorylation, and thus activation, by JAK2[39]. Although STAT1, STAT5, and STAT6 can be phosphorylated upon leptin treatment *in vitro*[15,36,40,41], only STAT3 activation has been observed *in vivo*, although this has only been determined in hypothalamus and blood mononuclear cells[42,43]. In addition to tyrosine phosphorylation of STAT3 mediated by binding of STAT3 to phospho-Y1138, STAT3 must be activated (phosphorylated) by the serine kinase ERK for nuclear translocation and full induction of gene expression[44]. One of the genes activated by leptin-induced STAT3 signaling, is SOCS3, which therefore represents a negative feedback action on the leptin receptor[37].

Phosphorylation of Y985 of ObRb by JAK2 leads to the phosphorylation of SH2 domain-containing proteins SHC and the tyrosine phosphatase SHP2[34-36]. The extent to which SHP2 inhibits JAK/STAT signaling is unclear. In most studies, SHP2 activation does not inhibit phosphorylation of STAT3[35,45-47], but mutation of Y985 does enhance STAT3 phosphorylation, suggesting an inhibitory role of SHP2[34]. SHP2 can dephosphorylate a tyrosine residue at position 974 of the receptor, but the role if any of this tyrosine in intracellular signaling has not been defined[48]. The phosphorylated SHC binds and activates Grb2, which in turn leads to activation of the MEK/ERK pathway[49]. Grb2 is also activated by SHP2[46] and may also be able to interact directly with JAK2[45].

Unlike Y985 and Y1138, the third intracellular tyrosine residue on ObRb, Y1077, appears to reside in a hydrophobic region of the receptor that would not be accessible to ligand binding and kinase activity, and therefore this residue appears to be less important for leptin signaling. Indeed, in one study when Y985 and Y1138 were mutated by site-directed mutagenesis, Y1077 did not become phosphorylated, showing that it is incapable of being independently activated[45]. Further, this tyrosine was not required for STAT3 or ERK activation *in vivo* in the hypothalamus[45]. However, Y1077 was shown to activate STAT5 in pancreatic cells *in vitro*[36], suggesting that it may have a role in mediating at least some of the actions of leptin.

Although ObRb is sometimes referred to as the "signaling isoform," there is evidence of signaling by other isoforms, particularly ObRa (also called the "short isoform" before the discovery of isoforms c-f). For example, in cells transfected with ObRa and not any other ObR isoform, leptin treatment induces activation of JAK2, erbB2, IRS1 and ERK/MAPK[29,30,50], although ERK activation is not as great as that induced by ObRb[30]. JAK2 can activate ERK without phosphorylation of receptor Y985, suggesting a mechanism different from the ERK activation pathway in ObRb[46]. Leptin treatment increased expression of c-fos, c-jun and jun-B via ObRa in transfected CHO cells[51], but failed to induce c-fos expression in COS cells transiently transfected with ObRa[30]. The ability of ObRa to induce immediate-early gene expression *in vivo* is unknown.

4. TISSUE DISTRIBUTION OF LEPTIN RECEPTORS

Leptin receptors are nearly ubiquitously expressed (Table 2; references 52-82). ObRa is expressed in almost every tissue that has been examined[83,84]. ObRb expression, by contrast, is abundant only in the hypothalamus, but is expressed at lower levels elsewhere.

Tissue	ObR long	ObR short	ObR soluble	References
Adipose	Yes	a, c		52, 53
Adrenal gland				54, 55
Medulla	No	Yes		
Cortex	Yes	Yes		
Bone	Yes	a, c	Yes	56
Brain	Yes	a, c	Yes	57
Endothelial	Yes			58, 59
Fetal	Yes	Yes		60, 61
Heart	Yes	a	Yes	62
Hematopoetic stem cells	Yes			63
Hypothalamus	Yes	a		64
Immune Cells				65-66
Monocytes	Yes	Yes		
Natural killer	Yes	Yes		
Neutrophils	No	Yes		
Thymocytes	Yes			
Intestine	Yes	Yes		67
Kidney		Yes		68
Liver	Yes	a,c	Yes	69
Lung	Yes	Yes		70
Mammary	Yes	Yes		71
Muscle	No	a		72
Ovary	Yes	Yes		73
Pancreas	Yes	Yes		74
Peripheral nerves	Yes	a	Yes	75
Pituitary	Yes	Yes		76
Placenta	Yes	Yes	Yes	8, 77
Salivary gland	Yes	Yes		78
Skin	Yes	a		79
Taste buds	Yes	a		80
Testis	Yes	a,c	Yes	81
Thyroid	Yes			82

Table 2. Localization of leptin receptor isoforms in mammals. The specific short isoform (a, c, etc.) is given where known. References are not necessarily inclusive.

Initial studies using RNase protection assays and RT-PCR on extracts of whole tissues, also identified the rest of the brain, adrenal, fat, heart, lymph nodes, lungs and spleen as tissues in which ObRb accounted for more than 5% of ObR expression[83,84]. That these receptors may mediate physiological functions is suggested by the fact that expression of the receptor has in some cases been found to be regulated and to change under certain circumstances. For example, expression of multiple forms of the receptor increase in placenta during the course of pregnancy in several species, including rat[85], baboon[86], mouse[8] and bat[8].

In addition to leptin receptor expression in normal tissues, functional leptin receptors may play a role in a variety of cancers including adipocyte[87], adrenal[88], breast[89], bladder[90], endometrial[91], liver[92], leukemia[93], ovarian[94], pituitary[95] and prostate[96] cancers. Evidence for this hypothesis stems from the observation that leptin receptors are expressed in the above cancers, and leptin induces proliferation in at least some human cancer cells *in vitro*[97].

5. ISOFORM-SPECIFIC FUNCTIONS OF LEPTIN RECEPTORS

The widespread expression of leptin receptors in tissues throughout the mammalian body suggests that in addition to its well-characterized role in regulating appetite and metabolic rate via actions in the hypothalamus, leptin receptors may mediate numerous other physiological functions, and indeed this turns out to be the case. Many of these functions are covered elsewhere in this volume. In this review, we will focus on select functions that have been attributed to specific receptor isoforms. The physiological importance of ObRb is the best established. The *db/db* mouse mutation is caused by a single substitution that creates a splice site that results in the production of almost no ObRb[98]. Thus, it is essentially an ObRb knockout mouse. The gross phenotype of the *db/db* mouse is indistinguishable from that of the leptin-deficient *ob/ob* mouse; it is obese, hyperglycemic, hyperinsulinemic and infertile[1]. Neuron-specific transgenic expression of ObRb in *db/db* mice has demonstrated that many, but not all ObRb functions occur in neuronal tissue[99]. Neuronal expression of ObRb corrected almost completely for adiposity, fertility, thermal regulation, and glucose regulation in *db/db* mice. Of note, however, is that the regulation of leptin secretion is not normal in *db/db* mice expressing neuronal ObRb, suggesting that ObRb expression on adipocytes may be important in regulating leptin secretion.

A mouse model called the LepR1138 mouse has been created with a single substitution at Y1138 of ObRb, which prevents phosphorylation of STAT3, and presumably inhibits SOCS3 phosphorylation, but is otherwise intact[100]. This mouse is obese and hyperphagic, indicating the importance of the ObRb-mediated STAT3 pathway in mediating effects of leptin. More specifically, the appetite-regulating peptides proopiomelanocortin and agouti-related peptide are abnormally expressed, but neuropeptide Y is unaffected in the Y1138 mutants. STAT3 signaling appears to mediate most, but not all of weight-regulating actions of ObRb, as these mice weigh 10% (males) - 20% (females) less than *db/db* mice. The Lepr1138 mice are hyperglycemic, but only about half as much as *db/db* mice. Similarly, changes in thermoregulation, thyroid function and locomotor activity exist, but are less severe in the Lepr1138 mice than in *db/db* mice[101]. The Lepr1138 mice are actually longer than normal mice, in contrast to the short *ob/ob* and *db/db* mice. Thus, leptin activation of STAT3 actually inhibits linear growth, at least in this strain of mouse.

The STAT3 pathway is less important for the regulation of reproduction than for the regulation of energy balance[100]. Female Lepr1138 mice have normal estrous cycles, unlike female *db/db* mice, although their cycles begin at a slightly later age than in normal mice. Ovulation and corpus luteum function appear normal, but overall fecundity may be reduced; only 3 of 7 Lepr1138 mice bore young in this study[100]. Further research is needed to determine whether this is significantly less than in normal mice, and whether it is due to specific effects on the reproductive axis or to changes in activity due to impaired energy balance.

One or more of the short receptor isoforms is involved in transporting leptin across the blood brain barrier, but they are not the only, or possibly even the primary, transport mechanism. ObRa and ObRc are highly expressed in the choroid plexus[2,102,103] and in brain capillary endothelium[103,104]. ObRf has a similar distribution in the rat, but is less abundant than ObRa and c[103]. The putative transport activity of ObRa is not a function of its location in neural tissue, *per se*. Both ObRa and c are capable of binding and internalizing leptin in transfected CHO cells[105], while ObRa-transfected kidney cells, but not untransfected controls, transport leptin from the apical to the basolateral side[106].

The data on the relative importance of leptin receptors in leptin transport in intact animals are less clear. In Koletsky rats, which have no functional leptin receptors, leptin concentrations in the cerebrospinal fluid are normal, whereas plasma leptin concentrations are sharply elevated[107]. However, in young Koletsky rats, the plasma leptin concentration is well below the saturating concentration for the leptin transport system in normal rats[107,108]. Intravenously injected leptin also crosses the blood brain barrier at a reduced rate in Koletsky rats[109]. Thus, leptin transport may occur in the genetic absence of leptin receptors, but it is reduced. Similarly, the brains of Koletsky rats perfused with radiolabeled leptin show specific leptin transport into the brain at a rate identical to that of normal rats, but this transport was saturated at a lower concentration in the leptin receptor null rats[108]. The New Zealand obese mouse model is characterized by peripheral, but not central, leptin resistance[110]. Leptin transport into the brain is reduced in this mouse, but this is not associated with decreased expression of ObRa or ObRc[103], suggesting the existence of another transporter.

In contrast, in an ObR-knockout mouse which lacks all leptin receptor isoforms, leptin transport *in vivo* was sharply reduced, and remaining leptin transport appeared to be non-specific[103]. In support of the idea that ObR contributes to the portion of blood-brain barrier transport that is regulated is the finding that a high fat diet induces ObRa expression[111]. Other studies, however, have failed to find any change in expression of ObR short forms at the blood brain barrier in response to a brief fast or a high fat diet, despite changes in leptin transport[103,112].

The soluble leptin receptor, ObRe, acts as a binding protein for leptin in the plasma in humans and mice[113,114]. It was initially proposed that the soluble receptor may contribute to elevated plasma leptin levels during pregnancy or obesity by inhibiting binding of leptin to its target cell receptors, as has been established for other hormone-binding proteins. *In vitro*, leptin bound to ObRe cannot activate ObRb, although the presence of this complex does not interfere with the ability of equal concentrations of free leptin to bind ObRb[115,116]. However, the overall effect of ObRe *in vivo*, is to *enhance* leptin activity. Infusion of soluble receptor enhances the effectiveness of leptin treatment in leptin null *ob/ob* mice[117]. This may simply be due to higher plasma leptin concentrations resulting from the predicted decreased leptin clearance from the circulation. Overexpression of the soluble receptor leads to elevated plasma leptin concentrations, without increasing adipose leptin expression[117]. By contrast, decreased soluble leptin receptor concentrations are present in obesity, a leptin resistant state[118-121], and fasting and weight loss both increase plasma ObRe concentrations in mice and humans[122,123].

6. LEPTIN RECEPTORS AND HUMAN HEALTH

Leptin receptors have been found to play a role in several aspects of human health. Not surprisingly, they are most associated with energy homeostasis, but there are other conditions in which leptin receptor function appears to be important. The genetics of obesity and leptin will be reviewed in more depth in another chapter. However, it should be noted that leptin receptor alleles have been associated with obesity in humans. A mutation which results in loss of the transmembrane and intracellular domains of the receptor has been identified, and is associated with a phenotype that includes morbid obesity and infertility[124]. Thus, leptin receptor mutation in humans results in a phenotype as severe as that seen in mouse models.

Polymorphisms in the leptin receptor gene which typically affect the extracellular portion of the receptor and which do not result in such severe loss of function are more common[125,126]. The Q223R mutation has been particularly well studied[127]. It has been associated with obesity, weight gain, increased body fat and increased abdominal fat[126,128-131], although no association with obesity was seen in other studies[127,132,133]. In a group of Pima Indians, Q223R was associated with altered energy expenditure and abdominal adipocyte size, but did not have a significant effect on total body fat[134]. In a study of Japanese men, Q223R was associated with elevated low density lipoprotein levels and reduced effectiveness of the cholesterol-lowering drug Simvistatin[135].

In addition to the involvement of leptin receptors in obesity, elevated soluble leptin receptor concentrations are associated with sleep apnea, independent of BMI[136]. Significantly lower soluble leptin concentrations are observed in women with endometriosis[137]. As discussed above, leptin receptors are expressed in many tumor cell types. In addition, the leptin receptor polymorphism Q223R, in combination with a mutation in leptin itself, has been associated with an increased incidence of non-Hodgkins lymphoma[138]. The Q223R variant is also associated with increased bone mineral density[139], whereas the A861G variant is correlated with the severity of spine ossification[140].

Finally, leptin receptors are also important in animal production. In pigs, leptin receptor gene polymorphisms have been identified that are associated with litter size, backfat thickness and feed efficiency[141,142]. In dairy cattle, a leptin receptor polymorphism has been associated with leptin concentrations in late pregnancy[143]. Leptin receptors have also been cloned in the chicken and turkey, but associations between specific polymorphisms and production traits have not yet been identified[144,145].

ACKNOWLEDGEMENTS

The authors thank Ms. Kristy Townsend for a critical review. This work was partially supported by NSF grant IBN0446057 to EPW and NIH grant F32 HD045116 to LCS.

ABBREVIATIONS NOT DEFINED IN THE TEXT

BMI   body mass index
CHO   Chinese hamster ovary (cells)
ERK   extracellular signal regulated kinase
GRB2   growth factor receptor-bound protein 2
IRS1   insulin receptor substrate 1
MEK   MAPK (mitogen-activated protein kinase)/ERK kinase
SH2   src homology domain 2
SHC   SH2 domain-containing protein
SHP2   SH2 domain-containing phosphotyrosine phosphatase 2
Q, R, G, A, F, W, S, Y: glutamine, arginine, glycine, alanine, phenylalanine, tryptophan, serine, tyrosine

REFERENCES

1. D. L. Coleman, Obese and diabetes: two mutant genes causing diabetes-obesity syndromes in mice. *Diabetologia,* **14**, 141-8 (1978).
2. Y. Zhang, R. Proenca, M. Maffei, M. Barone, L. Leopold, and J. M. Friedman, Positional cloning of the mouse obese gene and its human homologue, *Nature,* **372**, 425-432 (1994).
3. L. A. Tartaglia, M. Dembski, X. Weng, N. Deng, J. Culpepper, R. Devos, G. J. Richards, L. A. Campfield, F. T. Clark, J. Deeds, C. Muir, S. Sanker, A. Moriarty, K. J. Moore, J. S. Smutko, G. G. Mays, E. A. Wool, C. A. Monroe, and R. I. Tepper, Identification and expression cloning of a leptin receptor, OB-R. *Cell,* **83**, 1263-71 (1995).
4. W. K. Chung, L. Power-Kehoe, M. Chua, and R. L. Leibel, Mapping of the OB receptor to 1p in a region of nonconserved gene order from mouse and rat to human. *Genome Res,* **6**, 431-8 (1996).
5. Z. T. Ruiz-Cortes, T. Men, M. F. Palin, B. R. Downey, D. A. Lacroix, and B. D. Murphy, Porcine leptin receptor: molecular structure and expression in the ovary. *Mol Reprod Dev,* **56**, 465-74 (2000).
6. M. Pfister-Genskow, H. Hayes, A. Eggen, and M.D. Bishop, The leptin receptor (LEPR) gene maps to bovine chromosome 3q33. *Mamm Genome,* **8**, 227 (1997).
7. S. C. Chua, W. K. Chung, X. S. Wu-Peng, Y. Zhang, S. M. Liu, L. Tartaglia, L. and R. L. Leibel, Phenotypes of mouse diabetes and rat fatty due to mutations in the OB (leptin) receptor. *Science,* **271**, 994-6 (1996).
8. J. Zhao, K. L. Townsend, L. C. Schulz, T. H. Kunz, C. Li, and E. P. Widmaier, Leptin receptor expression increases in placenta, but not hypothalamus, during gestation in *Mus musculus* and *Myotis lucifugus. Placenta,* **25**, 712-22 (2004).
9. K. Nakashima, M. Narazaki, and T. Taga, Leptin receptor (OB-R) oligomerizes with itself but not with its closely related cytokine signal transducer gp130. *FEBS Lett,* **403**, 79-82 (1997).
10. J. A. Cioffi, A. W. Shafer, T. J. Zupancic, J. Smith-Gbur, A. Mikhail, D. Platika, and H. R. Snodgrass, Novel B219/OB receptor isoforms: possible role of leptin in hematopoiesis and reproduction. *Nat Med,* **2**, 585-9 (1996).
11. S. C. Chua, I. K. Koutras, L. Han, S. M. Liu, J. Kay, S. J. Young, W. K. Chung, and R. L. Leibel, Fine structure of the murine leptin receptor gene: splice site suppression is required to form two alternatively spliced transcripts. *Genomics,* **45**, 264-70 (1997).
12. M. Maamra, M. Bidlingmaier, M. C. Postel-Vinay, Z. Wu, C. J. Strasburger, and R. J. Ross, Generation of human soluble leptin receptor by proteolytic cleavage of membrane-anchored receptors. *Endocrinology,* **142**, 4389-93 (2001).
13. H. Ge, L. Huang, T. Pourbahrami, T. and C. Li, Generation of soluble leptin receptor by ectodomain shedding of membrane-spanning receptors *in vitro* and *in vivo. J Biol Chem,* **277**, 45898-903 (2002).
14. M. Y. Wang, Y. T. Zhou, C. B. Newgard, C.B. and R. H. Unger, A novel leptin receptor isoform in rat. *FEBS Lett,* **392**, 87-90 (1996).
15. N. Ghilardi, S. Ziegler, A. Wiestner, R. Stoffel, M. H. Heim, and R. C. Skoda, Defective STAT signaling by the leptin receptor in diabetic mice. *Proc Natl Acad Sci U S A,* **93**, 6231-5 (1996).
16. T. M. Fong, R. R. Huang, M. R. Tota, C. Mao, T. Smith, J. Varnerin, V. V. Karpitskiy, J. E. Krause, and L. H. Van der Ploeg, Localization of leptin binding domain in the leptin receptor. *Mol Pharmacol,* **53**, 234-40 (1998).

17. M. Haniu, T. Arakawa, E. J. Bures, Y. Young, J. O. Hui, M. F. Rohde, A. A. Welcher, and T. Horan, Human leptin receptor. Determination of disulfide structure and N-glycosylation sites of the extracellular domain. *J Biol Chem,* **273**, 28691-9 (1998).
18. T. Hiroike, J. Higo, H. Jingami, H. and H. Toh, Homology modeling of human leptin/leptin receptor complex. *Biochem Biophys Res Commun,* **275**, 154-8 (2000).
19. L. Zabeau, D. Defeau, J. Van der Heyden, H. Iserentant, J. Vandekerckhove, J. and J. Tavernier, Functional analysis of leptin receptor activation using a Janus kinase/signal transducer and activator of transcription complementation assay. *Mol Endocrinol,* **18**, 150-61 (2004).
20. H. Iserentant, F. Peelman, D. Defeau, J. Vandekerckhove, L. Zabeau, L. and J. Tavernier, J. Mapping of the interface between leptin and the leptin receptor CRH2 domain. *J Cell Sci,* **118**, 2519-27 (2005).
21. Y. Sandowski, N. Raver, E. E. Gussakovsky, S. Shochat, O. Dym, O. Livnah, M. Rubinstein, R. Krishna, and A. Gertler, Subcloning, expression, purification, and characterization of recombinant human leptin-binding domain. *J Biol Chem,* **277**, 46304-9 (2002).
22. R. Devos, Y. Guisez, J. Van der Heyden, D. W. White, M. Kalai, M. Fountoulakis, and G. Plaetinck, Ligand-independent dimerization of the extracellular domain of the leptin receptor and determination of the stoichiometry of leptin binding. *J Biol Chem,* **272**, 18304-10 (1997).
23. P. Mistrik, F. Moreau, and J. M. Allen, BiaCore analysis of leptin-leptin receptor interaction: evidence for 1:1 stoichiometry. *Anal Biochem,* **327**, 271-7 (2004).
24. C. Couturier, and R. Jockers, Activation of the leptin receptor by a ligand-induced conformational change of constitutive receptor dimers. *J Biol Chem,* **278**, 26604-11 (2003).
25. E. Biener, M. Charlier, K. V. Ramanujan, N. Daniel, A. Eisenberg, C. Bjorbaek, B. Herman, A. Gertler, and J. Djiane, Quantitative FRET imaging of leptin receptor oligomerization kinetics in single cells. *Biol Cell,* (2005).
26. D. W. White, and L. A. Tartaglia, Evidence for ligand-independent homo-oligomerization of leptin receptor (OB-R) isoforms: a proposed mechanism permitting productive long-form signaling in the presence of excess short-form expression. *J Cell Biochem,* **73**, 278-88 (1999).
27. D. W. White, K. K. Kuropatwinski, R. Devos, H. Baumann, H. and L. A. Tartaglia, Leptin receptor (OB-R) signaling. Cytoplasmic domain mutational analysis and evidence for receptor homo-oligomerization. *J Biol Chem,* **272**, 4065-71 (1997).
28. M. G. Myers, Jr., Leptin receptor signaling and the regulation of mammalian physiology, *Rec Prog Horm Res*, **59**, 287-304 (2004).
29. A. Eisenberg, E. Biener, M. Charlier, R. V. Krishnan, J. Djiane, B. Herman, B. and A. Gertler, Transactivation of erbB2 by short and long isoforms of leptin receptors. *FEBS Lett,* **565**, 139-42 (2004).
30. C. Bjorbaek, S. Uotani, B. da Silva, B. and J. S. Flier, Divergent signaling capacities of the long and short isoforms of the leptin receptor. *J Biol Chem,* **272**, 32686-95 (1997).
31. I. Sobhani, A. Bado, C. Vissuzaine, M. Buyse, S. Kermorgant, J. P. Laigneau, S. Attoub, T. Lehy, D. Henin, M. Mignon, and M. J. Lewin, Leptin secretion and leptin receptor in the human stomach. *Gut,* **47**, 178-83 (2000).
32. G. Bahrenberg, I. Behrmann, A. Barthel, P. Hekerman, P. C. Heinrich, H. G. Joost, and W. Becker, Identification of the critical sequence elements in the cytoplasmic domain of leptin receptor isoforms required for Janus kinase/signal transducer and activator of transcription activation by receptor heterodimers. *Mol Endocrinol,* **16**, 859-72 (2002).

33. J. Kloek, W. Akkermans, and G. M. Beijersbergen van Henegouwen, Derivatives of 5-aminolevulinic acid for photodynamic therapy: enzymatic conversion into protoporphyrin. *Photochem Photobiol,* **67**, 150-4 (1998).
34. L. R. Carpenter, T. J. Farruggella, A. Symes, M. L. Karow, G. D. Yancopoulos, and N. Stahl, Enhancing leptin response by preventing SH2-containing phosphatase 2 interaction with Ob receptor. *Proc Natl Acad Sci U S A,* **95**, 6061-6 (1998).
35. C. Li, and J. M. Friedman, Leptin receptor activation of SH2 domain containing protein tyrosine phosphatase 2 modulates Ob receptor signal transduction. *Proc Natl Acad Sci U S A,* **96**, 9677-82 (1999).
36. P. Hekerman, J. Zeidler, S. Bamberg-Lemper, H. Knobelspies, D. Lavens, J. Tavernier, H. G. Joost, and W. Becker, Pleiotropy of leptin receptor signalling is defined by distinct roles of the intracellular tyrosines. *Febs J,* **272**, 109-19 (2005).
37. C. Bjorbaek, K. El-Haschimi, J. D. Frantz, and J. S. Flier, The role of SOCS-3 in leptin signaling and leptin resistance. *J Biol Chem,* **274**, 30059-65 (1999).
38. S. Eyckerman, D. Broekaert, A. Verhee, J. Vandekerckhove, and J. Tavernier, Identification of the Y985 and Y1077 motifs as SOCS3 recruitment sites in the murine leptin receptor. *FEBS Lett,* **486**, 33-7 (2000).
39. J. E. Darnell, Jr., I. M. Kerr, I.M. and G. R. Stark, Jak-STAT pathways and transcriptional activation in response to IFNs and other extracellular signaling proteins. *Science,* **264**, 1415-21 (1994).
40. C. I. Rosenblum, M. Tota, D. Cully, T. Smith, R. Collum, S. Qureshi, J. F. Hess, M. S. Phillips, P. J. Hey, A. Vongs, T. M. Fong, L. Xu, H. Y. Chen, R. G. Smith, C. Schindler, and L. H. Van der Ploeg, Functional STAT 1 and 3 signaling by the leptin receptor (OB-R); reduced expression of the rat fatty leptin receptor in transfected cells. *Endocrinology,* **137**, 5178-81 (1996).
41. H. Baumann, K. K. Morella, D. W. White, M. Dembski, P. S. Bailon, H. Kim, C. F. Lai, and L. A. Tartaglia, The full-length leptin receptor has signaling capabilities of interleukin 6-type cytokine receptors. *Proc Natl Acad Sci U S A,* **93**, 8374-8 (1996).
42. C. Vaisse, J. L. Halaas, C. M. Horvath, J. E. Darnell, Jr., M. Stoffel, and J. M. Friedman, Leptin activation of Stat3 in the hypothalamus of wild-type and ob/ob mice but not db/db mice. *Nat Genet,* **14**, 95-7 (1996).
43. J. L. Chan, S. J. Moschos, J. Bullen, K. Heist, X. Li, Y. B. Kim, B. B. Kahn, and C. S. Mantzoros, Recombinant methionyl human leptin administration activates signal transducer and activator of transcription 3 signaling in peripheral blood mononuclear cells in vivo and regulates soluble tumor necrosis factor-alpha receptor levels in humans with relative leptin deficiency. *J Clin Endocrinol Metab,* **90**, 1625-31 (2005).
44. L. O'Rourke, L. and P. R. Shepherd, Biphasic regulation of extracellular-signal-regulated protein kinase by leptin in macrophages: role in regulating STAT3 Ser727 phosphorylation and DNA binding. *Biochem J,* **364**, 875-9 (2002).
45. A. S. Banks, S. M. Davis, S. H. Bates, and M. G. Myers, Jr., Activation of downstream signals by the long form of the leptin receptor. *J Biol Chem,* **275**, 14563-72 (2000).
46. C. Bjorbaek, R. M. Buchholz, S. M. Davis, S. H. Bates, D. D. Pierroz, H. Gu, B. G. Neel, M. G. Myers, Jr., and J. S. Flier, Divergent roles of SHP-2 in ERK activation by leptin receptors. *J Biol Chem,* **276**, 4747-55 (2001).
47. S. L. Dunn, M. Bjornholm, S. H. Bates, Z. Chen, M. Seifert, and M. G. Myers, Jr., Feedback inhibition of leptin receptor/Jak2 signaling via Tyr1138 of the leptin receptor and suppressor of cytokine signaling 3. *Mol Endocrinol,* **19**, 925-38 (2005).

48. A. Lothgren, M. McCartney, E. Rupp Thuresson, and S. R. James, A model of activation of the protein tyrosine phosphatase SHP-2 by the human leptin receptor. *Biochim Biophys Acta,* **1545**, 20-9 (2001).
49. O. Gualillo, S. Eiras, D. W. White, C. Dieguez, C. and F. F. Casanueva, Leptin promotes the tyrosine phosphorylation of SHC proteins and SHC association with GRB2. *Mol Cell Endocrinol,* **190**, 83-9 (2002).
50. T. Yamashita, T. Murakami, S. Otani, M. Kuwajima, and K. Shima, Leptin receptor signal transduction: OBRa and OBRb of fa type. *Biochem Biophys Res Commun,* **246**, 752-9 (1998).
51. T. Murakami, T. Yamashita, M. Iida, M. Kuwajima, and K. Shima, A short form of leptin receptor performs signal transduction. *Biochem Biophys Res Commun,* **231**, 26-9 (1997).
52. G. Fruhbeck, M. Aguado, and J. A. Martinez, In vitro lipolytic effect of leptin on mouse adipocytes: evidence for a possible autocrine/paracrine role of leptin. *Biochem Biophys Res Commun,* **240**, 590-4 (1997).
53. I. Aprath-Husmann, K. Rohrig, H. Gottschling-Zeller, T. Skurk, D. Scriba, M. Birgel, and H. Hauner, Effects of leptin on the differentiation and metabolism of human adipocytes. *Int J Obes Relat Metab Disord,* **25**, 1465-70 (2001).
54. G. Y. Cao, R. V. Considine, and R. B. Lynn, Leptin receptors in the adrenal medulla of the rat. *Am J Physiol,* **273**, E448-52 (1997).
55. L. K. Malendowicz, G. Neri, A. Markowska, A. Hochol, G. G. Nussdorfer, and M. Majchrzak, Effects of leptin and leptin fragments on steroid secretion of freshly dispersed rat adrenocortical cells. *J Steroid Biochem Mol Biol,* **87**, 265-8 (2003).
56. Y. J. Lee, J. H. Park, S. K. Ju, K. H. You, J. S. Ko, and H. M. Kim, Leptin receptor isoform expression in rat osteoblasts and their functional analysis. *FEBS Lett,* **528**, 43-7 (2002).
57. X. M. Guan, J. F. Hess, H. Yu, P. J. Hey, and L. H. van der Ploeg, Differential expression of mRNA for leptin receptor isoforms in the rat brain. *Mol Cell Endocrinol,* **133**, 1-7 (1997).
58. M. R. Sierra-Honigmann, A. K. Nath, C. Murakami, G. Garcia-Cardena, A. Papapetropoulos, W. C. Sessa, L. A. Madge, J. S. Schechner, M. B. Schwabb, P. J. Polverini, and J. R. Flores-Riveros, Biological action of leptin as an angiogenic factor. *Science,* **281**, 1683-6 (1998).
59. J. D. Knudson, U. D. Dincer, C. Zhang, A. N. Swafford Jr, R. Koshida, A. Picchi, M. Focardi, G. M. Dick, and J. D. Tune, Leptin Receptors are Expressed in Coronary Arteries and Hyperleptinemia Causes Significant Coronary Endothelial Dysfunction. *Am J Physiol Heart Circ Physiol,* (2005).
60. N. Hoggard, L. Hunter, J. S. Duncan, L. M. Williams, P. Trayhurn, J. G. Mercer, Leptin and leptin receptor mRNA and protein expression in the murine fetus and placenta. *Proc Natl Acad Sci U S A,* **94**, 11073-8 (1997).
61. S. C. Chen, J. J. Cunningham, and R. J. Smeyne, Expression of OB receptor splice variants during prenatal development of the mouse. *J Recept Signal Transduct Res,* **20**, 87-103 (2000).
62. D. M. Purdham, M. X. Zou, V. Rajapurohitam, and M. Karmazyn, Rat heart is a site of leptin production and action. *Am J Physiol Heart Circ Physiol,* **287**, H2877-84 (2004).
63. B. D. Bennett, G. P. Solar, J. Q. Yuan, J. Mathias, G. R. Thomas, and W. Matthews, A role for leptin and its cognate receptor in hematopoiesis. *Curr Biol,* **6**, 1170-80 (1996).

64. H. Zarkesh-Esfahani, A. G. Pockley, Z. Wu, P. G. Hellewell, A. P. Weetman, and R. J. Ross, Leptin indirectly activates human neutrophils via induction of TNF-alpha. *J Immunol*, **172**, 1809-14 (2004).
65. Y. Zhao, R. Sun, L. You, C. Gao, and Z. Tian, Expression of leptin receptors and response to leptin stimulation of human natural killer cell lines. *Biochem Biophys Res Commun*, **300**, 247-52 (2003).
66. B. Siegmund, J. A. Sennello, J. Jones-Carson, F. Gamboni-Robertson, H. A. Lehr, A. Batra, I. Fedke, M. Zeitz, and G. Fantuzzi, Leptin receptor expression on T lymphocytes modulates chronic intestinal inflammation in mice. *Gut*, **53**, 965-72 (2004).
67. M. Breidert, S. Miehlke, A. Glasow, Z. Orban, M. Stolte, G. Ehninger, E. Bayerdorffer, O. Nettesheim, U. Halm, A. Haidan, and S. R. Bornstein, Leptin and its receptor in normal human gastric mucosa and in Helicobacter pylori-associated gastritis. *Scand J Gastroenterol*, **34**, 954-61 (1999).
68. H. Hama, A. Saito, T. Takeda, A. Tanuma, Y. Xie, K. Sato, J. J. Kazama, and F. Gejyo, Evidence indicating that renal tubular metabolism of leptin is mediated by megalin but not by the leptin receptors. *Endocrinology*, **145**, 3935-40 (2004).
69. P. Cohen, G. Yang, X. Yu, A. A. Soukas, C. S. Wolfish, J. M. Friedman, and C. Li, Induction of leptin receptor expression in the liver by leptin and food deprivation. *J Biol Chem*, **280**, 10034-9 (2005).
70. T. Tsuchiya, H. Shimizu, T. Horie, and M. Mori, Expression of leptin receptor in lung: leptin as a growth factor. *Eur J Pharmacol*, **365**, 273-9 (1999).
71. K. Laud, I. Gourdou, L. Belair, D. H. Keisler, and J. Djiane, Detection and regulation of leptin receptor mRNA in ovine mammary epithelial cells during pregnancy and lactation. *FEBS Lett*, **463**, 194-8 (1999).
72. S. H. Bates, J. V. Gardiner, R. B. Jones, S. R. Bloom, and C. J. Bailey, Acute stimulation of glucose uptake by leptin in l6 muscle cells. *Horm Metab Res*, **34**, 111-5 (2002).
73. N. K. Ryan, K. H. Van der Hoek, S. A. Robertson, and R. J. Norman, Leptin and leptin receptor expression in the rat ovary. *Endocrinology*, **144**, 5006-13 (2003).
74. V. Emilsson, Y. L. Liu, M. A. Cawthorne, N. M. Morton, and M. Davenport, Expression of the functional leptin receptor mRNA in pancreatic islets and direct inhibitory action of leptin on insulin secretion. *Diabetes*, **46**, 313-6 (1997).
75. C. Peiser, J. Springer, D. A. Groneberg, G. P. McGregor, A. Fischer, and R. E. Lang, Leptin receptor expression in nodose ganglion cells projecting to the rat gastric fundus. *Neurosci Lett*, **320**, 41-4 (2002).
76. K. D. Dieterich, and H. Lehnert, Expression of leptin receptor mRNA and the long form splice variant in human anterior pituitary and pituitary adenoma. *Exp Clin Endocrinol Diabetes*, **106**, 522-5 (1998).
77. J. Challier, M. Galtier, T. Bintein, A. Cortez, J. Lepercq, and S. Hauguel-de Mouzon, Placental leptin receptor isoforms in normal and pathological pregnancies. *Placenta*, **24**, 92-9 (2003).
78. J. Bohlender, M. Rauh, J. Zenk, and M. Groschl, Differential distribution and expression of leptin and the functional leptin receptor in major salivary glands of humans. *J Endocrinol*, **178**, 217-23 (2003).
79. B. Stallmeyer, H. Kampfer, M. Podda, R. Kaufmann, J. Pfeilschifter, and S. Frank, A novel keratinocyte mitogen: regulation of leptin and its functional receptor in skin repair. *J Invest Dermatol*, **117**, 98-105 (2001).
80. N. Shigemura, H. Miura, Y. Kusakabe, A. Hino, and Y. Ninomiya, Expression of leptin receptor (Ob-R) isoforms and signal transducers and activators of

transcription (STATs) mRNAs in the mouse taste buds. *Arch Histol Cytol,* **66**, 253-60 (2003).
81. M. Tena-Sempere, L. Pinilla, F. P. Zhang, L. C. Gonzalez, I. Huhtaniemi, F. F. Casanueva, C. Dieguez, and E. Aguilar, Developmental and hormonal regulation of leptin receptor (Ob-R) messenger ribonucleic acid expression in rat testis. *Biol Reprod,* **64**, 634-43 (2001).
82. K. W. Nowak, P. Kaczmarek, P. Mackowiak, A. Ziolkowska, G. Albertin, W. J. Ginda, M. Trejter, G. G. Nussdorfer, and L. K. Malendowicz, Rat thyroid gland expresses the long form of leptin receptors, and leptin stimulates the function of the gland in euthyroid non-fasted animals. *Int J Mol Med,* **9**, 31-4 (2002).
83. N. Hoggard, J. G. Mercer, D. V. Rayner, K. Moar, P. Trayhurn, and L. M. Williams, Localization of leptin receptor mRNA splice variants in murine peripheral tissues by RT-PCR and in situ hybridization. *Biochem Biophys Res Commun,* **232**, 383-7 (1997).
84. B. Lollmann, S. Gruninger, A. Stricker-Krongrad, and M. Chiesi, Detection and quantification of the leptin receptor splice variants Ob-Ra, b, and, e in different mouse tissues. *Biochem Biophys Res Commun,* **238**, 648-52 (1997).
85. J. T. Smith, and B. J. Waddell, Leptin receptor expression in the rat placenta: changes in ob-ra, ob-rb, and ob-re with gestational age and suppression by glucocorticoids. *Biol Reprod,* **67**, 1204-10 (2002).
86. D. E. Edwards, R. P. Bohm, Jr., J. Purcell, M. S. Ratterree, K. F. Swan, V. D. Castracane, and M. C. Henson, Two isoforms of the leptin receptor are enhanced in pregnancy-specific tissues and soluble leptin receptor is enhanced in maternal serum with advancing gestation in the baboon. *Biol Reprod,* **71**, 1746-52 (2004).
87. A. M. Oliveira, A. G. Nascimento, and R. V. Lloyd, Leptin and leptin receptor mRNA are widely expressed in tumors of adipocytic differentiation. *Mod Pathol,* **14**, 549-55 (2001).
88. A. Glasow, S. R. Bornstein, G. P. Chrousos, J. W. Brown, and W. A. Scherbaum, Detection of Ob-receptor in human adrenal neoplasms and effect of leptin on adrenal cell proliferation. *Horm Metab Res,* **31**, 247-51 (1999).
89. M. Ishikawa, J. Kitayama, and H. Nagawa, Enhanced expression of leptin and leptin receptor (OB-R) in human breast cancer. *Clin Cancer Res,* **10**, 4325-31 (2004).
90. S. S. Yuan, Y. F. Chung, H. W. Chen, K. B. Tsai, H. L. Chang, C. H. Huang, and J. H. Su, Aberrant expression and possible involvement of the leptin receptor in bladder cancer. *Urology,* **63**, 408-13 (2004).
91. S. S. Yuan, K. B. Tsai, Y. F. Chung, T. F. Chan, Y. T. Yeh, L. Y. Tsai, and J. H. Su, Aberrant expression and possible involvement of the leptin receptor in endometrial cancer. *Gynecol Oncol,* **92**, 769-75 (2004).
92. X. J. Wang, S. L. Yuan, Q. Lu, Y. R. Lu, J. Zhang, Y. Liu, and W. D. Wang, Potential involvement of leptin in carcinogenesis of hepatocellular carcinoma. *World J Gastroenterol,* **10**, 2478-81 (2004).
93. M. Konopleva, A. Mikhail, Z. Estrov, S. Zhao, D. Harris, G. Sanchez-Williams, S. M. Kornblau, J. Dong, K. O. Kliche, S. Jiang, H. R. Snodgrass, E. H. Estey, and M. Andreeff, Expression and function of leptin receptor isoforms in myeloid leukemia and myelodysplastic syndromes: proliferative and anti-apoptotic activities. *Blood,* **93**, 1668-76 (1999).
94. J. H. Choi, S. H. Park, P. C. Leung, and K. C. Choi, Expression of leptin receptors and potential effects of leptin on the cell growth and activation of mitogen-activated protein kinases in ovarian cancer cells. *J Clin Endocrinol Metab,* **90**, 207-10 (2005).
95. L. Jin, B. G. Burguera, M. E. Couce, B. W. Scheithauer, J. Lamsan, N. L. Eberhardt,

E. Kulig, and R. V. Lloyd, Leptin and leptin receptor expression in normal and neoplastic human pituitary: evidence of a regulatory role for leptin on pituitary cell proliferation. *J Clin Endocrinol Metab,* **84**, 2903-11 (1999).
96. P. Somasundar, K. A. Frankenberry, H. Skinner, G. Vedula, D. W. McFadden, D. Riggs, B. Jackson, R. Vangilder, S. M. Hileman, and L. C. Vona-Davis, Prostate cancer cell proliferation is influenced by leptin. *J Surg Res,* **118**, 71-82 (2004).
97. M. Cauzac, D. Czuba, J. Girard, and S. Hauguel-de Mouzon, Transduction of leptin growth signals in placental cells is independent of JAK-STAT activation. *Placenta,* **24**, 378-84 (2003).
98. H. Chen, O. Charlat, L. A. Tartaglia, E. A. Woolf, X. Weng, S. J. Ellis, N. D. Lakey, J. Culpepper, K. J. Moore, R. E. Breitbart, G. M. Duyk, R. I. Tepper, and J. P. Morgenstern, Evidence that the diabetes gene encodes the leptin receptor: identification of a mutation in the leptin receptor gene in db/db mice. *Cell,* **84**, 491-5 (1996).
99. S. C. Chua, S. M. Liu, Q. Li, A. Sun, W. F. DeNino, S. B. Heymsfield, and X. E. Guo, Transgenic complementation of leptin receptor deficiency. II. Increased leptin receptor transgene dose effects on obesity/diabetes and fertility/lactation in lepr-db/db mice. *Am J Physiol Endocrinol Metab,* **286**, E384-92 (2004).
100. S. H. Bates, W. H. Stearns, T. A. Dundon, M. Schubert, A. W. Tso, Y. Wang, A. S. Banks, H. J. Lavery, A. K. Haq, E. Maratos-Flier, B. G. Neel, M. W. Schwartz, and M. G. Myers, Jr., STAT3 signalling is required for leptin regulation of energy balance but not reproduction. *Nature,* **421**, 856-9 (2003).
101. S. H. Bates, T. A. Dundon, M. Seifert, M. Carlson, E. Maratos-Flier, and M. G. Myers, Jr., LRb-STAT3 signaling is required for the neuroendocrine regulation of energy expenditure by leptin. *Diabetes,* **53**, 3067-73 (2004).
102. H. Fei, H. J. Okano, C. Li, G. H. Lee, C. Zhao, R. Darnell, and J. M. Friedman, Anatomic localization of alternatively spliced leptin receptors (Ob-R) in mouse brain and other tissues. *Proc Natl Acad Sci U S A,* **94**, 7001-5 (1997).
103. S. M. Hileman, D. D. Pierroz, H. Masuzaki, C. Bjorbaek, K. El-Haschimi, W. A. Banks, and J. S. Flier, Characterizaton of short isoforms of the leptin receptor in rat cerebral microvessels and of brain uptake of leptin in mouse models of obesity. *Endocrinology,* **143**, 775-83 (2002).
104. C. Bjorbaek, J. K. Elmquist, P. Michl, R. S. Ahima, A. van Bueren, A. L. McCall, and J. S. Flier, Expression of leptin receptor isoforms in rat brain microvessels. *Endocrinology,* **139**, 3485-91 (1998).
105. S. Uotani, C. Bjorbaek, J. Tornoe, and J. S. Flier, Functional properties of leptin receptor isoforms: internalization and degradation of leptin and ligand-induced receptor downregulation. *Diabetes,* **48**, 279-86 (1999).
106. S. M. Hileman, J. Tornoe, J. S. Flier, and C. Bjorbaek, Transcellular transport of leptin by the short leptin receptor isoform ObRa in Madin-Darby Canine Kidney cells. *Endocrinology,* **141**, 1955-61 (2000).
107. X. S. Wu-Peng, S. C. Chua, N. Okada, S. M. Liu, M. Nicolson, and R. L. Leibel, Phenotype of the obese Koletsky (f) rat due to Tyr763Stop mutation in the extracellular domain of the leptin receptor (Lepr): evidence for deficient plasma-to-CSF transport of leptin in both the Zucker and Koletsky obese rat. *Diabetes,* **46**, 513-8 (1997).
108. W. A. Banks, M. L. Niehoff, D. Martin, and C. L. Farrell, Leptin transport across the blood-brain barrier of the Koletsky rat is not mediated by a product of the leptin receptor gene. *Brain Res,* **950**, 130-6 (2002).

109. A. J. Kastin, W. Pan, L. M. Maness, R. J. Koletsky, and P. Ernsberger, Decreased transport of leptin across the blood-brain barrier in rats lacking the short form of the leptin receptor. *Peptides,* **20**, 1449-53 (1999).
110. J. L. Halaas, and J. M. Friedman, Leptin and its receptor. *J Endocrinol,* **155**, 215-6 (1997).
111. R. J. Boado, P. L. Golden, N. Levin, and W. M. Pardridge, Up-regulation of blood-brain barrier short-form leptin receptor gene products in rats fed a high fat diet. *J Neurochem,* **71**, 1761-4 (1998).
112. K. El-Haschimi, D. D. Pierroz, S. M. Hileman, C. Bjorbaek, and J. S. Flier, Two defects contribute to hypothalamic leptin resistance in mice with diet-induced obesity. *J Clin Invest,* **105**, 1827-32 (2000).
113. A. Lammert, W. Kiess, A. Bottner, A. Glasow, and J. Kratzsch, Soluble leptin receptor represents the main leptin binding activity in human blood. *Biochem Biophys Res Commun,* **283**, 982-8 (2001).
114. A. Lammert, G. Brockmann, U. Renne, W. Kiess, A. Bottner, J. Thiery, and J. Kratzsch, Different isoforms of the soluble leptin receptor in non-pregnant and pregnant mice. *Biochem Biophys Res Commun,* **298**, 798-804 (2002).
115. G. Yang, H. Ge, A. Boucher, X. Yu, and C. Li, Modulation of direct leptin signaling by soluble leptin receptor. *Mol Endocrinol,* **18**, 1354-62 (2004).
116. O. Zastrow, B. Seidel, W. Kiess, J. Thiery, E. Keller, A. Bottner, and J. Kratzsch, The soluble leptin receptor is crucial for leptin action: evidence from clinical and experimental data. *Int J Obes Relat Metab Disord,* **27**, 1472-8 (2003).
117. L. Huang, Z. Wang, and C. Li, Modulation of circulating leptin levels by its soluble receptor. *J Biol Chem,* **276**, 6343-9 (2001).
118. P. Monteleone, M. Fabrazzo, A. Tortorella, A. Fuschino, and M. Maj, Opposite modifications in circulating leptin and soluble leptin receptor across the eating disorder spectrum. *Mol Psychiatry,* **7**, 641-6 (2002).
119. V. Ogier, O. Ziegler, L. Mejean, J. P. Nicolas, and A. Stricker-Krongrad, Obesity is associated with decreasing levels of the circulating soluble leptin receptor in humans. *Int J Obes Relat Metab Disord,* **26**, 496-503 (2002).
120. F. M. van Dielen, C. van 't Veer, W. A. Buurman, and J. W. Greve, Leptin and soluble leptin receptor levels in obese and weight-losing individuals. *J Clin Endocrinol Metab,* **87**, 1708-16 (2002).
121. P. Cinaz, A. Bideci, M. O. Camurdan, A. Guven, and S. Gonen, Leptin and soluble leptin receptor levels in obese children in fasting and satiety states. *J Pediatr Endocrinol Metab,* **18**, 303-7 (2005).
122. J. L. Chan, S. Bluher, N. Yiannakouris, M. A. Suchard, J. Kratzsch, and C. S. Mantzoros, Regulation of circulating soluble leptin receptor levels by gender, adiposity, sex steroids, and leptin: observational and interventional studies in humans. *Diabetes,* **51**, 2105-12 (2002).
123. M. Laimer, C. F. Ebenbichler, S. Kaser, A. Sandhofer, H. Weiss, H. Nehoda, F. Aigner, and J. R. Patsch, Weight loss increases soluble leptin receptor levels and the soluble receptor bound fraction of leptin. *Obes Res,* **10**, 597-601 (2002).
124. K. Clement, C. Vaisse, N. Lahlou, S. Cabrol, V. Pelloux, D. Cassuto, M. Gourmelen, C. Dina, J. Chambaz, J. M. Lacorte, A. Basdevant, P. Bougneres, Y. Lebouc, P. Froguel, and B. Guy-Grand, A mutation in the human leptin receptor gene causes obesity and pituitary dysfunction. *Nature,* **392**, 398-401 (1998).
125. A. Takahashi-Yasuno, H. Masuzaki, T. Miyawaki, N. Matsuoka, Y. Ogawa, T. Hayashi, K. Hosoda, Y. Yoshimasa, G. Inoue, and K. Nakao, Association of Ob-R gene polymorphism and insulin resistance in Japanese men. *Metabolism,* **53**, 650-4 (2004).

126. C. T. van Rossum, B. Hoebee, M. A. van Baak, M. Mars, S. W. Saris, and J. C. Seidell, Genetic variation in the leptin receptor gene, leptin, and weight gain in young Dutch adults. *Obes Res,* **11**, 377-86 (2003).
127. R. V. Considine, E. L. Considine, C. J. Williams, T. M. Hyde, and J. F. Caro, The hypothalamic leptin receptor in humans: identification of incidental sequence polymorphisms and absence of the db/db mouse and fa/fa rat mutations. *Diabetes,* **45**, 992-4 (1996).
128. N. Yiannakouris, M. Yannakoulia, L. Melistas, J. L. Chan, D. Klimis-Zacas, and C. S. Mantzoros, The Q223R polymorphism of the leptin receptor gene is significantly associated with obesity and predicts a small percentage of body weight and body composition variability. *J Clin Endocrinol Metab,* **86**, 4434-9 (2001).
129. Y. C. Chagnon, J. H. Wilmore, I. B. Borecki, J. Gagnon, L. Perusse, M. Chagnon, G. R. Collier, A. S. Leon, J. S. Skinner, D. C. Rao, and C. Bouchard, Associations between the leptin receptor gene and adiposity in middle-aged Caucasian males from the HERITAGE family study. *J Clin Endocrinol Metab,* **85**, 29-34 (2000).
130. J. M. Guizar-Mendoza, N. Amador-Licona, S. E. Flores-Martinez, M. G. Lopez-Cardona, R. Ahuatzin-Tremary, and J. Sanchez-Corona, Association analysis of the Gln223Arg polymorphism in the human leptin receptor gene, and traits related to obesity in Mexican adolescents. *J Hum Hypertens,* (2005).
131. M. Wauters, I. Mertens, M. Chagnon, T. Rankinen, R. V. Considine, Y. C. Chagnon, L. F. Van Gaal, and C. Bouchard, Polymorphisms in the leptin receptor gene, body composition and fat distribution in overweight and obese women. *Int J Obes Relat Metab Disord,* **25**, 714-20 (2001).
132. K. Silver, J. Walston, W. K. Chung, F. Yao, V. V. Parikh, R. Andersen, L. J. Cheskin, D. Elahi, D. Muller, R. L. Leibel, and A. R. Shuldiner, The Gln223Arg and Lys656Asn polymorphisms in the human leptin receptor do not associate with traits related to obesity. *Diabetes,* **46**, 1898-900 (1997).
133. M. Heo, R. L. Leibel, K. R. Fontaine, B. B. Boyer, W. K. Chung, M. Koulu, M. K. Karvonen, U. Pesonen, A. Rissanen, M. Laakso, M. I. Uusitupa, Y. Chagnon, C. Bouchard, P. A. Donohoue, T. L. Burns, A. R. Shuldiner, K. Silver, R. E. Andersen, O. Pedersen, S. Echwald, T. I. Sorensen, P. Behn, M. A. Permutt, K. B. Jacobs, R. C. Elston, D. J. Hoffman, E. Gropp, and D. B. Allison, A meta-analytic investigation of linkage and association of common leptin receptor (LEPR) polymorphisms with body mass index and waist circumference. *Int J Obes Relat Metab Disord,* **26**, 640-6 (2002).
134. N. Stefan, B. Vozarova, A. Del Parigi, V. Ossowski, D. B. Thompson, R. L. Hanson, E. Ravussin, and P. A. Tataranni, The Gln223Arg polymorphism of the leptin receptor in Pima Indians: influence on energy expenditure, physical activity and lipid metabolism. *Int J Obes Relat Metab Disord,* **26**, 1629-32 (2002).
135. A. Takahashi-Yasuno, H. Masuzaki, T. Miyawaki, Y. Ogawa, N. Matsuoka, T. Hayashi, K. Hosoda, G. Inoue, Y. Yoshimasa, and K. Nakao, Leptin receptor polymorphism is associated with serum lipid levels and impairment of cholesterol lowering effect by simvastatin in Japanese men. *Diabetes Res Clin Pract,* **62**, 169-75 (2003).
136. D. Manzella, M. Parillo, T. Razzino, P. Gnasso, S. Buonanno, A. Gargiulo, M. Caputi, and G. Paolisso, Soluble leptin receptor and insulin resistance as determinant of sleep apnea. *Int J Obes Relat Metab Disord,* **26**, 370-5 (2002).
137. M. Muy-Rivera, Y. Ning, I. O. Frederic, S. Vadachkoria, D. A. Luthy, and M. A. Williams, Leptin, soluble leptin receptor and leptin gene polymorphism in relation to preeclampsia risk. *Physiol Res,* **54**, 167-74 (2005).

109. A. J. Kastin, W. Pan, L. M. Maness, R. J. Koletsky, and P. Ernsberger, Decreased transport of leptin across the blood-brain barrier in rats lacking the short form of the leptin receptor. *Peptides,* **20**, 1449-53 (1999).
110. J. L. Halaas, and J. M. Friedman, Leptin and its receptor. *J Endocrinol,* **155**, 215-6 (1997).
111. R. J. Boado, P. L. Golden, N. Levin, and W. M. Pardridge, Up-regulation of blood-brain barrier short-form leptin receptor gene products in rats fed a high fat diet. *J Neurochem,* **71**, 1761-4 (1998).
112. K. El-Haschimi, D. D. Pierroz, S. M. Hileman, C. Bjorbaek, and J. S. Flier, Two defects contribute to hypothalamic leptin resistance in mice with diet-induced obesity. *J Clin Invest,* **105**, 1827-32 (2000).
113. A. Lammert, W. Kiess, A. Bottner, A. Glasow, and J. Kratzsch, Soluble leptin receptor represents the main leptin binding activity in human blood. *Biochem Biophys Res Commun,* **283**, 982-8 (2001).
114. A. Lammert, G. Brockmann, U. Renne, W. Kiess, A. Bottner, J. Thiery, and J. Kratzsch, Different isoforms of the soluble leptin receptor in non-pregnant and pregnant mice. *Biochem Biophys Res Commun,* **298**, 798-804 (2002).
115. G. Yang, H. Ge, A. Boucher, X. Yu, and C. Li, Modulation of direct leptin signaling by soluble leptin receptor. *Mol Endocrinol,* **18**, 1354-62 (2004).
116. O. Zastrow, B. Seidel, W. Kiess, J. Thiery, E. Keller, A. Bottner, and J. Kratzsch, The soluble leptin receptor is crucial for leptin action: evidence from clinical and experimental data. *Int J Obes Relat Metab Disord,* **27**, 1472-8 (2003).
117. L. Huang, Z. Wang, and C. Li, Modulation of circulating leptin levels by its soluble receptor. *J Biol Chem,* **276**, 6343-9 (2001).
118. P. Monteleone, M. Fabrazzo, A. Tortorella, A. Fuschino, and M. Maj, Opposite modifications in circulating leptin and soluble leptin receptor across the eating disorder spectrum. *Mol Psychiatry,* **7**, 641-6 (2002).
119. V. Ogier, O. Ziegler, L. Mejean, J. P. Nicolas, and A. Stricker-Krongrad, Obesity is associated with decreasing levels of the circulating soluble leptin receptor in humans. *Int J Obes Relat Metab Disord,* **26**, 496-503 (2002).
120. F. M. van Dielen, C. van 't Veer, W. A. Buurman, and J. W. Greve, Leptin and soluble leptin receptor levels in obese and weight-losing individuals. *J Clin Endocrinol Metab,* **87**, 1708-16 (2002).
121. P. Cinaz, A. Bideci, M. O. Camurdan, A. Guven, and S. Gonen, Leptin and soluble leptin receptor levels in obese children in fasting and satiety states. *J Pediatr Endocrinol Metab,* **18**, 303-7 (2005).
122. J. L. Chan, S. Bluher, N. Yiannakouris, M. A. Suchard, J. Kratzsch, and C. S. Mantzoros, Regulation of circulating soluble leptin receptor levels by gender, adiposity, sex steroids, and leptin: observational and interventional studies in humans. *Diabetes,* **51**, 2105-12 (2002).
123. M. Laimer, C. F. Ebenbichler, S. Kaser, A. Sandhofer, H. Weiss, H. Nehoda, F. Aigner, and J. R. Patsch, Weight loss increases soluble leptin receptor levels and the soluble receptor bound fraction of leptin. *Obes Res,* **10**, 597-601 (2002).
124. K. Clement, C. Vaisse, N. Lahlou, S. Cabrol, V. Pelloux, D. Cassuto, M. Gourmelen, C. Dina, J. Chambaz, J. M. Lacorte, A. Basdevant, P. Bougneres, Y. Lebouc, P. Froguel, and B. Guy-Grand, A mutation in the human leptin receptor gene causes obesity and pituitary dysfunction. *Nature,* **392**, 398-401 (1998).
125. A. Takahashi-Yasuno, H. Masuzaki, T. Miyawaki, N. Matsuoka, Y. Ogawa, T. Hayashi, K. Hosoda, Y. Yoshimasa, G. Inoue, and K. Nakao, Association of Ob-R gene polymorphism and insulin resistance in Japanese men. *Metabolism,* **53**, 650-4 (2004).

126. C. T. van Rossum, B. Hoebee, M. A. van Baak, M. Mars, S. W. Saris, and J. C. Seidell, Genetic variation in the leptin receptor gene, leptin, and weight gain in young Dutch adults. *Obes Res*, **11**, 377-86 (2003).
127. R. V. Considine, E. L. Considine, C. J. Williams, T. M. Hyde, and J. F. Caro, The hypothalamic leptin receptor in humans: identification of incidental sequence polymorphisms and absence of the db/db mouse and fa/fa rat mutations. *Diabetes*, **45**, 992-4 (1996).
128. N. Yiannakouris, M. Yannakoulia, L. Melistas, J. L. Chan, D. Klimis-Zacas, and C. S. Mantzoros, The Q223R polymorphism of the leptin receptor gene is significantly associated with obesity and predicts a small percentage of body weight and body composition variability. *J Clin Endocrinol Metab*, **86**, 4434-9 (2001).
129. Y. C. Chagnon, J. H. Wilmore, I. B. Borecki, J. Gagnon, L. Perusse, M. Chagnon, G. R. Collier, A. S. Leon, J. S. Skinner, D. C. Rao, and C. Bouchard, Associations between the leptin receptor gene and adiposity in middle-aged Caucasian males from the HERITAGE family study. *J Clin Endocrinol Metab*, **85**, 29-34 (2000).
130. J. M. Guizar-Mendoza, N. Amador-Licona, S. E. Flores-Martinez, M. G. Lopez-Cardona, R. Ahuatzin-Tremary, and J. Sanchez-Corona, Association analysis of the Gln223Arg polymorphism in the human leptin receptor gene, and traits related to obesity in Mexican adolescents. *J Hum Hypertens*, (2005).
131. M. Wauters, I. Mertens, M. Chagnon, T. Rankinen, R. V. Considine, Y. C. Chagnon, L. F. Van Gaal, and C. Bouchard, Polymorphisms in the leptin receptor gene, body composition and fat distribution in overweight and obese women. *Int J Obes Relat Metab Disord*, **25**, 714-20 (2001).
132. K. Silver, J. Walston, W. K. Chung, F. Yao, V. V. Parikh, R. Andersen, L. J. Cheskin, D. Elahi, D. Muller, R. L. Leibel, and A. R. Shuldiner, The Gln223Arg and Lys656Asn polymorphisms in the human leptin receptor do not associate with traits related to obesity. *Diabetes*, **46**, 1898-900 (1997).
133. M. Heo, R. L. Leibel, K. R. Fontaine, B. B. Boyer, W. K. Chung, M. Koulu, M. K. Karvonen, U. Pesonen, A. Rissanen, M. Laakso, M. I. Uusitupa, Y. Chagnon, C. Bouchard, P. A. Donohoue, T. L. Burns, A. R. Shuldiner, K. Silver, R. E. Andersen, O. Pedersen, S. Echwald, T. I. Sorensen, P. Behn, M. A. Permutt, K. B. Jacobs, R. C. Elston, D. J. Hoffman, E. Gropp, and D. B. Allison, A meta-analytic investigation of linkage and association of common leptin receptor (LEPR) polymorphisms with body mass index and waist circumference. *Int J Obes Relat Metab Disord*, **26**, 640-6 (2002).
134. N. Stefan, B. Vozarova, A. Del Parigi, V. Ossowski, D. B. Thompson, R. L. Hanson, E. Ravussin, and P. A. Tataranni, The Gln223Arg polymorphism of the leptin receptor in Pima Indians: influence on energy expenditure, physical activity and lipid metabolism. *Int J Obes Relat Metab Disord*, **26**, 1629-32 (2002).
135. A. Takahashi-Yasuno, H. Masuzaki, T. Miyawaki, Y. Ogawa, N. Matsuoka, T. Hayashi, K. Hosoda, G. Inoue, Y. Yoshimasa, and K. Nakao, Leptin receptor polymorphism is associated with serum lipid levels and impairment of cholesterol lowering effect by simvastatin in Japanese men. *Diabetes Res Clin Pract*, **62**, 169-75 (2003).
136. D. Manzella, M. Parillo, T. Razzino, P. Gnasso, S. Buonanno, A. Gargiulo, M. Caputi, and G. Paolisso, Soluble leptin receptor and insulin resistance as determinant of sleep apnea. *Int J Obes Relat Metab Disord*, **26**, 370-5 (2002).
137. M. Muy-Rivera, Y. Ning, I. O. Frederic, S. Vadachkoria, D. A. Luthy, and M. A. Williams, Leptin, soluble leptin receptor and leptin gene polymorphism in relation to preeclampsia risk. *Physiol Res*, **54**, 167-74 (2005).

138. C. F. Skibola, E. A. Holly, M. S. Forrest, A. Hubbard, P. M. Bracci, D. R. Skibola, C. Hegedus, and M. T. Smith, Body mass index, leptin and leptin receptor polymorphisms, and non-hodgkin lymphoma. *Cancer Epidemiol Biomarkers Prev,* **13**, 779-86 (2004).
139. J. M. Koh, D. J. Kim, J. S. Hong, J. Y. Park, K. U. Lee, S. Y. Kim, and G. S. Kim, Estrogen receptor alpha gene polymorphisms Pvu II and Xba I influence association between leptin receptor gene polymorphism (Gln223Arg) and bone mineral density in young men. *Eur J Endocrinol,* **147**, 777-83 (2002).
140. M. Tahara, A. Aiba, M. Yamazaki, Y. Ikeda, S. Goto, H. Moriya, and A. Okawa, The extent of ossification of posterior longitudinal ligament of the spine associated with nucleotide pyrophosphatase gene and leptin receptor gene polymorphisms. *Spine,* **30**, 877-80 (2005).
141. C. C. Chen, T. Chang, and H. Y. Su, Characterization of porcine leptin receptor polymorphisms and their association with reproduction and production traits. *Anim Biotechnol,* **15**, 89-102 (2004).
142. M. Mackowski, K. Szymoniak, M. Szydlowski, M. Kamyczek, R. Eckert, M. Rozycki, and M. Switonski, Missense mutations in exon 4 of the porcine LEPR gene encoding extracellular domain and their association with fatness traits. *Anim Genet,* **36**, 135-7 (2005).
143. S. C. Liefers, R. F. Veerkamp, M. F. te Pas, C. Delavaud, Y. Chilliard, and T. van der Lende, A missense mutation in the bovine leptin receptor gene is associated with leptin concentrations during late pregnancy. *Anim Genet,* **35**, 138-41 (2004).
144. G. Horev, P. Einat, T. Aharoni, Y. Eshdat, and M. Friedman-Einat, Molecular cloning and properties of the chicken leptin-receptor (CLEPR) gene. *Mol Cell Endocrinol,* **162**, 95-106 (2000).
145. M. P. Richards, and S. M. Poch, Molecular cloning and expression of the turkey leptin receptor gene. *Comp Biochem Physiol B Biochem Mol Biol,* **136**, 833-47 (2003).

Chapter 3

LEPTIN AND OBESITY

Lauren N. Bell[1,2] and Robert V. Considine[1,2]
[1]*Department of Cellular and Integrative Physiology,* [2]*Department of Medicine, Indiana University, Indianapolis, IN*

Abstract: Serum leptin levels are increased in obesity in proportion to the amount of body fat. Gender and fat distribution into subcutaneous or visceral adipose tissue depots contribute to greater serum leptin in women than men of equivalent fat mass. Serum leptin circulates in the plasma in association with a binding protein comprised of the extracellular domain of the leptin receptor. The postprandial surge in insulin and glucose stimulate leptin synthesis and a diurnal pattern in serum leptin. Hexosamine biosynthesis and adipocyte size contribute to greater leptin synthesis in adipocytes of obese subjects. Leptin resistance describes the inability of leptin to reduce food intake and decrease body weight in obese subjects with elevated leptin levels. Selective leptin resistance results in some systems remaining responsive to the elevated leptin in obesity. Selective leptin resistance contributes to obesity related hypertension and may contribute to other metabolic complications in obesity.

Key words: Adipocytes; body mass index; caloric restriction; gender; hexosamines; leptin binding proteins; leptin resistance; lipostasis theory; SOCS proteins.

1. INTRODUCTION

Kennedy[1] first suggested in the lipostasis theory that a satiety factor might be produced in proportion to the amount of body fat present in the body. This peripherally produced signal would then be compared to a "setpoint" in the brain, and modifications to energy intake and expenditure made to maintain a constant amount of adipose tissue. Subsequent parabiosis experiments in rodents supported the tenets of the lipostasis theory in that the serum "satiety signal" was at a higher concentration in obese animals than in lean animals[2,3]. These early studies predicted the existence of leptin, which was found in 1994 by Friedman's group in a search for the single gene defect causing obesity in *ob/ob* mice[4].

Since the discovery of leptin a significant amount has been learned about the regulation of energy intake and energy expenditure, and the role of leptin in these processes. This chapter will summarize what is known about the relationship between serum leptin in obesity, with a particular emphasis on findings in humans. We will also discuss the concept of leptin resistance as an explanation for the inability of leptin to prevent excess weight gain, and the contribution of selective leptin resistance to development of co-morbidities in obesity.

2. SERUM LEPTIN IS INCREASED IN OBESITY

The amount of adipose tissue in the body is the primary determinant of the serum leptin concentration. As shown in Figure 1, there is a strong positive correlation between adiposity, represented as percent body fat, and serum leptin across a wide range of body weights in human subjects. Reasonably similar correlations are obtained with other measures of adiposity such as body mass index (BMI) or fat mass. Leptin is also significantly correlated with body fat in children and newborns[5,6]. Although serum leptin is elevated with increasing fat mass in the general population, there is a considerable degree of variation in serum leptin at any given fat mass. Factors that contribute to the variation in serum leptin are gender, differential distribution of adipose tissue into the visceral or subcutaneous depots and insulin/glucose metabolism.

2.1 Effect of Gender and Fat Distribution

Women have significantly higher serum leptin concentrations than men of equivalent body weight[7,8]. The simplest explanation for this observation is that women have a greater amount of body fat than men of equivalent weight or body mass index. However, in comparing men and women with equivalent fat mass, women still have significantly higher serum leptin concentrations[9]. One factor contributing to this difference between men and women is the deposition of body fat into different adipose tissue depots. Females have greater amounts of subcutaneous adipose tissue in contrast to males, who tend to have greater visceral adipose tissue mass, particularly in obesity. As discussed in detail below, *LEP* gene expression and leptin secretion are greater from subcutaneous than visceral adipocytes[9-13], thus

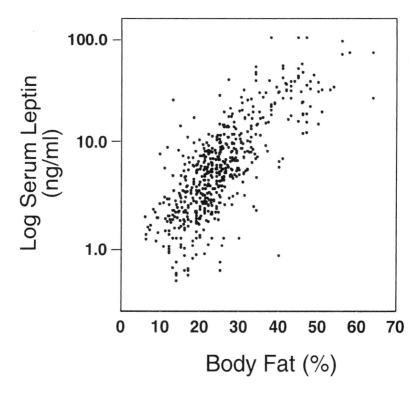

Figure 1. Relationship between percent body fat and serum leptin in adults. Reprinted from reference 41 with permission from *The American Diabetes Association.* Copyright © 1996.

more leptin is released into the blood from the greater subcutaneous adipose tissue mass in females.

A second factor contributing to greater serum leptin in females are the gonadal steroids. In vivo and in vitro studies have suggested that testosterone and estrogens can regulate leptin synthesis and release from adipose tissue independently of their effects to influence deposition of adipose tissue into the subcutaneous or visceral depots. In general, androgenic hormones reduce leptin synthesis while estrogens increase leptin synthesis in adipose tissue[9]. Evidence in support of a suppressive effect of testosterone on serum leptin is derived from studies of pubertal development in males, in which serum leptin levels decrease as testosterone increases[14], and during testosterone therapy in hypogonadal men, which also reduces serum leptin[15,16]. Administration of testosterone decreases leptin in female-to-male transsexuals[17] and leptin secretion is decreased from visceral adipose tissue pieces of lean humans exposed to dihydrotestosterone for 48 hours[18,19]. In support of a stimulating effect of estrogens on serum leptin are the observations that estrogen administration (along with anti-androgens) increases leptin in male-to-female transsexuals[17] and that in vitro estradiol increases leptin production release from visceral adipose tissue pieces[18,19]. The mechanism(s) through which gonadal steroids directly regulate leptin synthesis and release from adipocytes remain to be fully elucidated.

2.2 Insulin and Glucose Influence Serum Leptin

With a pattern of consistent food intake (three regularly scheduled meals a day in humans), serum leptin levels measured in the early morning following an overnight fast tend to remain fairly constant. Over a 24 h period serum leptin exhibits a diurnal pattern with the peak in serum leptin at ~0200 h in both lean and obese individuals[20,21,22]. A 6 h shift in meal times moves the leptin peak by 6 h and day/night reversal results in peak leptin at 1400 h[21]. These observations suggest that the nocturnal leptin peak is entrained to food intake and that glucose and insulin are significant regulators of serum leptin. Evidence to support a role for insulin and glucose in regulating serum leptin is derived from observations that hyperinsulinemic-euglycemic clamps of differing duration increase serum leptin[23,24] and that feeding high fat/low carbohydrate meals, which result in smaller postprandial excursions in insulin and glucose than meals of standard carbohydrate content, reduce serum leptin[25].

It has been suggested that insulin and glucose may influence serum leptin levels through regulation of hexosamine (UDP-GlcNAc) biosynthesis in adipocytes[26]. Infusion of glucosamine, uridine or free fatty acids during a hyperinsulinemic-euglycemic clamp in rats increased tissue UDP-GlcNAc and serum leptin[27]. In transgenic mice overexpressing glutamine:fructose amidotransferase, the rate-limiting enzyme in UDP-GlcNAc biosynthesis, *Lep* mRNA in adipose tissue and serum leptin were increased[28]. UDP-GlcNAc is elevated 3.2-fold in the subcutaneous adipose tissue of obese humans and a significant positive correlation between BMI and adipose tissue UDP-GlcNAc has been reported[29]. In vitro, stimulation of UDP-GlcNAc synthesis in human subcutaneous adipocytes increases leptin secretion and inhibition of UDP-GlcNAc synthesis decreases leptin release[29]. Taken together, these findings suggest that hexosamine biosynthesis in the adipocyte may link serum insulin and glucose with leptin production.

2.3 Serum Leptin Binding Protein

Leptin circulates in the blood in association with a binding protein comprised of the extracellular domain of the leptin receptor[30,31,32]. In rodents an mRNA encoding the soluble leptin receptor has been detected[33]; however, in humans the soluble receptor is generated by proteolytic cleavage of membrane-bound receptors[34]. One site for release of leptin binding protein is adipose tissue itself[35]. In vitro, release of free leptin and leptin bound to its binding protein are greater from subcutaneous adipose tissue explants from obese subjects[34]. The amount of leptin binding protein in serum is higher in men than women, and decreases with increasing adiposity independently of gender[36]. Most leptin in lean subjects is bound with little free hormone detectable in the blood[30,31,32]. Together, the reduction in soluble leptin receptor with increasing adiposity and the increase in leptin synthesis result in greater free leptin in obese subjects.

Leptin binding protein prolongs the half-life of leptin in the circulation[32,37] and sequesters leptin from its receptor to reduce leptin signaling[38,39]. Thus, the higher "free" leptin levels in obese subjects are appropriate if leptin is to signal to the central nervous system of the increased energy stores in the body.

3. SERUM LEPTIN AS A SIGNAL OF REDUCTION IN ENERGY INTAKE

Weight loss and weight gain, which result in changes in the amount of adipose tissue, alter *LEP* mRNA in adipocytes and serum leptin levels. An increase in adipose tissue mass with weight gain results in a significant increase in circulating leptin while a decrease in fat mass with weight loss reduces serum leptin[40,41]. These observations thus support the concept that leptin provides a signal to the central nervous system of the size of energy stores in the body. However, extreme changes in energy intake such as fasting reduce serum leptin, suggesting a role for the hormone in coordinating the neuroendocrine response to caloric deprivation[42]. Such a response would include initiation of food seeking behavior to increase energy intake, and activation of processes to reduce energy expenditure, both to insure survival should the fast be prolonged.

Serum leptin levels are rapidly decreased with short-term fasting (24-72 h) in both animals[43] and humans[44,45,46]. The rapid fall in leptin with fasting is disproportionately greater than the small reduction in adipose tissue mass that occurs over the same time period. Thus it is reasonable to suggest that serum leptin during fasting serves as a peripheral signal to the central nervous system that caloric restriction is occurring, rather than as a signal of current energy stores in the body. Evidence that leptin coordinates the neuroendocrine response to fasting was originally derived through replacement experiments in rodents[43]. In these studies recombinant leptin was administered to 48 h fasted mice to achieve serum leptin levels similar to that observed during the fed state. In untreated mice fasting reduced thyroid and reproductive hormone levels, and increased glucocortiocoids. Preventing the starvation-induced fall in leptin substantially blunted reductions in gonadal and thyroid hormones and attenuated the increase in glucocorticoids. More recently, Chan et al[46] have demonstrated that replacement of leptin during complete caloric restriction in men can prevent the fasting-induced reduction in testosterone and partially prevent the suppression of the hypothalamic pituitary thyroid axis. Taken together, these observations establish a role for leptin in regulating hypothalamic-pituitary function in both rodents and humans in response to caloric restriction. The effect of leptin on hypothalamic-pituitary function is discussed in detail in Chapter 6.

Infusion of glucose during short-term fasting to maintain blood sugar at 90 mg/dl prevents the fall in serum leptin[44,45]. This observation suggests that the fall in glucose or insulin with fasting may be the nutritional signal that is recognized by adipose tissue resulting in reduced leptin secretion.

4. REGULATION OF LEPTIN SYNTHESIS IN ADIPOCYTES

The amount of *LEP* mRNA is significantly elevated in isolated adipocytes from obese individuals as illustrated in Figure 2. In most studies both in vivo and in vitro, changes in *LEP* gene expression correlate with parallel changes in the amount of leptin secretion. These findings suggest that regulation of leptin synthesis is achieved primarily at the transcriptional level, although two studies suggest that insulin may regulate translation of leptin[47,48]. Several factors likely contribute to the increase in synthesis and release of leptin from adipocytes of obese subjects.

Adipocyte size appears to be an important determinant of leptin synthesis. *LEP* mRNA is greater in large adipocytes than in small adipocytes isolated from the same piece of adipose tissue[49,50] and leptin secretion is strongly correlated with fat cell volume[51]. As adipocytes are on average larger in obese subjects, adipocyte size contributes to the greater serum leptin levels observed in obesity. Hexosamine biosynthesis has been suggested to link adipocyte size and leptin synthesis[29,52].

TNFα is produced by adipocytes and is elevated in the adipose tissue of obese subjects[53]. However, a role for TNFα in up-regulating leptin synthesis is controversial. In cultured rodent adipocytes[54], and isolated subcutaneous and omental adipocytes from morbidly obese humans[55], TNFα treatment results in a significant time- and dose-dependent inhibition of leptin production. On the contrary, in vivo TNFα administration acutely increases

Leptin and obesity

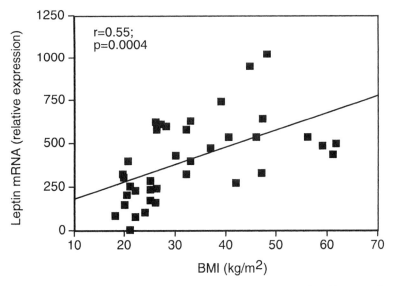

Figure 2. Relationship between BMI and *LEP* mRNA levels in isolated human subcutaneous adipocytes. *LEP* gene expression is significantly increased in adipocytes isolated from obese male and female subjects (BMI>30 kg/m^2) compared to that in lean subjects (BMI<30 kg/m^2). Greater amounts of *LEP* mRNA in obese adipocytes can be attributed to the larger adipocytes present in obesity.

serum leptin[56] and survivors of acute sepsis exhibit increased leptin levels[57]. The discrepancy between the in vivo and in vitro findings may result from an effect of TNFα to induce other hormones or cytokines which stimulate leptin synthesis in vivo.

Cortisol is a potent simulus for leptin synthesis and secretion from adipocytes in vivo and in vitro[58,13,others]. Local synthesis of cortisol from inactive metabolites by 11β-hydroxysteroid dehydrogenase is likely an important source of cortisol regulating leptin synthesis in adipose tissue[59]. The mechanism through which glucocorticoids regulate leptin synthesis in adipocytes is not completely understood as the glucocorticoid response element on the *LEP* gene promoter is not needed for dexamethasone to stimulate promoter activity[60].

5. LEPTIN RESISTANCE IN OBESITY

Inactivating mutations in either the *LEP* gene or leptin receptor gene that result in obesity are extremely rare in humans, and have been identified in only a handful of families throughout the world[61,62,63]. Rather, serum leptin levels are elevated in obese individuals due to the greater amount of adipose tissue (Fig. 1). These observations have led to the hypothesis that obesity is a state of "leptin resistance" in which there is an excess of serum leptin present, but the body does not effectively respond to these increased levels by reducing food intake or body weight[8,64].

The concept of leptin resistance is based on the postulate that an increase in serum leptin, resulting from deposition of adipose tissue, will initiate processes in the central nervous system to increase energy expenditure and decrease energy intake, reducing body energy stores to the original size. A significant amount of work has shown that administration of exogenous leptin to animals and leptin-deficient humans can reduce body fat[65-70]. It has also been demonstrated that the fall in serum leptin with caloric restriction is a signal to the brain to increase energy intake and reduce energy expenditure[42,43]. Taken together, these observations suggest that a leptin resistant state in obese humans might result if the leptin signal to the brain was not properly received or propagated, which despite elevated serum levels would lead to energy conservation and increased food intake.

Defects at two points within the leptin endocrine pathway have been suggested to contribute to leptin resistance. The first defect involves access of leptin to the brain. Leptin is detectable in cerebrospinal fluid[71,72] and regulated transport of leptin across the blood brain barrier has been demonstrated[73]. Cerebrospinal fluid leptin levels are positively correlated with BMI, but the ratio of CSF leptin to circulating leptin decreases with increasing BMI, indicating that transport of leptin across the blood brain barrier is limited[71,72]. In addition, blood brain barrier transport of leptin is decreased by high-fat diets[74,75] and triglycerides[76], suggesting that such transport defects could play a role in development of obesity. However, transport of the leptin across the blood brain barrier may not be necessary for leptin action. The arcuate nucleus of the hypothalamus is located close to the median eminence, where the blood brain barrier is incomplete. Thus leptin likely has direct access to neurons within the arcuate nucleus, which is the major target nucleus for leptin binding in the brain.

A defect in leptin signal transduction in hypothalamic neurons is a second possible explanation for leptin resistance. Once leptin has bound to its receptor in the arcuate nucleus, expression of neuropeptides that inhibit food intake is increased while expression of neuropeptides that stimulate food intake is suppressed (see Chapter 4). Several studies have indicated that the ability of leptin to activate the appropriate hypothalamic signaling is impaired with diet-induced obesity[74,75,77]. One group of proteins that may be involved in inhibition of leptin signaling is the suppressors of cytokine signaling (SOCS) proteins. These early genes are activated by the JAK/STAT signal transduction pathway and act in a negative feedback manner to limit cytokine signaling[78]. SOCS-3 expression is induced by leptin in the hypothalamus and is a potent inhibitor of leptin receptor initiated JAK/STAT signaling in cultured cell lines[79]. Increased hypothalamic SOCS-3 expression has been found in some rodent models of obesity[79], supporting the possibility that greater SOCS-3 levels in leptin-target neurons may cause leptin resistance in these animals.

A second molecule that has been shown to inhibit leptin receptor signaling is the protein tyrosine phosphatase PTP1B. In Cos-7 cells expressing leptin receptor, co-expression of PTP1B inhibited tyrosyl phosphorylation of JAK2 and STAT3[80]. Fibroblasts engineered to express leptin receptor but lacking PTP1B have enhanced leptin signaling[80]. PTP1B knockout animals are resistant to obesity and have enhanced leptin-induced hypothalamic STAT3 phosphorylation[80,81] suggesting that PTP1B can regulate leptin signaling in vivo.

Two clinical trials in which recombinant leptin was used to treat common obesity support the concept of leptin resistance in humans. In the first trial, which included both lean and obese adults, recombinant human leptin self-administered daily caused modest weight loss after 24 weeks of treatment[82]. Although weight loss was highly variable by subject, in general greater weight loss was achieved with higher doses of recombinant leptin. In a second trial administering pegylated recombinant leptin in obese men, there was a reduction in appetite but no significant decrease in body weight with 12 weeks of therapy[83]. It is important to note that in this second study serum leptin levels were only elevated with treatment at two timepoints over the 12 week treatment period, thus suggesting that weight loss was not achieved because insufficient leptin was given. Taken together, these two studies demonstrate that leptin resistance in humans exists, but that this resistance can be overcome with sufficiently high doses of leptin. However, it is possible that the central mechanisms regulating energy intake may become resistant to the higher concentrations of leptin achieved with therapy, initiating a vicious cycle in which therapy must then be continuously increased to overcome the development of resistance to ever increasing levels of serum leptin.

6. SELECTIVE LEPTIN RESISTANCE AND METABOLIC COMPLICATIONS IN OBESITY

Leptin resistance was originally proposed to explain the observation that greater levels of the endogenous hormone did not reduce food intake or prevent body weight gain in obese humans. However, as discussed in other chapters in this volume, a significant amount of work has shown that leptin is a pleiotropic hormone regulating many physiologic processes in the body in addition to energy intake and expenditure. In many cases the ability of leptin to regulate these other systems does not appear to be impaired, and in fact, the high serum leptin levels resulting from the inability of the hormone to prevent excess adipose tissue deposition may contribute to some of the metabolic complications of obesity.

Leptin increases energy expenditure through activation of sympathetic nervous system outflow to thermogenic brown adipose tissue[84]. Leptin also increases sympathetic outflow to non-thermogenic tissues including the kidney and adrenals[84,85]. The kidney has a major role in control of blood pressure and sympathetic stimulation of the kidney activates processes to increase blood pressure[86]. Studies in obese agouti mice[87,88] and in diet-induced obese mice[89] have shown that the ability of leptin to activate the sympathetic nervous system through central mechanisms and increase blood pressure is preserved in these mouse models, despite the fact that leptin is less efficacious in reducing food intake and body weight. The reduction in leptin-induced phosphorylation of STAT3 as a measure of leptin resistance in diet-induced obese mice has also recently been reported to vary across hypothalamic and extrahypothalamic nuclei[77]. Taken together, these observations support the concept of selective leptin resistance in the central nervous system and suggest that hyperleptinemia is a contributing factor to hypertension in obesity.

Leptin receptors have been found on many tissues and cells outside of the central nervous system[90]. Expression of Ob-Ra (short receptor isoform) is most abundant but a signaling mechanism for this receptor isoform is not well defined. Low levels of Ob-Rb (long receptor isoform) expression are also detected in many tissues and leptin-induced activation of the JAK/STAT pathway has been demonstrated. Thus leptin can regulate tissue function directly and independently of effects mediated through the central nervous system.

Leptin appears to have direct effects on components of the circulation. Leptin promotes platelet aggregation and thrombosis in response to vascular injury[91,92], and to induce oxidative stress in several different endothelial cell models in vitro[93,94]. Obesity is associated with accelerated atherothrombosis and increased systemic oxidative stress. It is therefore reasonable to suggest that the high leptin levels found in obesity may have pathologic effects on the vasculature, especially if the vasculature does not become leptin resistant in obese subjects. Future studies will be needed to fully understand the effect of leptin and leptin resistance on vascular function.

Unger has proposed that a major function of leptin in peripheral tissues is to prevent excess deposition of lipids and subsequent development of lipotoxicity[95]. Leptin reduces lipids in non-adipose tissues such as muscle and liver by upregulating fatty acid oxidation and inhibiting lipogenesis.

These effects of leptin are partially mediated by a direct effect of the hormone at the tissue level[96,97]. Unger further postulates that lipotoxicity occurs when tissues become resistant to the ability of leptin to reduce lipid storage. Loss of the leptin response in peripheral tissues has been suggested to result from down regulation of leptin receptors in liver[98] and induction of SOCS-3 expression in muscle and adipose tissue[99,100,101]. Obesity is characterized as a state of low-grade inflammation and many cytokines induce expression of SOCS proteins as part of the feedback loop limiting their activity[102]. Interestingly, insulin has also been shown to induce SOCS-3 expression[103]. Thus, an increase in SOCS-3 expression in peripheral tissues, which may contribute to development of leptin resistance, may occur through several possible mechanisms.

Leptin has direct effects on rodent adipocytes, the most studied of which is the induction of lipolysis[104,105,106]. Leptin has no lipolytic effect on adipocytes obtained from *db/db* mice or *fa/fa* rats, which have defective leptin receptors. STAT3 in adipose tissue is phosphorylated three minutes after intravenous leptin injection, but not intracerebroventricular leptin administration, providing additional evidence for leptin signaling through Ob-Rb on adipocytes[107]. It has recently been observed that leptin at fairly high concentrations (50 nM) can impair insulin signaling in rat adipocytes in vitro, an effect that appears to result from induction of SOCS-3 expression[108]. This work has been interpreted to suggest that SOCS-3 is increased to prevent down-regulation of leptin production by adipocytes in obese subjects. Thus leptin resistance in adipocytes may contribute to insulin resistance in adipose tissue of very obese subjects.

7. SUMMARY

Leptin is synthesized and released into the circulation in proportion to the amount of body fat. Other factors that determine serum leptin levels at steady state are gender and body fat distribution. Elevated serum leptin in obesity results from the greater fat mass in the body and greater leptin synthesis in adipocytes of obese subjects. Adipocyte size, hexosamine biosynthesis mediated by insulin stimulated glucose uptake, and elevated production of cortisol in adipose tissue all contribute to the increase in leptin synthesis by adipocytes in obesity. Leptin resistance in the hypothalamic nuclei regulating food intake and energy expenditure has been suggested to explain the observation that elevated leptin levels in obesity do not reduce food intake or body weight. However, leptin resistance in the central nervous system appears to be selective, with leptin-induced activation of the sympathetic nervous system intact and contributing to hypertension in obese subjects. Leptin resistance in peripheral tissues, or the lack of such resistance, also has a role in development of co-morbidities in obesity. Future work should focus on increasing our understanding of the effects of leptin on the central nervous system and directly on peripheral tissues, keeping in mind that leptin resistance in each instance may be either beneficial or pathologic.

ACKNOWLEDGEMENTS

Work of the authors cited in this chapter was supported in part by grants from the National Institutes of Health (DK51140 and M01 RR00750 [Indiana University General Clinical Research Center]), the American Diabetes Association and the Showalter Trust. Lauren N. Bell is supported in part by the Indiana University Diabetes and Obesity Research Training Program (NIH DK064466).

REFERENCES

1. G.C. Kennedy, The role of depot fat in the hypothalamic control of food intake in the rat. *Proc R Soc B*, **140**:578-592 (1953).
2. G.R. Hervey, The effects of lesions in the hypothalamus in parabiotic rats. *J Physiol*, **145**:336-352 (1959).
3. D.L. Coleman, Obese and diabetes: two mutant genes causing diabetes-obesity syndromes in mice. *Diabetologia*, **14**:141-148 (1978).
4. Y. Zhang, R. Proenca, M. Maffei, M. Barone, L. Leopold and J.M. Friedman, Positional cloning of the mouse obese gene and its human homologue. *Nature*, **372**:425-432 (1994).
5. R.V. Considine and J.F. Caro, Leptin and the regulation of body weight. *Int J Biochem Cell Biol*, **29**:1255-1272 (1997).
6. W.F. Blum, P. Englaro, A.M. Attanasio, W. Kiess and W. Rascher, Human and clinical perspectives on leptin. *Proc Nutr Soc*, **57**:477-485 (1998).
7. M. Maffei, J. Halaas, E. Ravussin, R.E. Pratley, G.H. Lee, Y. Zhang, H. Fei, S. Kim, R. Lallone, S. Ranganathan, P.A. Kern and J.M. Friedman, Leptin levels in human and rodent: measurement of plasma leptin and ob RNA in obese and weight-reduced subjects. *Nat Med*, **1**:1155-1161 (1995).
8. R.V. Considine, M.K. Sinha, M.L. Heiman, A. Kriauciunas, T.W. Stephens, M.R. Nyce, J.P. Ohannesian, C.C. Marco, L.J. McKee, T.L. Bauer and J.F. Caro, Serum immunoreactive-leptin concentrations in normal-weight and obese humans. *N Engl J Med*, **334**:292-295 (1996).
9. M. Rosenbaum and R.L. Leibel, Clinical Review 107. Role of gonadal steroids in the sexual dimorphisms in body composition and circulating concentrations of leptin. *J Clin Endocrinol Metab*, **84**:1784-1789 (1999).
10. C.T. Montague, J.B. Prins, L. Sanders, J.E. Digby and S. O'Rahilly, Depot and sex-specific differences in human leptin mRNA expression. *Diabetes*, **46**:342-347 (1997).

11. A.M. Lefebvre, M. Laville, N. Veg, J.P. Riou, L. van Gaal, J. Auwerx and H. Vidal, Depot-specific differences in adipose tissue gene expression in lean and obese subjects. *Diabetes*, **47**:98-103 (1998).
12. V. Van Harmelen, S. Reynisdotir, P. Eriksson, A. Thorne, J. Hoffstedt, F. Lonnqvist and P. Arner, Leptin secretion from subcutaneous and visceral adipose tissue of women. *Diabetes*, **47**:913-917 (1998).
13. L.B. Williams, R.L. Fawcett, A.S. Waechter, P. Zhang, B.E. Kogon, R.M. Jones, M. Inman, J. Huse and R.V. Considine, Leptin production in adipocytes from morbidly obese subjects: stimulation by dexamethasone, inhibition with troglitazone and influence of gender. *J Clin Endocrinol Metab*, **85**:2678-2684 (2000).
14. C.S. Mantzoros, J.S. Flier and A.D. Rogol, A longitudinal assessment of hormonal and physical alterations during normal puberty in boys. V. Rising leptin levels may signal the onset of puberty. *J Clin Endocrinol Metab*, **82**:1066-1070 (1997).
15. R. Sih, J.E. Morley, F.E. Kaiser, H.M. Perry III, P. Patrick and C. Ross, Testosterone replacement in older hypogonadal men: a 12-month randomized controlled trial. *J Clin Endocrinol Metab*, **82**:1661-1667 (1997).
16. F. Jockenhovel, W.F. Blum, E. Vogel, P. Englaro, D. Muller-Wieland, D. Reinwein, W. Rascher and W Krone, Testosterone substitution normalizes elevated serum leptin levels in hypogonadal men. *J Clin Endocrinol Metab*, **82**:2510-2513 (1997).
17. J.M. Elbers, H. Asscheman, J.C. Seidell, M. Frolich, A.E. Meinders and L.J. Gooren, Reversal of the sex difference in serum leptin levels upon cross-sex hormone administration in transsexuals. *J Clin Endocrinol Metab*, **82**:3267-3270 (1997).
18. X. Casabiell, V. Pineiro, R. Peino, M. Lage, J.P. Camina, R. Gallego, L.G. Vallejo, C. Dieguez and F.F. Casanueva, Gender differences in both spontaneous and stimulated leptin secretion by human omental adipose tissue in vitro: dexamethasone and estradiol stimulate leptin release in women, but not in men. *J Clin Endocrinol Metab*, **83**:2149-2155 (1998).
19. V. Pineiro, X. Casabiell, R. Peino, M. Lage, J.P. Camina, C. Menendez, J. Baltar, C. Dieguez and F.F. Casanueva, Dihydrotestosterone, stanozol, androstenedione and dehydroepiandrosterone sulphate inhibit leptin secretion in female but not male samples of omental adipose tissue in vitro: lack of effect of testosterone. *J Endocrinol*, **160**:425-432 (1999).
20. M. Sinha, J.P. Ohannesian, M.L. Heiman, A. Kriauciunas, T.W. Stephens, S. Magosin, C. Marco and J.F. Caro, Nocturnal rise of leptin in lean, obese, and non-insulin-dependent diabetes mellitus subjects. *J Clin Invest*, **97**:1344-1347 (1996).
21. D.A. Schoeller, L.K. Cella, M.K. Sinha and J.F. Caro, Entrainment of the diurnal rhythm of plasma leptin to meal timing. *J Clin Invest*, **100**:1882-1887 (1997).
22. J. Licinio, C. Mantzoros, A.B. Negrao, G. Cizza, M.L. Wong, P.B. Bongiorno, G.P. Chrousos, B. Karp, C. Allen, J.S. Flier and P.W. Gold, Human leptin levels are pulsatile and inversely related to pituitary-adrenal function. *Nature Med*, **3**:575-579 (1997).
23. T. Utriainen, R. Malmstrom, S. Makimattila and H. Yki-Jarvinen, Supraphysiological hyperinsulinemia increases plasma leptin concentrations after 4 h in normal subjects. *Diabetes*, **45**:1364-1366 (1996).
24. M.F. Saad, A. Khan, A. Sharma, R. Michael, M.G. Road-Gabriel, R. Boyadjian, S.D. Jinagouda, G.M. Steil and V. Kamdar, Physiological insulinemia acutely modulates plasma leptin. *Diabetes*, **47**:544-549 (1998).

25. P.J. Havel, R. Townsend, L. Chaump and K. Teff, High fat meals reduce 24 h circulating leptin concentration in women. *Diabetes*, **48**:334-341 (1999).
26. L. Rossetti, Perspective: hexosamines and nutrient sensing. *Endocrinol*, **141**:1922-1925 (2000).
27. J. Wang, R. Liu, M. Hawkins, N. Barzilai and L. Rossetti, A nutrient-sensing pathway regulates leptin gene expression in muscle and fat. *Nature*, **393**:684-688 (1998).
28. D.A. McClain, T. Alexander, R.C. Cooksey and R.V. Considine, Hexosamines stimulate leptin production in transgenic mice. *Endocrinol*, **141**:1999-2002 (2000).
29. R.V. Considine, R.C. Cooksey, L.B. Williams, R.L. Fawcett, P. Zhang, W.T. Ambrosius, R.M. Whitfield, R.M. Jones, M. Inman, J. Huse and D.A. McClain, Hexosamines regulate leptin production in human subcutaneous adipocytes. *J Clin Endo Metab*, **85**:3551-3556 (2000).
30. M.K. Sinha, I. Opentanova, J.P. Ohannesian, J.W. Kolaczynski, M.L. Heiman, J. Hale, G.W. Becker, R.R. Bowsher, T.W. Stephens and J.F. Caro, Evidence of free and bound leptin in human circulation. Studies in lean and obese subjects and during short-term fasting. *J Clin Invest*, **98**:1277-1282 (1996).
31. K.L. Houseknecht, C.S. Mantzoros, R. Kuliawat, E. Hadro, J.S. Flier and B.B. Kahn, Evidence for leptin binding to proteins in serum of rodents and humans: modulation with obesity. *Diabetes*, **45**:1638-1643 (1996).
32. N. Lahlou, K. Clement, J.C. Carel, C. Vaisse, C. Lotton, Y. Le Bihan, A. Basdevant, Y. Lebouc, P. Froguel, M. Roger and B. Guy-Grand, Soluble leptin receptor in serum of subjects with complete resistance to leptin: relation to fat mass. *Diabetes*, **49**:1347-1352 (2000).
33. G.H. Lee, R. Proenca, J.M. Montez, K.M. Carroll, J.G. Darvishzadeh, J.I. Lee and J.M. Friedman, Abnormal splicing of the leptin receptor in *diabetic* mice. *Nature*, **379**:632-635 (1996).
34. M. Maamra, M. Bidlingmaier, M.C. Postel-Vinay, Z. Wu, C.J. Strasburger and R.J. Ross, Generation of human soluble leptin receptor by proteolytic cleavage of membrane-anchored receptors. *Endocrinol*, **142**:4389-4393 (2001).
35. G. Brabant, H. Nave, B. Mayr, M. Behrend, V. van Harmelen and P. Arner, Secretion of free and protein-bound leptin from subcutaneous adipose tissue of lean and obese women. *J Clin Endocrinol Metab*, **87**:3966-3970 (2002).
36. J.L. Chan, S. Bluher, N. Yiannakouris, M.A. Suchard, J. Kratzsch and C.S. Mantzoros, Regulation of circulating soluble leptin receptor levels by gender, adiposity, sex steroids, and leptin: observational and interventional studies in humans. *Diabetes*, **51**:2105-2112 (2002).
37. L. Huang, Z. Wang and C. Li, Modulation of circulating leptin levels by its soluble receptor. *J Biol Chem*, **276**:6343-6349 (2001).
38. O. Zastrow, B. Seidel, W. Kiess, J. Thiery, E. Keller, A. Bottner and J. Kratzsch, The soluble leptin receptor is crucial for leptin action: evidence from clinical and experimental data. *Int J Obes Relat Metab Disord*, **27**:1472-1478 (2003).
39. G. Yang, H. Ge, A. Boucher, X. Yu and C. Li, Modulation of direct leptin signaling by soluble leptin receptor. *Mol Endocrinol*, **18**:1354-1362 (2004).
40. J.M. Friedman, Leptin, leptin receptors, and the control of body weight. *Nutr Rev*, **56**:S38-S48 (1998).
41. J.F. Caro, M.K. Sinha, J.W. Kolaczynski, P.L. Zhang and R.V. Considine, Leptin: the tale of an obesity gene. *Diabetes*, **45**:1455-1462 (1996).
42. J.S. Flier, What's in a name? In search of leptin's physiologic role. *J Clin Endocrinol Metab*, **83**:1407-1413 (1998).

43. R.S. Ahima, D. Prabakaran, C. Mantzoros, D. Qu, B. Lowell, E. Maratos-Flier and J.S. Flier, Role of leptin in the neuroendocrine response to fasting. *Nature*, **382**:250-252 (1996).
44. J.W. Kolaczynski, R.V. Considine, J. Ohannesian, C. Marco, I. Opentanova, M.R. Nyce, M. Myint and J.F. Caro, Responses of leptin to short-term fasting and refeeding in humans: a link with ketogenesis but not ketones themselves. *Diabetes*, **45**:1511-1515 (1996).
45. G. Boden, X. Chen, M. Mozzoli and I. Ryan, Effect of fasting on serum leptin in normal human subjects. *J Clin Endocrinol Metab*, **81**:3419-3423 (1996).
46. J.L. Chan, K. Heist, A.M. DePaoli, J.D. Veldhuis and C.S. Mantzoros, The role of falling leptin levels in the neuroendocrine and metabolic adaptation to short-term starvation in healthy men. *J Clin Invest*, **111**:1409-1421 (2003).
47. V.A. Barr, D. Malide, M.J. Zarnowski, S.I. Taylor and S.W. Cushman, Insulin stimulates both leptin secretion and production by white adipose tissue. *Endocrinol*, **138**:4463-4472 (1997).
48. R.L. Bradley and B. Cheatham, Regulation of ob gene expression and leptin secretion by insulin and dexamethasone in rat adipocytes. *Diabetes*, **48**:272-278 (1999).
49. B.S. Hamilton, D. Paglia, A.Y.M. Kwan and M. Deitel, Increased obese mRNA expression in omental fat cells from massively obese humans. *Nat Med*, **1**:953-956 (1995).
50. K.Y. Guo, P. Halo, R.L. Leibel and Y. Zhang, Effects of obesity on the relationship of leptin mRNA expression and adipocyte size in anatomically distinct fat depots in mice. *Am J Physiol Regul Integr Comp Physiol*, **287**:R112-R119 (2004).
51. F. Lonnqvist, L. Nordfors, M. Jansson, A. Thorne, M. Schalling and P. Arner, Leptin secretion from adipose tissue of women. Relationship to plasma levels and gene expression. *J Clin Invest*, **99**:2398-2404 (1997).
52. P. Zhang, E.S. Klenk, M.A. Lazzaro, L.B. Williams and R.V. Considine, Hexosamines regulate leptin production in 3T3-L1 adipocytes through transcriptional mechanisms. *Endocrinol*, **143**:99-106 (2002).
53. G.S. Hotamisligil, P. Arner, J.F. Caro, R.L. Atkinson and B.M. Spiegelman, Increased adipose tissue expression of tumor necrosis factor-alpha in human obesity and insulin resistance. *J Clin Invest*, **95**:2409-2415 (1995).
54. E.A. Medina, K.L. Stanhope, T.M. Mizuno, C.V. Mobbs, F. Gregoire, N.E. Hubbard, K.L. Erickson and P.J. Havel, Effects of tumor necrosis factor alpha on leptin secretion and gene expression:relationship to changes of glucose metabolism in isolated rat adipocytes. *Int J Obes Relat Metab Disord*, **23**:896-903 (1999).
55. R.L. Fawcett, A.S. Waechter, L.B. Williams, P. Zhang, R. Louie, R.M. Jones, M. Inman, J. Huse and R.V. Considine, TNFα inhibits leptin production in subcutaneous and omental adipocytes from morbidly obese humans. *J Clin Endocrinol Metab*, **85**:530-535 (2000).
56. M.S. Zumbach, M.W. Boehme, P. Wahl, W. Stremmel, R. Ziegler and P.P. Nawroth, Tumor necrosis factor increases serum leptin levels in humans. *J Clin Endocrinol Metab*, **82**:4080-4082 (1997).
57. S.R. Bornstein, J. Licinio, R. Tauchnitz, L. Engelmann, A.B. Negrao, P. Gold and G.P. Chrousos, Plasma leptin levels are increased in survivors of acute sepsis: associated loss of diurnal rhythm, in cortisol and leptin secretion. *J Clin Endocrinol Metab*, **83**:280-283 (1998).

58. H. Larsson and B. Ahren, Short-term dexamethasone treatment increases plasma leptin independently of changes in insulin sensitivity in healthy women. *J Clin Endocrinol Metab*, **81**:4428-4432 (1996).
59. D.J. Wake and B.R. Walker, 11 beta-hydroxysteroid dehydrogenase type 1 in obesity and the metabolic syndrome. *Mol Cell Endocrinol*, **215**:45-54 (2004).
60. P. De Vos, A.M. Lefebvre, I. Shrivo, J.C. Fruchart and J. Auwerx, Glucocorticoids induce the expression of the leptin gene through a non-classical mechanism of transcriptional activation. *Eur J Biochem*, **253**:619-626 (1998).
61. C.T. Montague, I.S. Farooqi, J.P. Whitehead, M.A. Soos, H. Rau, N.J. Wareham, C.P. Sewter, J.E. Digby, S.N. Mohammed, J.A. Hurst, C.H. Cheetham, A.R. Early, A.H. Barnett, J.B. Prins and S. O'Rahilly, Congenital leptin deficiency is associated with severe early-onset obesity in humans. *Nature*, **387**:903-908 (1997).
62. A. Strobel, T. Issad, L. Camoin, M. Ozata and A.D. Strosberg, A leptin missense mutation associated with hypogonadism and morbid obesity. *Nat Genet*, **18**:213-215 (1998).
63. K. Clement, C. Vaisse, N. Lahlou, S. Cabrol, V. Pelloux, D. Cassuto, M. Gourmelen, C. Dina, J. Chambaz, J.M. Lacorte, A. Basdevant, P. Bougneres, Y. Lebouc, P. Froguel and B. Guy-Grand, A mutation in the human leptin receptor gene causes obesity and pituitary dysfunction. *Nature*, **392**:398-401 (1998).
64. R.C. Frederich, A. Hamann, S. Anderson, B. Lollmann, B.B. Lowell and J.S. Flier, Leptin levels reflect body lipid content in mice: evidence for diet-induced resistance to leptin action. *Nat Med*, **1**:1311-1314 (1995).
65. M.A. Pelleymounter, M.J. Cullen, M.B. Baker, R. Hecht, D. Winters, T. Boone and F. Collins, Effects of the *obese* gene product on body weight regulation in ob/ob mice. *Science*, **269**:540-543 (1995).
66. J.L. Halaas, K.S. Gajiwala, M. Maffei, S.L. Cohen, B.T. Chait, D. Rabinowitz, R.L. Lallone, S.K. Burley and J.M. Friedman, Weight-reducing effects of the plasma protein encoded by the obese gene. *Science*, **269**:543-546 (1995).
67. L.A. Campfield, F.J. Smith, Y. Guisez, R. Devos and P. Burn, Recombinant mouse OB protein: evidence for a peripheral signal linking adiposity and central neural networks. *Science*, **269**:546-549 (1995).
68. T.W. Stephens, M. Basinski, P.K. Bristow, J.M. Bue-Valleskey, S.G. Burgett, L. Craft, J. Hale, J. Hoffman, H.M. Hsiung, A. Kriauciunas, W. MacKellar, P.R. Rosteck Jr., B. Schoner, D. Smith, F.C. Tinsley, X.Y. Zhang and M. Heiman, The role of neuropeptide Y in the antiobesity action of the obese gene product. *Nature*, **377**:530-532 (1995).
69. D.S. Weigle, T.R. Bukowski, D.C. Foster, S. Holderman, J.M. Kramer, G. Lasser, C.E. Lofton-Day, D.E. Prunkard, C. Raymond and J.L. Kuijper, Recombinant ob protein reduces feeding and body weight in the ob/ob mouse. *J Clin Invest*, **96**:2065-2070 (1995).
70. M.W. Schwartz, D.G. Baskin, T.R. Bukowski, J.L. Kuijper, D. Foster, G. Lasser, D.E. Prunkard, D. Porte Jr., S.C. Woods, R.J. Seeley and D.S. Weigle, Specificity of leptin action on elevated blood glucose levels and hypothalamic neuropeptide Y gene expression in ob/ob mice. *Diabetes*, **45**:531-535 (1996).
71. J.F. Caro, J.W. Kolaczynski, M.R. Nyce, J.P. Ohannesian, I. Opentanova, W.H. Goldman, R.B. Lynn, P.L. Zhang, M.K. Sinha and R.V. Considine, Decreased cerebrospinal fluid serum leptin ratio in obesity: a possible mechanism for leptin resistance. *Lancet*, **348**:159-161 (1996).

72. M.W. Schwartz, E. Peskind, M. Raskind, E.J. Boyko and D. Porte Jr., Cerebrospinal fluid leptin levels: relationship to plasma levels and to adiposity in humans. *Nat Med*, **2**:589-593 (1996).
73. W.A. Banks, A.J. Kastin, W. Huang, J.B. Jaspan and L.M. Maness, Leptin enters the brain by a saturable system independent of insulin. *Peptides*, **17**:305-311 (1996).
74. M. Van Heek, D.S. Compton, C.F. France, R.P. Tedesco, A.B. Fawzi, M.P. Graziano, E.J. Sybertz, C.D. Strader and H.R. Davis Jr., Diet-induced obese mice develop peripheral, but not central, resistance to leptin. *J Clin Invest*, **99**:385-390 (1997).
75. K. El-Haschimi, D.D. Pierroz, S.M. Hileman, C. Bjorbaek and J.S. Flier, Two defects contribute to hypothalamic leptin resistance in mice with diet-induced obesity. *J Clin Invest*, **105**:1827-1832 (2000).
76. W.A. Banks, A.B. Coon, S.M. Robinson, A. Moinuddin, J.M. Schultz, R. Nakaoke and J.E. Morley, Triglycerides induce leptin resistance at the blood-brain barrier. *Diabetes*, **53**:1253-1260 (2004).
77. H. Munzberg, J.S. Flier and C. Bjorbaek, Region-specific leptin resistance within the hypothalamus of diet-induced-obese mice. *Endocrinol*, **145**:4880-4889 (2004).
78. X.P. Chen, J.A. Losman and P. Rothman, SOCS proteins, regulators of intracellular signaling. *Immunity*, **13**:287-290 (2000).
79. C. Bjorbaek, J.K. Elmquist, J.D. Frantz, S.E. Shoelson and J.S. Flier, Identification of SOCS-3 as a potential mediator of central leptin resistance. *Mol Cell*, **191**:619-625 (1998).
80. J.M. Zabolotny, K.K. Bence-Hanulec, A. Stricker-Krongrad, F. Haj, Y. Wang, Y. Minokoshi, Y. Kim, J.K. Elmquist, L.A. Tartaglia, B.B. Kahn and B.G. Neel, PTP1B regulates leptin signal transduction in vivo. *Dev Cell*, **2**:489-495 (2002).
81. A. Cheng, N. Uetani, P.D. Simoncic, V.P. Chaubey, A. Lee-Loy, C.J. McGlade, B.P. Kennedy and M.L. Tremblay, Attenuation of leptin action and regulation of obesity by protein tyrosine phosphatase 1B. *Dev Cell*, **2**:497-503 (2002).
82. S.B. Heymsfield, A.S. Greenberg, K. Fujioka, R.M. Dixon, R Kusher, T. Hunt, J.A. Lubina, J. Patane, B. Self, P. Hunt and M. McCamish, Recombinant leptin for weight loss in obese and lean adults. *JAMA*, **282**:1568-1575 (1999).
83. C.J. Hukshorn, W.H.M. Saris, S. Westerterp-Plantenga, A.R. Farid, F.J. Smith, L.A. Campfield, Weekly subcutaneous pegylated recombinant native human leptin (PEG-OB) administration in obese men. *J Clin Endocrinol Metab*, **85**:4003-4009 (2000).
84. W.G. Haynes, D.A. Morgan, S.A. Walsh, A.L. Mark and W.I. Sivitz, Receptor-mediated regional sympathetic nerve activation by leptin. *J Clin Invest*, **100**:270-278 (1997).
85. J.C. Dunbar, Y. Hu and H. Lu, Intracerebroventricular leptin increases lumbar and renal sympathetic nerve activity and blood pressure in normal rats. *Diabetes*, **46**:2040-2043 (1997).
86. G.F. DiBona, The sympathetic nervous system and hypertension: recent developments. *Hypertension*, **43**:147-150 (2004).
87. A.L. Mark, R.A. Shaffer, M.L. Correia, D.A. Morgan, C.D. Sigmund and W.G. Haynes, Contrasting blood pressure effects of obesity in leptin-deficient ob/ob mice and agouti yellow obese mice. *J Hypertens*, **17**:1949-1953 (1999).
88. M. Aizawa-Abe, Y. Ogawa, H. Masuzaki, K. Ebihara, N. Satoh, H. Iwai, N. Matsuoka, T. Hayashi, K. Hosoda, G. Inoue, Y. Yoshimasa and K. Nakao,

Pathophysiological role of leptin in obesity-related hypertension. *J Clin Invest*, **105**:1243-1252 (2000).
89. K. Rahmouni, D.A. Morgan, G.M. Morgan, A.L. Mark and W.G. Haynes, Role of selective leptin resistance in diet-induced obesity hypertension. *Diabetes*, **54**:2012-2018 (2005).
90. C. Bjorbaek and B.B. Kahn, Leptin signaling in the central nervous system and the periphery. *Recent Prog Horm Res*, **59**:305-331 (2004).
91. M. Nakata, T. Yada, N. Soejima and I. Maruyama, Leptin promotes aggregation of human platelets via the long form of its receptor. *Diabetes*, **48**:426-429 (1999).
92. S. Konstantinides, K. Shafer, S. Koschnick and D.J. Loskutoff, Leptin-dependent platelet aggregation and arterial thrombosis suggests a mechanism for atherothrombotic disease in obesity. *J Clin Invest*, **108**:1533-1540 (2001).
93. A. Bouloumie, T. Marumo, M. Lafontan and R. Busse, Leptin induces oxidative stress in human endothelial cells. *FASEB J*, **13**:1231-1238 (1999).
94. S.I. Yamagishi, D. Edelstein, X.L. Du, Y. Kaneda, M. Guzman and M. Brownlee, Leptin induces mitochondrial superoxide production and monocyte chemoattractant protein-1 expression in aortic endothelial cells by increasing fatty acid oxidation via protein kinase A. *J Biol Chem*, **276**:25096-25100 (2001).
95. R.H. Unger, Longevity, lipotoxicity and leptin: the adipocyte defense against feasting and famine. *Biochimie*, **87**:57-64 (2005).
96. Y. Lee, M.Y. Wang, T. Kakuma, Z.W. Wang, E. Babcock, K. McCorkle, M. Higa, Y.T. Zhou and R.H. Unger, Liporegulation in diet-induced obesity. The antisteatotic role of hyperleptinemia. *J Biol Chem*, **276**:5629-5635 (2001).
97. R.B. Ceddia, Direct metabolic regulation in skeletal muscle and fat tissue by leptin: implications for glucose and fatty acids homeostasis. *Int J Obes Relat Metab Disord*, Epub ahead of print (2005).
98. G. Brabant, G. Muller, R. Horn, C. Anderwald, M. Roden and H. Nave, Hepatic leptin signaling in obesity. *FASEB J*, **19**:1048-1050 (2005).
99. Z. Wang, Y.T. Zhou, T. Kakuma, Y. Lee, S.P. Kalra, P.S. Kalra, W. Pan and R.H. Unger, Leptin resistance of adipocytes in obesity: role of suppressors of cytokine signaling. *Biochem Biophys Res Commun*, **277**:20-26 (2000).
100. J. Rieusset, K. Bouzakri, E. Chevillotte, N. Ricard, D. Jacquet, J.P. Bastard, M. Laville and H. Vidal, Suppressor of cytokine signaling 3 expression and insulin resistance in skeletal muscle of obese and type 2 diabetic patients. *Diabetes*, **53**:2232-2241 (2004).
101. H. Shi, I. Tzameli, C. Bjorbaek and J.S. Flier, Suppressor of cytokine signaling 3 is a physiological regulator of adipocyte insulin signaling. *J Biol Chem*, **279**:34744-34740 (2004).
102. D.L. Krebs and D.J. Hilton, SOCS proteins: negative regulators of cytokine signaling. *Stem Cells*, **19**:378-387 (2001).
103. B. Emanuelli, P. Peraldi, C. Filloux, D. Sawka-Verhelle, D. Hilton and E. Van Obberghen, SOCS-3 is an insulin-induced negative regulator of insulin signaling. *J Biol Chem*, **275**:15985-15991 (2000).
104. G. Fruhbeck, M. Aguado and J.A. Martinez, In vitro lipolytic effect of leptin on mouse adipocytes: evidence for a possible autocrine/paracrine role of leptin. *Biochem Biophys Res Commun*, **240**:590-594 (1997).
105. C.A. Siegrist-Kaiser, V. Pauli, C.E. Juge-Aubry, O. Boss, A. Pernin, W.W. Chin, I. Cusin, F. Rohner-Jeanrenaud, A.G. Burger, J. Zapf and C.A. Meier, Direct effects of leptin on brown and white adipose tissue. *J Clin Invest*, **100**:2858-2864 (1997).

106. M.Y. Wang, Y. Lee and R.H. Unger, Novel form of lipolysis induced by leptin. *J Biol Chem*, **274**:17541-17544 (1999).
107. Y.B. Kim, S. Uotani, D.D. Pierroz, J.S. Flier and B.B. Kahn, In vivo administration of leptin activates signal transduction directly in insulin-sensitive tissue: overlapping but distinct pathways from insulin. *Endocrinol*, **141**:2328-2339 (2000).
108. C. Perez, C. Fernandez-Galaz, T. Fernandez-Agullo, C. Arribas, A. Andres, M. Ros and J.M. Carrascosa, Leptin impairs insulin signaling in rat adipocytes. *Diabetes*, **53**:347-353 (2004).

Chapter 4

LEPTIN AND NEUROENDOCRINOLOGY

Abhiram Sahu
Department of Cell Biology and Physiology, University of Pittsburgh School of Medicine, S829 Scaife Hall, 3550 Terrace Street, Pittsburgh, PA

Abstract: The hormone leptin, a long sought satiety factor secreted mainly from adipocytes that relays the status of fat store to the hypothalamus, has emerged as one of the most important peripheral signals involved in the variety of neuroendocrine functions, including the regulation of food intake and body weight. Because the hypothalamus is a major site for integration of central and peripheral signals for the maintenance of energy homeostasis and many other physiological functions, most if not all, of the neuroendocrine functions of leptin are transduced primarily at the level of the hypothalamus. Leptin action in the hypothalamus for the maintenance of body weight is mediated by several orexigenic and anorectic signal producing neurons residing in the arcuate–paraventricular-lateral hypothalamus axis. Leptin not only modifies gene expression and release of the neuropeptides, but also modifies post- synaptic action of the neural signals and synaptic plasticity in the hypothalamus. In addition to the classical JAK2 (Janus kinase2)-STAT3 (signal transducer and activator of transcription 3) pathway, the phosphatidylinositol-3-kinase (PI3K)-phosphodiesterase-3B (PDE3B)–cAMP pathway plays a critical role in mediating leptin receptor signaling in the hypothalamus. A crosstalk between these two pathways may be important in leptin signaling in the hypothalamus. Defective hypothalamic STAT3 signaling, most likely due to an increase in suppressor of cytokine signaling-3, appears to play a role in the development of central leptin resistance in diet-induced obese (DIO) animals. Leptin signaling in the hypothalamus via STAT3 is also important in glucose homeostasis and reproduction. However, the development of leptin resistance in the neuropeptide Y, proopiomelanocortin and neurotensin neurons following chronic central leptin infusion is associated with normal STAT3, but a defective PI3K-PDE3B-cAMP pathway of leptin signaling in the hypothalamus. Future investigations on the role of the PI3K-PDE3B-cAMP pathway and its interaction with STAT3 and other pathways of leptin signaling in mediating various neuroendocrine functions are of significant importance to further our understanding on leptin biology.

Key words: Leptin, hypothalamus, energy homeostasis, leptin resistance, STAT3, PI3K, PDE3B, cAMP, feeding, obesity

1. INTRODUCTION

The discovery of the hormone leptin, which is mainly produced by adipocytes, has greatly enhanced our understanding on neuroendocrine mechanisms involved in various physiological functions including reproduction, food intake and body weight regulation. Most importantly, we are beginning to understand the complex neuroendocrine mechanisms underlying the development of obesity. Obesity is a major health hazard in humans. It is not restricted to the western societies anymore, but it qualifies as a worldwide health epidemic. Various genetic (monogenic, susceptible gene) and environmental (diet, exercise, social factors, chemicals, etc) factors are involved in the development of obesity[1]. Remarkably, in most humans body weight is maintained in stable condition. Positive energy balance as a result of less energy expenditure as compared to energy intake leads to the storage of energy in the form of fat. Continuous increases in fat mass eventually lead to obesity. Although energy homeostasis is maintained by multiple mechanisms including that which gathers the body's nutritional status and make appropriate behavioral and metabolic responses, it is widely accepted that a complex circuitry involving both central and peripheral factors working primarily in the brain, particularly in the hypothalamus, regulates body weight. In fact, the idea that some factors originating in the periphery relay the status of body fat stores to the brain originated with Kennedy, almost 50 years ago[2]. The findings that lesions in the hypothalamic ventromedial (VMH) and paraventricular (PVN) nuclei caused hyperphagia and obesity, and that in the lateral hypothalamus (LH) resulted in hypophagic response in rat, prompted Kennedy in 1953 to hypothesize that the hypothalamus senses some peripheral factors that provide the information about the body fat stores, and the hypothalamus would then transduce this information to change food intake to compensate for changes in body fat content[2]. Subsequent demonstration by Hervey using parabiosis experiments in rats that, when one of the parabiotic partners was made obese by a lesion in the VMH, the intact partner became anorexic and lean,[3] suggesting that some blood-borne factor produced by the increased fat mass acted to induce satiety in the intact partner. In addition, its lack of effect in the lesioned animals also suggested that the action of this factor(s) in the hypothalamus was essential for the maintenance of normal body weight.

In the 1970s, using parabiosis experiments with *ob/ob* and *db/db* mice, Douglas Coleman concluded that the blood-borne factor was encoded in the *ob* gene and the receptor for this factor was encoded in the *db* gene[4]. Finally in 1994, Jeffrey Friedman's team discovered the product of the *ob* gene as a 16 kD protein and it was named leptin[5]. Subsequently, in 1995, Tartaglia's group cloned the leptin receptor[6]. Expectedly, leptin signals nutritional status to key regulatory centers in the hypothalamus and it has emerged as an important signal regulating energy homeostasis[7-15]. Over the last decade it has been evident that besides its obligatory role in the neuroendocrinology of energy homeostasis, leptin also plays an important role in various other physiological functions such as neuroendocrinology of reproduction, bone formation and cardiovascular systems, etc. This chapter focuses on the mechanisms of leptin action in the hypothalamus in relation to neuroendocrinology of energy homeostasis. Other neuroendocrine functions of leptin will be described briefly.

2. LEPTIN AND NEUROENDOCRINOLOGY OF FOOD INTAKE AND BODY WEIGHT REGULATION

2.1 Hypothalamus as a Primary Site of Leptin Action in Body Weight Regulation and Energy Homeostasis

From the lesion studies by Hetherington and Ranson[16], and by Anand and Brobeck[17], it was established that within the brain, the hypothalamus is the primary center for regulation of food intake and body weight. Furthermore, a large body of evidence suggest that neural circuitry comprised of both orexigenic (appetite stimulant) and anorectic (appetite suppressant) signals residing in the hypothalamus plays a critical role in normal food intake and body weight regulation in the individual.[8-10, 14,15] This circuitry senses the status of body energy stores from peripheral signals, such as leptin and insulin, and modifies its activity accordingly. Several lines of evidence have clearly established that the leptin signal to the hypothalamus is obligatory for normal food intake and body weight regulation. For example, central injection of leptin is more effective than peripheral injection in reducing food intake and body weight[12], and within the hypothalamus, leptin is most effective in the arcuate nucleus (ARC) and ventromedial nucleus (VMN) in reducing food intake and body weight.[18, 19] The long-form of the leptin receptor (Ob-Rb) that is thought to be crucial for intracellular leptin signal transduction is localized in various hypothalamic sites including the ARC, VMN, dorsomedial (DMN), paraventricular (PVN) and lateral hypothalamic (LH) nuclei that have been implicated in food intake and body weight regulation[20]. In addition, central or peripheral administrations of leptin modify the activity of several neurons in these hypothalamic sites[1-10, 14, 15]; and lesions in the hypothalamus makes the animals become obese and resistant to exogenous leptin[21]. While deletion of leptin receptor in the hypothalamus results in the development of obesity[22], the ARC specific leptin receptor gene therapy in rats lacking functional leptin receptor results in an amelioration of the obese phenotype[23]. Finally, inhibition of leptin signaling in the hypothalamus due to mutation in leptin receptors is the cause of obesity in *db/db* mice and Zucker *fa/fa* rats[24, 25]; and leptin can cross the blood-brain barrier[26]. Recent evidence also suggests that leptin action in the hypothalamus is critical for normal glucose homeostasis. For example, leptin receptor activation in the ARC of Lepr$^{neo/neo}$ mice (these mice are homozygous for Lepr-null allele and thus similar to Lepr $^{db/db}$ mice) improved glucose homeostasis[27]. Therefore, any alteration in leptin action in the hypothalamus due either to a defect in leptin transport and or leptin resistance in leptin target neurons would lead to dysregulation of body weight and energy homeostasis seen in obesity.

2.2 Leptin Action on Hypothalamic Peptides Governing Energy Homeostasis

The hypothalamus produces an array of orexigenic and anorectic peptides that constitute a major part of the neural circuitry regulating ingestive behavior and body weight[8, 15, 28, 29]. Leptin target neurons are mainly localized in the ARC, LH and PVN areas that are known to be major sites of production and integration of neural signals involved in energy homeostasis. Cumulative evidence suggests that leptin's effects are mediated through the activity of several neuropeptidergic neurons, both orexigenic and anorectic in nature, in specific sites of the hypothalamus. In general, leptin decreases the activity of the orexigenic signal producing neurons and stimulates the activity of the anorectic signal producing neurons in the hypothalamus (Figure 1). Leptin sensitive neurons include those that produce neuropeptide Y (NPY), agouti-related protein (AgRP), melanin concentrating hormone (MCH), galanin, orexin, α-melanocyte stimulating hormone (α-MSH), neurotensin (NT), corticotropin-releasing hormone (CRH), and cocaine- and amphetamine-regulated transcript (CART), etc. Because food intake is regulated not only by several peptidergic signals of central and peripheral origins (Table 1), it is also under the control of catecholamines and serotonins, leptin's action in the hypothalamus most likely involves its interaction with various orexigenic and anorectic signals.

Among the neuropeptidergic systems that are the targets of leptin, two neural types in the ARC, the NPY and pro-opiomelanocortin (POMC) neurons, have been studied extensively because of their critical opposite roles in food intake. NPY is the most potent endogenous orexigenic signal and continuous or repeated central infusion of NPY causes obesity. Furthermore, knocking out NPY in the *ob/ob* mice reduces food intake and obesity[30], suggesting contribution of NPY in the development of hyperphagia and obesity in *ob/ob* mice. NPY neurons coexpress agouti–related protein (AgRP), an orexigenic peptide and an endogenous antagonist of α-MSH at central melanocortin receptors.[8, 9] Expectedly, leptin decreases

Leptin action on hypothalamic signals governing feeding

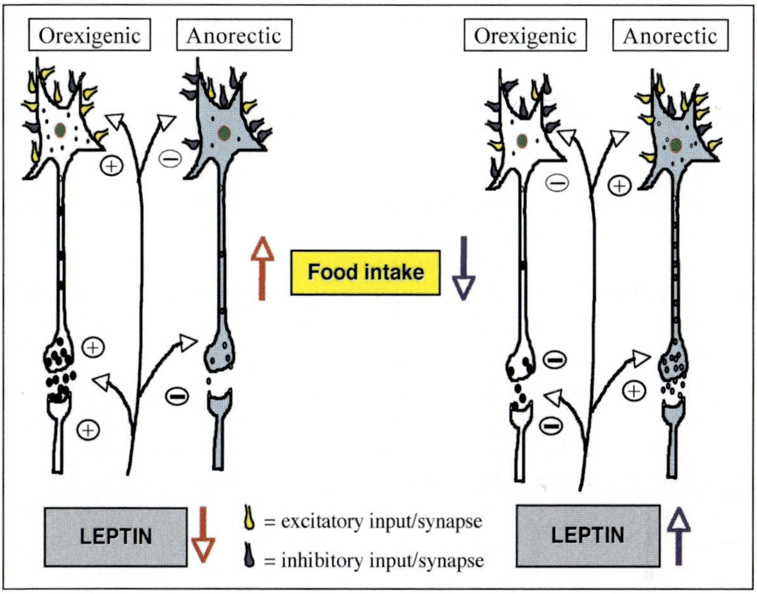

Figure 1. Schematic presentation of leptin action on hypothalamic peptides governing feeding. In this model, decrease in circulating leptin levels during fasting or deficiency in leptin action due to absence of leptin, leptin receptor mutation or leptin resistance would increase gene expression, peptide release, and action of orexigenic neuropeptides, such as NPY, MCH, GAL and orexin; and decrease synthesis, release of anorectic peptides, such as α-MSH, NT, CRH, etc. resulting in increased food intake. Similarly, increased circulating leptin levels would inhibit not only the synthesis and release of the orexigenic peptides, but it would modify the action of these peptides after being released, and enhance activity of anorectic peptides including synthesis, release and postsynaptic action, resulting in decreased food intake. We hypothesize that acute inhibition of food intake that occurs within an hour of leptin injection may be due to modification of postsynaptic action of orexigenic and anorectic neuropeptides. In addition, recent evidence (ref.55) suggests that leptin modifies synaptic plasticity in the hypothalamus as demonstrated by altered excitatory/inhibitory inputs on to orexigenic/anorectic signal producing neurons in response to leptin. Note that the number of inputs presented in this figure represents the situation, but they are arbitrary and do not reflect actual number of synapses/inputs. Modified from Sahu (2003)[14].

NPY/AgRP neuronal activity and NPY/AgRP neurons express Ob-Rb and signal-transducer and activator of transcription 3 (STAT3), suggesting a direct action of leptin on these neurons[9, 14]. Leptin also opposes the action of NPY on feeding and NPY may act antagonistically against anorectic effect of leptin[14]. Because of antagonism of melanocortin by AgRP, it appears that inhibition of AgRP may be an important mechanism by which leptin's anorectic effect is transduced at the level of hypothalamus.

Table 1. Peptidergic signals that stimulate or inhibit food intake

Stimulatory: Neuropeptide Y (NPY), Agouti-related protein (AGRP), Melanin concentrating hormone (MCH), Hypocretins/Orexins, Ghrelin, Galanin, Growth hormone-releasing hormone (GHRH), Dynorphin, β-Endorphin*, 26RFa (a member of RFamide peptide family), VGF   ***Inhibitory:***   Leptin, α-Melanocyte-stimulating hormone (a product of proopiomelanocortin gene, POMC), Cocaine-amphetamine-related peptide (CART), Neurotensin (NT), Cholecystokinin (CCK), Corticotropin-releasing hormone (CRH), Thyrotropin-releasing hormone (TRH), Prolactin-releasing peptide (PrRP), Calcitonin-gene related peptide (CGRP), Brain-derived neural factor (BDNF), Ciliary neurotrophic factor (CNTF), Glucagon-like peptide-1 (GLP-1), Galanin-like peptide (GALP), Peptide YY_{3-36}, Neuropeptide K (NPK), Neuromedin B and Neuromedin U, Neuropeptide B (NPB) and NPW, Somatostatin, Oxytocin, Bombesin, Motilin, Enterostatin, Anorectin, Amylin, Interleukin-1, Insulin, Insulin-like growth factor 1 (IGF-1) & IGF-11, Urocortin.

* Although pharmacological studies have demonstrated β-endorphin (β-End) to stimulate feeding in variety of animals, recent demonstration of hyperphagia and obesity in β-End knockout male mice suggests that endogenous β-End may have anorexic effect in regulating energy homeostasis (see ref. 129). Modified from Sahu (2004)[15].

The CNS melanocortin system has been examined extensively to understand the mechanism of leptin signaling in the hypothalamus because it exerts effects opposite to NPY. The endogenous melanocortin implicated most strongly in reducing food intake and body weight is α-MSH, a product of POMC neurons. α-MSH binds with high affinity to melanocortin receptor-3 (MC3) and MC4; which are highly expressed in the hypothalamus[31-33]. Mice lacking MC4 receptor become obese and MC4 receptor mutation causes obesity in mice and humans[31-34], and MC4 antagonist reverses the effect of leptin on feeding[9]. POMC neurons also express CART, a potent inhibitor of food intake[11, 35]. Leptin stimulates POMC/CART neuronal activity as expected. POMC/CART neurons express leptin receptors and STAT3; and leptin induces suppressor of cytokine signaling–3 (SOCS3) and c-Fos in these neurons, suggesting direct action of leptin on POMC/CART neurons[11]. Leptin action on POMC neurons may also involve reduction of γ-aminobutyric acid (GABA) and AgRP release from the NPY/AgRP neurons[36]. In addition, NPY/GABA cells innervate POMC neurons[37], suggesting interaction between NPY/GABA and POMC neurons. Altogether it appears that stimulation of POMC neurons by leptin is a result of direct action, as well as by inhibition of NPY/AgRP neurons. Because orexin, an orexigenic peptide, also excites GABAergic neurons in the ARC[38], it is possible that leptin's effect on POMC could be mediated indirectly by decreasing orexin neuronal activity. Furthermore, the finding of

Xu et al.[39] that brain-derived neurotrophic factor (BDNF), an inhibitor of food intake, regulates energy balance downstream of MC4 receptor suggests the involvement of BDNF in MC4 mediated leptin action in the hypothalamus. Recent studies further show that POMC neurons are glucose responsive and express K-ATP channels, and leptin activates K-ATP channel in POMC neurons[36]. These findings along with the demonstration that mutation in POMC gene results in obesity[34], provide further evidence in support of a significant role of POMC/CART neurons in mediating leptin's action in the hypothalamus.

Besides NPY/AgRP and POMC/CART neuronal systems, MCH, galanin (GAL), galanin-like peptide (GALP), orexin, thyroid-releasing hormone (TRH), NT, CRH and prolactin-releasing peptide (PrRP) producing neurons appear to mediate leptin action in the hypothalamus. Accordingly, leptin decreases or increases gene expression of orexigenic (MCH, GAL and orexin) and anorectic (GALP, NT, PrRP, TRH, CRH) peptide producing neurons, respectively[14, 15, 40, 41]. Leptin receptors have been localized, and leptin activates STAT3 in many of these neurons suggesting direct action of leptin. In addition, indirect actions of leptin on these neuronal systems via NPY/AgRP and or POMC/CART neurons have been documented. The findings that GALP neurons in the ARC express leptin receptors[42, 43], leptin increases GALP mRNA in *ob/ob* mice[44, 45] and fasted rats[46], and central injection of GALP decreases food intake and body weight in mice[47] suggest an important role of GALP in mediating leptin action in the hypothalamus. Furthermore, the effects of insulin on GALP neurons are similar to that seen after leptin[47], suggesting GALP neurons as targets of both leptin and insulin action[47]. A significant role of NT in mediating leptin action in the hypothalamus is supported by the observations that prior administration of NT antibody or specific NT antagonist blocks the anorectic effect of leptin[48], and that NT acts synergistically with leptin to reduce food intake[49]. Evidence also suggests that leptin inhibits the actions of MCH, galanin, and NPY on feeding[50]. Leptin action on hypothalamic NPY/AgRP and POMC neurons can be transduced indirectly by modifying the action of ghrelin, the only peripheral orexigenic signal of stomach origin[51]. Ghrelin and leptin functionally interact in that ghrelin blocks the effects of leptin on feeding and prior leptin administration attenuates the effects of ghrelin on feeding[52]. Leptin attenuates ghrelin-induced Ca++ increase in the NPY neurons[53]. Furthermore, ghrelin producing neurons are present in the hypothalamus and these neurons send efferents onto NPY/AgRP, POMC and CRH neurons[54]. Thus, regulation of ghrelin's effect on hypothalamic neurons, particularly NPY/AgRP neurons, may be one of the important mechanisms of leptin signaling in the hypothalamus.

Recent reports by Pinto et al.[55] and Bouret et al.[56] have provided a new dimension in understanding the mechanisms of leptin action in the hypothalamus in that they suggest a new role of leptin in modifying synaptic plasticity as well as axon guidance within the hypothalamus. Using *ob/ob* mice expressing a variant of green fluorescence protein (GFP) in the hypothalamic POMC and NPY neurons, Pinto et al. have demonstrated an increase in the excitatory inputs (excitatory postsynaptic currents, EPSCs), as assessed by electrophysiological recoding, to the NPY neurons and a parallel increase in the inhibitory inputs (inhibitory postsynaptic currents, IPSCs) to the POMC neurons in these mice. Ultrastructural studies showed reciprocal changes in excitatory and inhibitory synaptic inputs to the NPY and POMC neurons in *ob/ob* mice. Interestingly, leptin administration to the *ob/ob* mice normalized synaptic plasticity within 6 hours of injection. In addition, orexigenic peripheral hormone ghrelin rapidly (within 2 h) shifts input organization on POMC perikarya to support decreased cellular activity. These intriguing findings clearly indicate rapid synaptic re-arrangements by leptin as well as other metabolic signals such as ghrelin, and could be involved in hypothalamic regulation of food intake and energy homeostasis. It however remains to be determined whether synaptic plasticity shows diurnal rhythm in association with changes in food intake and metabolic factors including leptin, ghrelin, insulin, etc. Nevertheless, any dysregulation in synaptic plasticity could be involved in the development of central leptin resistance and obesity. The study by Bouret et al.[56] demonstrated that leptin is required for the normal innervation of the PVN, DMN and LH by the POMC and NPY/AgRP neurons of the ARC in that the density of innervation of these nuclei was significantly compromised in the *ob/ob* mice lacking leptin. Importantly, leptin replacement in the perinatal period but not in the adult completely restored the density of innervation to that seen in wild-type mice, suggesting a critical period during which leptin exerts its neurotrophic effect. These findings are in support of the concept that under- and over nutrition during the developmental period could have a long-lasting effect in the adult.

It is also becoming increasingly apparent that besides the hypothalamus, hindbrain plays an important role in transducing leptin action on food intake and body weight regulation. Leptin receptors are localized in the nucleus tractus solitarius (NTS)[57], leptin administration into the fourth ventricle reduces food intake and body weight gain[58], and peripheral administration of leptin activates neurons within the NTS[11]. There is also communication between the forebrain and hindbrain in mediating leptin action. For example, restoration of leptin signaling in the ARC by leptin receptor expression in Koletsky rats lacking leptin receptor normalized the effect of cholecystokinin (CCK) on the activation of neurons in the NTS and enhanced the satiety effect of CCK in these rats[59]. In addition, it is to be noted that besides the neurons of the ARC, the neurons in the PVN, particularly TRH, CRH, NT and oxytocin, play an important role in mediating leptin action in food intake and body weight regulation. These neurons not only are the direct targets of leptin, some of them link hypothalamic leptin action to caudal brain stem nuclei controlling meal size. In this regard, PVN oxytocin neurons are the prime candidate for this action of leptin[60]. Some of the oxytocin neurons of the PVN project directly to the NTS. Leptin administration into the 3rd ventricle induces cFos expression in the oxytocin neurons, and oxytocin antagonist not only reverses the effect of leptin on food intake but it also decreases potentiating effect of leptin on CCK activation of Fos expression in the NTS.

Overall, accumulated evidence including that cited above strongly suggest that leptin action in the hypothalamus is mediated by a large number of orexigenic and anorectic peptides in the ARC-PVN-PF/LH axis. It appears that leptin not only modifies synthesis and release of these neuropeptides, it also modifies the action of these peptides after they are secreted. Morphological connections and functional interactions seen between orexigenic and anorectic neurons[14, 61] suggest that leptin could alter (enhance or decrease) interactions between orexigenic and anorectic signals to fulfill its role in energy homeostasis. Recent demonstration of leptin-induced rapid changes in synaptic plasticity in the hypothalamus and a significant role of leptin in axonal guidance from the ARC neurons to the other hypothalamic areas during a critical developmental period have provided additional mechanisms by which leptin's action is transduced in the hypothalamus. Furthermore, leptin's overall effect on food intake and energy homeostasis is mediated by interactions of several first order (NPY/AgRP, POMC/CART) and second order (CRH, MCH, NT, oxytocin, GAL, etc.) neurons in the hypothalamus, and their communication with the hindbrain.

2.3 Leptin Signal Transduction in the Hypothalamus

Leptin receptor belongs to the family of class-1 cytokine receptor. Among six splice variants of the leptin receptor (Ob-R), the Ob-Rb, which is the long-form of the Ob-R, mediates leptin signaling in various tissues including the hypothalamus[25]. Ob-Rb is expressed in various hypothalamic sites including the ARC, VMN, DMN and PVN that have been implicated in energy homeostasis, and most of the leptin target neurons express leptin receptors[62]. Fasting, which causes a decrease in circulating leptin concentration, up-regulates leptin receptor expression and leptin binding in the hypothalamus[62]. Accumulated evidence also suggests that besides leptin, other factors, such as insulin may be involved in leptin receptor regulation[14].

2.3.1 Leptin Signaling through the Janus Kinase 2 (Jak2)-Stat3 Pathway

Leptin receptor signaling in the hypothalamus via activation of the JAK2–STAT3 pathway was established right after the discovery of leptin receptor[63]. In this pathway leptin binding to the receptor initiates a sequence of events involving phosphorylation of JAK2, receptor, and STAT3. After phosphorylation, STAT3 becomes dimerized and translocated to the nucleus where they bind and regulate expression from target promoter (Figure 2). Leptin activates STAT3 in the hypothalamus including the ARC, LH, VMN and DMN; indicating STAT3 as one of the major intracellular mediators of leptin signaling in the hypothalamus. Although STAT3 is expressed in several target neurons including NPY, POMC, galanin and orexin neurons, leptin induction of STAT3 has been documented only in the POMC neurons[64, 65]. In a series of investigations, Bates at al.[66, 67] demonstrated that in transgenic mice in which Tyr 1138 of Ob-Rb was replaced with a serine residue, STAT3 activation by leptin was impaired in association with development of obesity with reduced energy expenditure but without affecting reproduction. In addition, disruption of Ob-Rb-STAT3 signaling resulted in dysregulation of leptin action on the POMC without compromising the effects of leptin on NPY neurons, suggesting that inhibition of NPY neurons by leptin may be independent of STAT3 signaling. These authors have also shown that Ob-Rb-STAT3 signaling in the hypothalamus may be involved in regulation of glucose homeostasis by leptin[68]. However, a recent study with neuron-specific knock out of STAT3 (STAT3$^{N-/-}$ mice) showed that leptin-signaling through STAT3 is important for energy homeostasis, fertility and other neuroendocrine functions[69].

Leptin signaling through the JAK2-STAT3 pathway appears to be under the negative feedback control of SOCS3 protein. Over expression of SOCS3 reduces JAK-STAT signaling in mammalian cell lines by inhibiting leptin-induced JAK2 phosphorylation[70]; and leptin induces SOCS3 in the hypothalamus[71] and activates SOCS3 in NPY and POMC neurons[11]. The role of SOCS3 in leptin signaling in the hypothalamus has been recently appreciated from the studies using neuron-specific SOCS3 knockout mice and haplosufficient SOCS3 mice[72, 73]. Furthermore, SOCS3 also inhibits leptin signaling by binding to phosphorylated Tyr-985. SH2-containing phosphatase-2 (SHP-2), another mediator of leptin signaling, also competes with SOCS3 for p-Tyr-985 of Ob-Rb[74]. Thus, an alteration in any of these mechanisms could compromise inhibitory feedback action of SOCS3 during leptin signaling. Protein tyrosine phosphatase 1B (PTP1B), another negative regulator of leptin receptor signaling[75, 76], is localized in the hypothalamic areas where Ob-Rb is localized[76], and PTP1B knockout mice are resistant to diet-induced obesity (DIO) and more sensitive to leptin[77, 78], suggesting a significant role of PTP1B in leptin signaling in the hypothalamus. Unlike SOCS3, PTPIB compromises leptin receptor signaling primarily via dephosphorylation of JAK2[75]. Nevertheless, interactions among SHP2, SOCS3 and PTPIB could play a critical role during normal leptin signaling and that occurs during the development of leptin resistance[14].

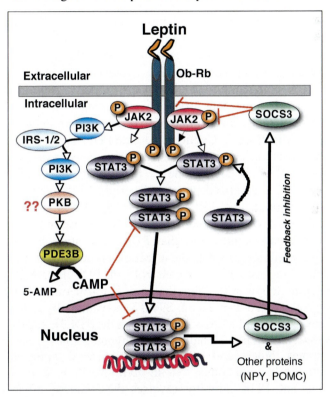

Figure 2. Schematic of leptin intracellular signal transduction in the hypothalamus. Leptin binding to its receptor (Ob-Rb) induces activation of Janus kinase (JAK), receptor dimerization, and JAK-mediated phosphorylation of the intracellular part of the receptor, followed by phosphorylation and activation of signal transducer and activators of transcription-3 (STAT3). Activated STAT3 dimerizes, translocates to the nucleus and tans-activates target genes, including suppressor of cytokine signaling-3 (SOCS3), neuropeptide Y (NPY) and proopiomelanocortin (POMC). Our evidence suggests that leptin also activates phosphatidylinositol 3-kinase (PI3K) and phosphodiesterase 3B (PDE3B) and reduces cAMP levels in the hypothalamus, and that the PI3K-PDE3B-cAMP pathway interacts with the JAK2-STAT3 of leptin signaling in the hypothalamus. Other potential signaling pathways including the involvement of SHP2-GRB2-Ras-Raf-MAPK/ERK pathway and PTP1B in regulating leptin action in the hypothalamus are left out of this scheme to avoid complication in the figure. Furthermore, the role of SHP2-GRB2-Ras-Raf-MAPK/ERK pathway in leptin signaling in the hypothalamus is not clearly understood. Also the role of cofactors and co-activators, such as p300/CBP and NcoA/SRC1a, in STAT3 transcriptional activity is yet to be established in the hypothalamus. Modified from Sahu (2004)[15].

2.3.2 Leptin Signaling through the Phosphatidylinositol-3 Kinase (PI3K)-Phosphodiesterase 3B (PDE3B)-cAMP Pathway

In several non-neuronal tissues, the insulin–like signaling pathway involving PI3K-dependent activation of phosphodiesterase-3B (PDE3B) and eventual reduction of cAMP mediates leptin action[79, 80]. Because intrahypothalamic cAMP injection increases food intake[81], central dibutyryl cAMP injection increases hypothalamic levels of NPY[82], and leptin modifies cAMP response element-mediated gene expression including that of NPY neurons in the hypothalamus[83], we hypothesized that regulation of cAMP by PDE3B plays an important role in mediating leptin action in the hypothalamus. Notably, intracellular cAMP levels are regulated by adenylyl cyclase and cAMP PDEs[84]. Cyclic nucleotide PDEs are a large super family of enzymes consisting currently of 20 different genes sub-grouped into 11 different families[85, 86]. PDE3B, one of the two members of type 3 PDE family of genes[85], is localized in several peripheral tissues and in the CNS including the hypothalamic ARC, VMN, DMN, PVN, LH and PFH areas[14, 87]. Our evidence that leptin induces PDE3B activity and reduces cAMP levels in the hypothalamus, and that PDE3 inhibition by cilostamide, a specific PDE3 inhibitor, reverses the effect of leptin on food intake and body weight clearly suggests a significant role of PDE3B-cAMP pathway in mediating leptin action in the hypothalamus[88]. Furthermore our observation of the reversal of leptin-induced STAT3 activation by cilostamide (see Figure 3) has established a cross talk between the PDE3B-cAMP and JAK2-STAT3 pathways of leptin signaling in the hypothalamus[88]. As seen in non-neuronal tissues, others and we have demonstrated leptin-induced PI3K activation in the hypothalamus[88, 89]. In addition, PI3K is localized in the hypothalamus and PI3K inhibitor reverses the anorectic effect of leptin[90]. Our preliminary study suggests PI3K as an upstream regulator of PDE3B signaling in the hypothalamus[91]. Overall, these findings all together indicate that a PI3K-PDE3B-cAMP pathway interacting with the JAK2-STAT3 pathway constitutes a critical component of leptin signaling in the hypothalamus (Figure 2). We hypothesize that defects in either one or both of the signaling pathways may be responsible for the development of leptin resistance seen in obesity. It is most likely that PI3K-PDE3B-cAMP signaling pathway may mediate leptin's action in the hypothalamus in general. Therefore, further understanding of this signal transduction pathway would be of significant importance in unraveling the molecular mechanisms of hypothalamic action of leptin in normal states and during the development of leptin resistance seen in obesity and related disorders.

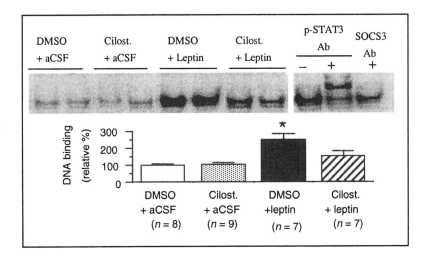

Figure 3. Cilostamide reverses the effect of leptin on STAT3 activation in the hypothalamus. Fasted (24 hr) rats were injected ICV with DMSO or cilostamide (10 µg) followed 30 min later by leptin (4 µg) or aCSF (artificial cerebrospinal fluid). DNA binding activity of STAT3 in the medial basal hypothalamus was determined by an electrophoretic mobility shift assay using a ^{32}P-labeled M67-SIE oligonucleotide probe. Top right, DNA binding activity is specific to p-STAT3 because a 'supershift' did not occur in the presence of anti-SOCS3 antibody. Bottom, results obtained by phosphor imaging and expressed as relative (%) to vehicle. Data are means ± SEM for the number (n) of animals in parentheses. *p < 0.05 as compared to all other groups. The reversal of STAT3 activation by PDE3B inhibition implies a crosstalk between the JAK2-STAT3 and PDE3B-cAMP pathways in transducing leptin action in the hypothalamus. (Adapted from ref. 88)

As seen for leptin action, insulin also stimulates PI3K in the hypothalamus, and PI3K inhibitor reverses the anorectic effect of insulin, suggesting that stimulation of PI3K may be a common pathway for both leptin and insulin signaling in the hypothalamus[92]. Furthermore, activation of PI3K has been proposed to mediate acute membrane effect of leptin and insulin including the activation of ATP-sensitive potassium channel in the hypothalamus[93, 94]. Because insulin stimulates STAT3 in the hypothalamus[95], it remains to be determined whether, like leptin signaling[88]; insulin signaling through STAT3 pathway also requires PDE3B activation-dependent reduction in cAMP levels. It is possible that PDE3B activation-dependent reduction in cAMP levels by leptin is responsible for modifying NPY gene expression and NPY's action on feeding. Likewise, inhibition of NPY neuronal activity by insulin[28, 96] may involve the activation of PI3K-PDE3B-cAMP pathway of intracellular signal transduction. In this regard, a recent study by Xu et al.[97] demonstrated that PI3K integrates the action of leptin and insulin at the levels of hypothalamic POMC neurons.

3. LEPTIN SIGNALING IN THE HYPOTHALAMUS DURING THE DEVELOPMENT OF DIET-INDUCED OBESITY

The majority of the obese patients have high circulating levels of leptin suggesting the state of leptin resistance. Although the mechanisms behind the development of leptin resistance is not clearly understood, decreased transport of leptin into the brain has been suggested as one of the mechanisms of central leptin resistance in obesity. In support of this view is the demonstration that the cerebrospinal fluid: plasma leptin ratio is lower in obese individuals compared to lean controls[98, 99], and that leptin administration shows very limited response in obese individuals[100]. Because diet-induced obese (DIO) rodents may represent the form of obesity seen in most humans, understanding the mechanisms underlying the development of DIO is of significant importance and as such, several DIO models are now being used to elucidate the mechanisms of leptin signaling during the development of DIO. The evidence that the anorectic effect of central leptin is reduced in DIO rats and mice[101, 102], and that defects in blood-brain transport are acquired during development of obesity[103, 104] and that central leptin gene therapy failed to overcome leptin resistance in DIO[105] strongly suggest that central leptin resistance plays a significant role in the development of DIO. Among the mechanisms behind the development of central leptin resistance, downregulation of leptin receptor expression and reduced receptor signaling through the STAT3 pathway appear to play a major role in DIO[14, 106, 107]. In line with this view are the findings that leptin-induced STAT3 activation is specifically reduced in the ARC of mice within a week of high-fat diet feeding[108], and that inbred DIO prone rats develop a defect in central leptin signaling through STAT3 activation before the onset of obesity[104]. Furthermore, disruption of STAT3 signaling in the hypothalamus causes obesity[66, 69].

Because SOCS3 is a negative regulator of cytokine signaling including that of leptin receptor signaling through the JAK2-STAT3 pathway, and because peripheral leptin increases SOCS3 expression in the hypothalamus and SOCS3 is expressed in leptin–sensitive neurons, SOCS3 is thought to be a potential mediator of central leptin resistance[71]. In support of this hypothesis are the findings that SOCS3 is increased in the ARC within a week of HFD feeding in mice[108], and that neuron-specific SOCS3 deletion[72] or haploinsufficiency in SOCS3[73] causes the development of resistance to DIO. In addition, two later studies have shown that leptin-induced STAT3 activity in the hypothalamus is enhanced in the SOCS3 deficient mice, providing further evidence in support of SOCS3 inhibition of STAT3 signaling in the hypothalamus. As described earlier (see section 2.3.2),

PI3K-PDE3B-cAMP pathway of leptin signaling plays a critical role in mediating leptin receptor signaling in the hypothalamus. Thus, it is quite likely that a defect in this pathway of signaling could occur and contribute to the development of DIO. Many studies have examined the changes in various leptin target neurons during DIO[14, 15]. There is some evidence for the possible development of leptin resistance in NPY/AgRP neurons during DIO[109, 110]. Future studies should examine how and when the changes, if any, in leptin sensitivity to these and other target neurons occur during the development of DIO.

4. LEPTIN SIGNALING DURING THE DEVELOPMENT OF LEPTIN RESISTANCE AFTER CHRONIC ELEVATION OF HYPOTHALAMIC LEPTIN TONE

The evidence of elevated leptin levels within 1 day of HFD feeding in rats[101] suggest that an extended period of exposure of the brain, especially the hypothalamus, to a high level of leptin may result in the development of central leptin resistance during DIO. We tested this hypothesis in a rat model of chronic central leptin infusion in which animals developed resistance to the satiety action of leptin[111]. In this rat model we observed that hypothalamic NPY, POMC and NT neurons developed leptin resistance following chronic leptin infusion in that during the initial period of leptin infusion, when food intake was decreased, these neurons remained sensitive to leptin; however, within 2 weeks of leptin infusion, when food intake was normalized, these neurons become insensitive to leptin[111, 112]. Despite leptin resistance in the NPY, POMC and NT neurons, the JAK2-STAT3 pathway of leptin signaling in the hypothalamus remained activated throughout the 16 d of leptin infusion in that leptin receptor phosphorylation, STAT3 phosphorylation and DNA binding activity of STAT3 were increased in leptin infused group as compared to that in vehicle infused control group[113]. However, increased JAK2 phosphorylation seen during the initial period was not evident on day 16 of leptin infusion. Notably, STAT3 pathway remained activated despite an increase in SOCS3 expression in the hypothalamus. In contrast, the PI3K-PDE3B-cAMP pathway of leptin signaling in the hypothalamus was impaired following chronic leptin infusion[114, 115]. Specifically, PI3K and PDE3B activities were increased and cAMP levels were decreased on day 2 but not day 16 of leptin infusion. These findings suggest a selective resistance in the PI3K-PDE3B-cAMP pathway of leptin signaling following chronic increase in hypothalamic leptin tone attained by central infusion of this peptide hormone. While future investigations should address whether PI3K-PDE3B-cAMP pathway of leptin signaling is impaired during the development of DIO, our unpublished observation suggests impairment in the PI3K pathway of leptin signaling in DIO mice.

Overall, critical evaluation of hypothalamic leptin signaling mechanisms during early part of high-fat diet (HFD) feeding when the animals do not show any sign of obesity should delineate whether the defect in any signaling pathway is the cause or an effect of DIO. Furthermore, an emphasis on hypothalamic region specific as well as neuron specific changes in the signaling mechanisms could be given priority in understanding complex mechanisms of central leptin resistance leading to the development of DIO.

5. OTHER NEUROENDOCRINE FUNCTIONS OF LEPTIN

One of the major roles of leptin is to regulate the adaptive neuroendocrine and metabolic response to alterations in nutritional state. Ahima et al.[116] in their elegant study, suggested that leptin's most important role might be to act as a signal of fasting. In support of this view are the findings that fasting associated abnormalities in neuroendocrine functions including suppression of the hypothalamic-pituitary-gonadal, and -thyroid axes and in immune functions, reduced energy expenditure, and increased appetite are similar to that seen in leptin deficient or leptin-insensitive rodents; and all these are advantageous adaptations in the context of starvation. Furthermore, as suggested by these authors, leptin deficiency in *ob/ob* mice may be perceived as a state of starvation. Remarkably, leptin treatments largely correct starvation-induced immune abnormalities[117] and blunt the activation of the HPA axis. In addition, leptin therapy prevents the dysfunction in reproductive, thyroid and growth hormone axes. However, leptin does not correct starvation–induced hyperphagia, hypoglycemia and hypoinsulinemia[117].

Cumulative evidence suggests that leptin may have an important role in reproductive neuroendocrinology. For example, leptin therapy restored puberty and fertility in *ob/ob* mice, and this action of leptin was not due to its body weight reducing effect because pair-feeding that maintained the body weight to that of leptin-treated group did not normalize reproductive failure seen in these animals[118]. Leptin or leptin receptor deficiency is associated with delayed or absence of puberty in humans, and leptin therapy to a girl with leptin deficiency resulted in initiation of puberty[119, 120]. Leptin treatment has been shown to advance puberty in mice[121, 122]. In human and higher primates, leptin's role in puberty is yet to be established[123]. It appears that leptin plays a permissive role in pubertal development and reproduction. Nevertheless, leptin's effect in the hypothalamus is important for its action on the reproductive axis. In this regard, intracerebroventricular administration of leptin antiserum prevents luteinizing hormone secretion[124], leptin stimulates hypothalamic luteinizing hormone releasing hormone (LHRH)[125], and leptin receptor gene therapy at the hypothalamic ARC and

MPOA areas has been shown to restore fertility in Koletsky rats[126]. Leptin action on reproductive axis may also involve stimulation of excitatory amino acids in the hypothalamus[127]. Since several leptin sensitive neuropeptidergic systems in the hypothalamus including the NPY, POMC, MCH and GAL producing neurons have been implicated in regulating LHRH neuronal functions[8], these neuronal systems are likely to mediate leptin action on reproduction. Besides its effect on energy homeostasis and reproduction, leptin's other neuroendocrine functions include its role in regulating TRH, growth hormone and prolactin secretion[122]. Furthermore, hypothalamic action of leptin may be important in regulating bone mass[128].

6. CONCLUSIONS AND FUTURE PERSPECTIVES

Although discovery of leptin was expected to be involved primarily in body weight regulation, it is now becoming increasingly clear that leptin has a multifaceted role in neuroendocrine regulation of various physiological functions including those that have been presented in this chapter. Evidently, energy homeostasis has been implicated as the prime neuroendocrine function of leptin acting at the level of the hypothalamus. Recent studies are engaged in dissecting out details of the neural circuitry, neural sites and specific signaling mechanisms in the hypothalamus and extra-hypothalamic regions including that in the hindbrain to understand the neuroendocrine physiology of leptin. In the process, leptin responsive neurons have been designated as the first order (NPY/AgRP, POMC/CART) or the second order neurons (MCH, orexin, NT, CRH, etc.) on the basis of their locations (ARC vs LH or PVN), physiological roles in energy homeostasis and other functions such as reproduction, and their responsiveness to various peripheral signals including insulin, ghrelin, CCK, etc. Leptin not only engages both orexigenic and anorectic peptide producing neurons in the ARC-PVN-LH axis, it also modifies postsynaptic actions of orexigenic and anorectic signals. Morphological communication and interactions between the orexigenic and anorectic signal producing neurons could be targets of leptin action in the hypothalamus. Evidence of rapid rewiring of the hypothalamic circuitry in response to leptin as well as other signals such as ghrelin has opened up a new chapter in understanding the hypothalamic mechanisms involved in food intake and body weight regulation. Interestingly, excitatory and inhibitory inputs to the orexigenic and anorectic peptide producing neurons are modified by leptin in such a way so that it can fulfill its obligatory role in energy homeostasis. Whether synaptic plasticity is involved in memorizing the body weight 'set point' in the hypothalamus remains to be seen. Besides the classical JAK2-STAT3 pathway, the PI3K-PDE3B-cAMP pathway has evolved as a critical component of the leptin signaling in the hypothalamus. Importantly, the PI3K-PDE3B-cAMP pathway appears to integrate leptin and insulin signaling in the hypothalamus. Defect in STAT3 pathway of leptin signaling has been documented in the hypothalamus of rats and mice on the high-fat diet, and increased SOCS3 appears to play an important role in the development of central leptin resistance seen in DIO. The evidence of 'selective leptin resistance' in the PI3K-PDE3B-cAMP pathway but not in the STAT3 pathway during the development of leptin resistance in the NPY, POMC and NT neurons following chronic elevation of the hypothalamic leptin tone by central leptin infusion further suggests the importance of this pathway of leptin signaling in the hypothalamus. Thus, it is most likely that an alteration in the PI3K-PDE3B-cAMP pathway would occur during the development of central leptin resistance and DIO. However, it is critical to demonstrate whether dysregulation of this pathway of leptin signaling, if it does happen, is a cause or an effect of DIO. In addition, it is important to document if the PI3K-PDE3B-cAMP pathway of leptin signaling is involved in other neuroendocrine functions of leptin such as in reproductive, thyroid and adrenal axes. It is quite possible that different signaling pathways in the hypothalamus are involved in different neuroendocrine functions of leptin.

ACKNOWLEDGEMENTS

The author's work was supported by National Institutes of Health Grants DK54484 and DK61499.

REFERENCES

1. P.G. Kopelman, Obesity as a medical problem, *Nature* **404**, 635-643 (2000).
2. G.C. Kennedy, The role of depot fat in the hypothalamic control of food intake in the rat, *Proc. Roy. Soc. Lond.* **140**, 579-592 (1953).
3. G. Hervey, The effects of lesions in the hypothalamus in parabiotic rats, *J. Physiol.* **145**, 3336-3352(1959).
4. D.L. Coleman, Obese and diabetes: two mutant genes causing diabetes-obesity syndromes in mice, *Diabetologia* **14**, 141-148 (1978).
5. Y. Zhang, R. Proenca, M. Maffei, M. Barone, L. Leopold, and J.M. Friedman, Positional cloning of the mouse obese gene and its human homologue, *Nature* **372**, 425-432 (1994).
6. L.A. Tartaglia, M. Dembski, X. Weng, N. Deng, J. Culpepper, R. Devos, G.J. Richards, L.A. Campfield, F.T. Clark, J. Deeds, C. Muir, S. Sanker, A. Moriarty, K.J. Moore, J.S. Smutko, G.G. Mays, E.A. Woolf, C.A. Monroe, and R.I. Tepper, Identification and expression cloning of a leptin receptor, OB-R, *Cell* **83**, 1263-1271(1995).
7. J.K. Elmquist, E. Maratos-Flier, C.B. Saper, and J.S. Flier, Unraveling the central nervous system pathways underlying responses to leptin, *Nat. Neurosci.* **1**, 445-450 (1998).
8. S.P. Kalra, M.G. Dube, S. Pu, B. Xu, T.L. Horvath, and P.S. Kalra, Interacting appetite-regulating pathways in the hypothalamic regulation of body weight, *Endocr. Rev.* **20**, 68-100 (1999).
9. M.W. Schwartz, S.C. Woods, D. Porte, Jr., R.J. Seeley, and D.G. Baskin, Central nervous system control of food intake, *Nature* **404**, 661-671(2000).
10. S.C. Woods, R.J. Seeley, D. Porte, Jr., and M.W. Schwartz, Signals that regulate food intake and energy homeostasis, *Science* **280**, 1378-1383 (1998).

11. J.M. Zigman, and J.K. Elmquist, Minireview: from anorexia to obesity- The Yin and yang of body weight control, *Endocrinology* **144**, 3749-3756 (2003).
12. L.A. Campfield, F.J. Smith, Y. Guisez, R. Devos, and P. Burn, Recombinant mouse OB protein: evidence for a peripheral signal linking adiposity and central neural networks, *Science* **269**, 546-549 (1995).
13. J.M. Friedman, and J.L. Halaas, Leptin and the regulation of body weight in mammals, *Nature* **395**, 763-770 (1998).
14. A. Sahu, Leptin signaling in the hypothalamus: emphasis on energy homeostasis and leptin resistance, *Front. Neuroendocrinol.* **24**, 225-253 (2003).
15. A. Sahu, Minireview: A hypothalamic role in energy balance with special emphasis on leptin. *Endocrinology* **145**, 2613-2620 (2004).
16. A.W. Hetherington, and S.W. Ranson, Hypothalamic lesions and adiposity in the rat, *Anat. Rec.* **78**, 149-172 (1940).
17. B.K. Anand, and J.R. Brobeck, Localization of feeding center in the hypothalamus of the rat, *Proc. Soc. Exp. Biol. Med.* **11**, 323-324 (1951).
18. R.J. Jacob, J. Dziura, M.B. Medwick, P. Leone, S. Caprio, M. During, G.I. Shulman, and R.S. Sherwin, The effect of leptin is enhanced by microinjection into the ventromedial hypothalamus, *Diabetes* **46**, 150-152 (1997).
19. N. Satoh, Y. Ogawa, T. Katsuura, M. Hayase, T. Tsuji, K. Imagawa, Y. Yoshimasa, S. Nighi, K. Hosoda, and K. Nakao, The arcuate nucleus s a primary site of satiety effect of leptin in rats, *Neurosci. Lett.* **224**, 149-152 (1997).
20. J.G. Mercer, N. Hoggard, L.M. Williams, C.B. Lawrence, L.T. Hannah, and P. Trayhurn, Localization of leptin receptor mRNA and the long form splice variant (Ob-Rb) in mouse hypothalamus and adjacent brain regions by in situ hybridization, *FEBS Lett.* **387**, 113-116 (1996).
21. N. Satoh, Y. Ogawa, G. Katsuura, T. Tsuji, H. Masuzaki, J. Hiraoka, T. Okazaki, M. Tamaki, M. Hayase, Y. Yoshimasa, S. Nishi, K. Hosoda, and K. Nakao, Pathophysiological significance of the obese gene product, leptin, in ventromedial hypothalamus (VMH)-lesioned rats: evidence for loss of its satiety effect in VMII-lesioned rats, *Endocrinology* **138**, 947-954 (1997).
22. P. Cohen, C. Zhao, X. Cai, J.M. Montez, S.C. Rohani, P. Feinstein, P. Mombaerts, and J.M. Friedman, Selective deletion of leptin receptor in neurons leads to obesity, *J. Clin. Invest.* **108**, 1113-1121 (2001).
23. G.J. Morton, K.D. Niswender, C.J. Rhodes, M.G. Myers Jr, J.E. Blevins, D.G. Baskin, and M.W. Schwartz, Arcuate nucleus-specific leptin receptor gene therapy attenuates the obesity phenotype of Koletsky (fa(k)/fa(k)) rats, *Endocrinology* **144**, 2016-2024 (2003).
24. S.C. Chua, Jr., W.K. Chung, X.S. Wu-Peng, Y. Zhang, S.M. Liu, L. Tartaglia, and R.L. Leibel, Phenotypes of mouse diabetes and rat fatty due to mutations in the OB (leptin) receptor, *Science* **271**, 994-996 (1996).
25. L.A. Tartaglia, The leptin receptor, *J. Biol. Chem.* **272**, 6093-6096 (1997).
26. W.A. Banks, A.J. Kastin, W. Huang, J.B. Jaspan, and L. M. Maness, Leptin enters the brain by a saturable system independent of insulin, *Peptides* **17**, 305-311 (1996).
27. R. Coppari, M. Ichinose, C.E. Lee, A.E. Pullen, C.D. Kenny, R.A. McGovern, V. Tang, S.M. Liu, T. Ludwig, S.C. Chua Jr, B.B. Lowell, and J.K. Elmquist, The hypothalamic arcuate nucleus: a key site for mediating leptin's effects on glucose homeostasis and locomotor activity. *Cell Metab.* **1**, 63-72 (2005).
28. A. Sahu, and S.P. Kalra, Neuropeptidergic regulation of feeding behavior: neuropeptide Y, *Trends Endocrinol. Metab.* **4**, 217-224 (1993).
29. J.J. Hillebrand, D. de Wied, and R.A. Adan, Neuropeptides, food intake and body weight regulation: a hypothalamic focus, *Peptides* **23**, 2283-2306 (2002).
30. J.C. Erickson, G. Hollopeter, and R.D. Palmiter, Attenuation of the obesity syndrome of ob/ob mice by the loss of neuropeptide Y, *Science* **274**, 1704-1707 (1996).
31. A.A. Butler, and R. D. Cone, The melanocortin receptors: lessons from knockout models, *Neuropeptide* **36**, 77-84 (2002).

32. R.D. Cone, Anatomy and regulation of the central melanocortin system, *Nature Neurosci.* **8**, 571-578 (2005).
33. R.D. Cone, The Central Melanocortin System and Energy Homeostasis, *Trends Endocrinol. Metab.* **10**, 211-216 (1999).
34. S. O'Rahilly, I.S. Farooqi, G.S. Yeo, and B.G. Challis, Minireview: human obesity-lessons from monogenic disorders, *Endocrinology* **144**, 3757-3764 (2003).
35. P. Kristensen, M.E. Judge, L. Thim, U. Ribel, K.N. Christjansen, B.S. Wulff, J.T. Clausen, P.B. Jensen, O.D. Madsen, N. Vrang, P.J. Larsen, and S. Hastrup, Hypothalamic CART is a new anorectic peptide regulated by leptin, *Nature* **393**, 72-76 (1998).
36. M.A. Cowley, J.L. Smart, M. Rubinstein, M.G. Cerdan, S. Diano, T.L. Horvath, R.D. Cone, and M.J. Low, Leptin activates anorexigenic POMC neurons through a neural network in the arcuate nucleus, *Nature* **411**, 480-484 (2001).
37. T.L. Horvath, F. Naftolin, S.P. Kalra, and C. Leranth, Neuropeptide-Y innervation of beta-endorphin-containing cells in the rat mediobasal hypothalamus: a light and electron microscopic double immunostaining analysis, *Endocrinology* **131**, 2461-2467 (1992).
38. D. Burdakov, B. Liss, and F.M. Ashcroft, Orexin excites GABAergic neurons of the arcuate nucleus by activating the sodium--calcium exchanger, *J. Neurosci.* **23**, 4951-4957 (2003).
39. B. Xu, E.H. Goulding, K. Zang, D. Cepoi, R.D. Cone, K.R. Jones, L.H. Tecott, and L.F. Reichardt, Brain-derived neurotrophic factor regulates energy balance downstream of melanocortin-4 receptor, *Nat. Neurosci.* **6**, 736-742 (2003).
40. A. Sahu, Evidence suggesting that galanin (GAL), melanin-concentrating hormone (MCH), neurotensin (NT), proopiomelanocortin (POMC) and neuropeptide Y (NPY) are targets of leptin signaling in the hypothalamus, *Endocrinology* **139**, 795-798 (1998).
41. M. Harris, C. Aschkenasi, C.F. Elias, A. Chandrankunnel, E.A. Nillni, C. Bjoorbaek, J.K. Elmquist, J.S. Flier, and A.N. Hollenberg, Transcriptional regulation of the thyrotropin-releasing hormone gene by leptin and melanocortin signaling, *J. Clin. Invest.* **107**, 111-120 (2001).
42. M. J. Cunningham, J. M. Scarlett, and R. A. Steiner, Cloning and distribution of galanin-like peptide mRNA in the hypothalamus and pituitary of the macaque, *Endocrinology* **143**, 755-763 (2002).
43. Y. Takatsu, H. Matsumoto, T. Ohtaki, S. Kumano, C. Kitada, H. Onda, O. Nishimura, and M. Fujino, Distribution of galanin-like peptide in the rat brain, *Endocrinology* **142**, 1626-1634 (2001).
44. A. Jureus, M. J. Cunningham, D. Li, L. L. Johnson, S. M. Krasnow, D. N. Teklemichael, D. K. Clifton, and R. A. Steiner, Distribution and regulation of galanin-like peptide (GALP) in the hypothalamus of the mouse, *Endocrinology* **142**, 5140-5144 (2001).
45. S. Kumano, H. Matsumoto, Y. Takatsu, J. Noguchi, C. Kitada, and T. Ohtaki, Changes in hypothalamic expression levels of galanin-like peptide in rat and mouse models support that it is a leptin-target peptide, *Endocrinology* **144**, 2634-2643 (2003).
46. A. Jureus, M. J. Cunningham, M. E. McClain, D. K. Clifton, and R. A. Steiner, Galanin-like peptide (GALP) is a target for regulation by leptin in the hypothalamus of the rat, *Endocrinology* **141**, 2703-2706 (2000).
47. M. L. Gottsch, D. K. Clifton, and R. A. Steiner, Galanin-like peptide as a link in the integration of metabolism and reproduction, *Trends Endocrinol. Metab.* **15**, 215-221 (2004).
48. A. Sahu, R.E. Carraway, and Y. P. Wang, Evidence that neurotensin mediates the central effect of leptin on food intake in rat, *Brain Res.* **888**, 343-347 (2001).
49. B. Beck, A. Stricker-Krongrad, S. Richy, and C. Burlet, Evidence that hypothalamic neurotensin signals leptin effects on feeding behavior in normal and fat-preferring rats, *Biochem. Biophys. Res. Commun.* **252**, 634-638 (1998).
50. A. Sahu, Leptin decreases food intake induced by melanin-concentrating hormone (MCH), galanin (GAL) and neuropeptide Y (NPY) in the rat, *Endocrinology* **139**, 4739-4742 (1998).

51. M. Nakazato, N. Murakami, Y. Date, M. Kojima, H. Matsuo, K. Kangawa, and S. Matsukura, A role for ghrelin in the central regulation of feeding, *Nature* **409**, 194-198 (2001).
52. M. Shintani, Y. Ogawa, K. Ebihara, M. Aizawa-Abe, F. Miyanaga, K. Takaya, T. Hayashi, G. Inoue, K. Hosoda, M. Kojima, K. Kangawa, and K. Nakao, Ghrelin, an endogenous growth hormone secretagogue, is a novel orexigenic peptide that antagonizes leptin action through the activation of hypothalamic neuropeptide Y/Y1 receptor pathway, *Diabetes* **50**, 227-232 (2001).
53. D. Kohno, H.Z. Gao, S. Muroya, S. Kikuyama, and T. Yada, Ghrelin directly interacts with neuropeptide-Y-containing neurons in the rat arcuate nucleus: Ca2+ signaling via protein kinase A and N-type channel-dependent mechanisms and cross-talk with leptin and orexin, *Diabetes* **52**, 948-956 (2003).
54. M.A. Cowley, R.G. Smith, S. Diano, M. Tschop, N. Pronchuk, K.L. Grove, C.J. Strasburger, M. Bidlingmaier, M. Esterman, M.L. Heiman, L.M. Garcia-Segura, E.A. Nillni, P. Mendez, M.J. Low, P. Sotonyi, J.M. Friedman, H. Liu, S. Pinto, W.F. Colmers, R.D. Cone, and T.L. Horvath, The distribution and mechanism of action of ghrelin in the CNS demonstrates a novel hypothalamic circuit regulating energy homeostasis, *Neuron* **37**, 649-661 (2003).
55. S. Pinto, A.G. Roseberry, H. Liu, S. Diano, M. Shanabrough, X. Cai, J.M. Friedman, and T.L. Horvath, Rapid rewiring of arcuate nucleus feeding circuits by leptin, *Science* **304**, 110-115 (2004).
56. S.G. Bouret, S.J. Draper, and R.B. Simerly, Trophic action of leptin on hypothalamic neurons that regulate feeding, *Science* **304**,108-110 (2004).
57. J.G. Mercer, K.M. Moar, and N. Hoggard, Localization of leptin receptor (Ob-R) messenger ribonucleic acid in the rodent hindbrain, *Endocrinology* **139**, 29-34 (1998).
58. H.J. Grill, M.W. Schwartz, J.M. Kaplan, J.S. Foxhall, J. Breininger, and D.G. Baskin, Evidence that the caudal brainstem is a target for the inhibitory effect of leptin on food intake, *Endocrinology* **143**, 239-246 (2002).
59. G.J. Morton, J.E. Blevins, D.L. Williams, K.D. Niswender, R.W. Gelling, C.J. Rhodes, D.G. Baskin, and M.W. Schwartz, Leptin action in the forebrain regulates the hindbrain response to satiety signals, *J. Clin. Invest.* 115:703-710 (2005).
60. J.E. Blevins, M.W. Schwartz, and D.G. Baskin, Evidence that paraventricular nucleus oxytocin neurons link hypothalamic leptin action to caudal brain stem nuclei controlling meal size. *Am. J. Physiol. Regul. Integr. Comp. Physiol.* **287**, R87-96 (2004).
61. A. Sahu, Interactions of neuropeptide Y, hypocretin-I (orexin A) and melanin-concentrating hormone on feeding in rats, *Brain Res.* **944**, 232-238 (2002).
62. B. Meister, Control of food intake via leptin receptors in the hypothalamus, *Vitam. Horm.* **59**, 265-304 (2000).
63. C. Vaisse, J.L. Halaas, C.M. Horvath, J.E. Darnell, Jr., M. Stoffel, and J.M. Friedman, Leptin activation of Stat3 in the hypothalamus of wild-type and ob/ob mice but not db/db mice. *Nat. Genet.* **14**, 95-97 (1996).
64. T. Hubschle, E. Thom, A. Watson, J. Roth, S. Klaus, and W. Meyerhof, Leptin-induced nuclear translocation of STAT3 immunoreactivity in hypothalamic nuclei involved in body weight regulation, *J. Neurosci.* **21**, 2413-2424 (2001).
65. H. Munzberg, L. Huo, E.A. Nillni, A.N. Hollenberg, and C. Bjorbaek, Role of signal transducer and activator of transcription 3 in regulation of hypothalamic proopiomelanocortin gene expression by leptin, *Endocrinology* **144**, 2121-2131 (2003).
66. S.H. Bates, W.H. Stearns, T.A. Dundon, M. Schubert, A.W. Tso, Y. Wang, A.S. Banks, H.J. Lavery, A.K. Haq, E. Maratos-Flier, B.G. Neel, M.W. Schwartz, and M.G. Myers, Jr., STAT3 signalling is required for leptin regulation of energy balance but not reproduction, *Nature* **421**, 856-859 (2003).
67. S.H. Bates, T.A. Dundon, M. Seifert, M. Carlson, E. Maratos-Flier, and M.G. Myers Jr., LRb-STAT3 signaling is required for the neuroendocrine regulation of energy expenditure by leptin. *Diabetes* **53**, 3067-3073 (2004).

68. S.H. Bates, R.N. Kulkarni, M. Seifert, and M.G. Myers Jr., Roles for leptin receptor/STAT3-dependent and -independent signals in the regulation of glucose homeostasis, *Cell Metab.* **1**, 169-178 (2005).
69. Q. Gao, M.J. Wolfgang, S. Neschen, K. Morino, T.L. Horvath, G.I. Shulman, and X.Y. Fu, Disruption of neural signal transducer and activator of transcription 3 causes obesity, diabetes, infertility, and thermal dysregulation, *Proc. Natl. Acad. Sci. USA* **101**, 4661-4666 (2004).
70. C. Bjorbaek, K. El-Haschimi, J.D. Frantz, and J.S. Flier, The role of SOCS-3 in leptin signaling and leptin resistance, *J. Biol. Chem.* **274**, 30059-30065 (1999).
71. C. Bjorbaek, J.K. Elmquist, J.D. Frantz, S.E. Shoelson, and J.S. Flier, Identification of SOCS-3 as a potential mediator of central leptin resistance, *Mol. Cell* **1**, 619-625 (1998).
72. H. Mori, R. Hanada, T. Hanada, D. Aki, R. Mashima, H. Nishinakamura, T. Torisu, K.R. Chien, H. Yasukawa, and A. Yoshimura, Socs3 deficiency in the brain elevates leptin sensitivity and confers resistance to diet-induced obesity, *Nat. Med.* **10**, 739-743 (2004).
73. J.K. Howard, B.J. Cave, L.J. Oksanen, I. Tzameli, C. Bjorbaek, and J.S. Flier, Enhanced leptin sensitivity and attenuation of diet-induced obesity in mice with haploinsufficiency of Socs3, *Nat. Med.* **10**, 734-738 (2004).
74. M.G. Myers Jr., Leptin receptor signaling and the regulation of mammalian physiology, *Recent Prog. Horm. Res.* **59**, 287-304 (2004).
75. A. Cheng, N. Uetani, P.D. Simoncic, V.P. Chaubey, A. Lee-Loy, C.J. McGlade, B.P. Kennedy, and M.L. Tremblay, Attenuation of leptin action and regulation of obesity by protein tyrosine phosphatase 1B, *Dev. Cell* **2**, 497-503 (2002).
76. J.M. Zabolotny, K.K. Bence-Hanulec, A. Stricker-Krongrad, Y. Haj F. Wang, Y. Minokoshi, Y.B. Kim, J.K. Elmquist, L.A. Tartaglia, B.B. Kahn, and B.G. Neel, PTP1B regulates leptin signal transduction in vivo, *Dev. Cell* **2**, 489-495 (2002).
77. M. Elchebly, P. Payette, E. Michaliszyn, W. Cromlish, S. Collins, A.L. Loy, D. Normandin, A. Cheng, J. Himms-Hagen, C.C. Chan, C. Ramachandran, M.J. Gresser, M.L. Tremblay, and B.P. Kennedy, Increased insulin sensitivity and obesity resistance in mice lacking the protein tyrosine phosphatase-1B gene, *Science* **283**, 1544-1548 (1999).
78. L.D. Klaman, O. Boss, O.D. Peroni, J.K. Kim, J.L. Martino, J.M. Zabolotny, N. Moghal, M. Lubkin, Y.B. Kim, A.H. Sharpe, A. Stricker-Krongrad, G.I. Shulman, B.G. Neel, and B.B. Kahn, Increased energy expenditure, decreased adiposity, and tissue-specific insulin sensitivity in protein-tyrosine phosphatase 1B-deficient mice, *Mol. Cell. Biol.* **20**, 5479-5489 (2000).
79. A.Z. Zhao, K.E. Bornfeldt, and J.A. Beavo, Leptin inhibits insulin secretion by activation of phosphodiesterase 3B, *J. Clin. Invest.* **102**, 869-873 (1998).
80. A.Z. Zhao, M.M. Shinohara, D. Huang, M. Shimizu, H. Eldar-Finkelman, E.G. Krebs, J.A. Beavo, and K.E. Bornfeldt, Leptin induces insulin-like signaling that antagonizes cAMP elevation by glucagon in hepatocytes, *J. Biol. Chem.* **275**, 11348-11354 (2000).
81. E.R. Gillard, A.M. Khan, H. Ahsanul, R.S. Grewal, B. Mouradi, and B.G. Stanley, Stimulation of eating by the second messenger cAMP in the perifornical and lateral hypothalamus. *Am. J. Physiol.* **273**, R107-112 (1997).
82. A. Akabayashi, C.T. Zaia, S.M. Gabriel, I. Silva, W.K. Cheung, and S.F. Leibowitz, Intracerebroventricular injection of dibutyryl cyclic adenosine 3',5'-monophosphate increases hypothalamic levels of neuropeptide Y, *Brain Res.* **660**, 323-328 (1994).
83. M. Shimizu-Albergine, D.L. Ippolito, and J.A. Beavo, Downregulation of fasting-induced cAMP response element-mediated gene induction by leptin in neuropeptide Y neurons of the arcuate nucleus, *J. Neurosci.* **21**, 1238-1246 (2001).
84. P.B. Daniel, W.H. Walker, and J.F. Habener, Cyclic AMP signaling and gene regulation, *Annu. Rev. Nutr.* **18**, 353-383 (1998).
85. J.A. Beavo, Cyclic nucleotide phosphodiesterases: functional implications of multiple isoforms. *Physiol. Rev.* **75**, 725-748 (1995).
86. S.H. Soderling, and J.A. Beavo, Regulation of cAMP and cGMP signaling: new phosphodiesterases and new functions, *Curr. Opin. Cell Biol.* **12**, 174-179 (2000).

87. R.R. Reinhardt, E. Chin, J. Zhou, M. Taira, T. Murata, V.C. Manganiello, and C.A. Bondy, Distinctive anatomical patterns of gene expression for cGMP-inhibited cyclic nucleotide phosphodiesterases, *J. Clin. Invest.* **95**, 1528-1538 (1995).
88. A.Z. Zhao, J.N. Huan, S. Gupta, R. Pal, and A. Sahu, A phosphatidylinositol 3-kinase phosphodiesterase 3B-cyclic AMP pathway in hypothalamic action of leptin on feeding. *Nat. Neurosci.* **5**, 727-728 (2002).
89. K.D. Niswender, G.J. Morton, W.H. Stearns, C.J. Rhodes, M.G. Myers, Jr., and M.W. Schwartz, Intracellular signaling- Key enzyme in leptin-induced anorexia, *Nature* **413**, 794-795 (2001).
90. K.D. Niswender, B. Gallis, J.E. Blevins, M.A. Corson, M.W. Schwartz, and D.G. Baskin, Immunocytochemical detection of phosphatidylinositol 3-kinase activation by insulin and leptin, *J. Histochem. Cytochem.* **51**, 275-283 (2003).
91. A. Sahu, and A.R. Metlakunta, Evidence suggesting phosphatidylinositol 3-Kinase as an upstream regulator of phosphodiesterase 3B mediated leptin signaling in the hypothalamus, *Abst. 34th Ann. Meet. Soc. Neurosci., San Diego, CA, October 23-27*, (2004).
92. K.D. Niswender, C.D. Morrison, D.J. Clegg, R. Olson, D.G. Baskin, M.G. Myers, Jr., R.J. Seeley, and M.W. Schwartz, Insulin activation of phosphatidylinositol 3-kinase in the hypothalamic arcuate nucleus: a key mediator of insulin-induced anorexia, *Diabetes* **52**, 227-231 (2003).
93. J. Harvey, and M.L. Ashford, Leptin in the CNS: much more than a satiety signal, *Neuropharmacology* **44**, 845-854 (2003).
94. D. Spanswick, M.A. Smith, V.E. Groppi, S.D. Logan, and M.L. Ashford, Leptin inhibits hypothalamic neurons by activation of ATP-sensitive potassium channels, *Nature* **390**, 521-525 (1997).
95. J.B. Carvalheira, R.M. Siloto, I. Ignacchitti, S.L. Brenelli, C.R. Carvalho, A. Leite, L.A. Velloso, J.A. Gontijo, and M.J. Saad, Insulin modulates leptin-induced STAT3 activation in rat hypothalamus, *FEBS Lett.* **500**, 119-124 (2001).
96. A. Sahu, M.G. Dube, C.P. Phelps, C.A. Sninsky, P.S. Kalra, and S.P. Kalra, Insulin and insulin-like growth factor II suppress neuropeptide Y release from the nerve terminals in the paraventricular nucleus: a putative hypothalamic site for energy homeostasis, *Endocrinology* **136**, 5718-5724 (1995).
97. A.W. Xu, C.B. Kaelin, K. Takeda, S. Akira, M.W. Schwartz, and G.S. Barsh, PI3K integrates the action of insulin and leptin on hypothalamic neurons, *J. Clin. Invest.* **115**, 951-958 (2005).
98. M.W. Schwartz, E. Peskind, M. Raskind, E.J. Boyko, and D. Porte, Jr., Cerebrospinal fluid leptin levels: relationship to plasma levels and to adiposity in humans, *Nat. Med.* **2**, 589-593 (1996).
99. J.F. Caro, J.W. Kolaczynski, M.R. Nyce, J.P. Ohannesian, I. Opentanova, W.H. Goldman, R.B. Lynn, P.L. Zhang, M.K. Sinha, and R.V. Considine, Decreased cerebrospinal-fluid/serum leptin ratio in obesity: a possible mechanism for leptin resistance, *Lancet* **348**, 159-161(1996).
100. S.B. Heymsfield, A.S. Greenberg, K. Fujioka, R.M. Dixon, R. Kushner, T. Hunt, J.A. Lubina, J. Patane, B. Self, P. Hunt, and M. Mccamish, Recombinant leptin for weight loss in obese and lean adults: a randomized, controlled, dose-escalation trial, *Jama.* **282**, 1568-1575 (1999).
101. B.E. Levin, and A.A. Dunn-Meynell, Reduced central leptin sensitivity in rats with diet-induced obesity. *Am. J. Physiol. Regul. Integr. Comp. Physiol.* **283**, R941-948 (2002).
102. H. Bowen, T.D. Mitchell, and R.B. Harris, Method of leptin dosing, strain, and group housing influence leptin sensitivity in high-fat-fed weanling mice, *Am. J. Physiol. Regul. Integr. Comp. Physiol.* **284**, R87-100 (2003).
103. W.A. Banks, and C.L. Farrell, 2003 Impaired transport of leptin across the blood-brain barrier in obesity is acquired and reversible, *Am. J. Physiol. Endocrinol. Metab.* **285**, E10-15 (2003).

104. B.E. Levin, A.A. Dunn-Meynell, and W.A. Banks, Obesity-prone rats have normal blood-brain barrier transport but defective central leptin signaling before obesity onset, *Am. J. Physiol. Regul. Integr. Comp. Physiol.* **286**, R143-150 (2004).
105. J. Wilsey, S. Zolotukhin, V. Prima, and P.J. Scarpace, Central leptin gene therapy fails to overcome leptin resistance associated with diet-induced obesity. *Am. J. Physiol. Regul. Integr. Comp. Physiol.* **285**, R1011-1020 (2003).
106. A. Sahu, L. Nguyen, and R.M. O'Doherty, Nutritional regulation of hypothalamic leptin receptor gene expression is defective in diet-induced obesity, *J. Neuroendocrinol.* **14**, 887-893 (2002) (see erratum in J Neuroendocrinol 15:104, 2003).
107. K. El-Haschimi, D.D. Pierroz, S.M. Hileman, C. Bjorbaek, and J.S. Flier, Two defects contribute to hypothalamic leptin resistance in mice with diet-induced obesity, *J. Clin. Invest.* **105**, 1827-1832 (2000).
108. H. Munzberg, J.S. Flier, and C. Bjorbaek, Region-specific leptin resistance within the hypothalamus of diet-induced obese mice, *Endocrinology* **145**, 4880-4889 (2004).
109. M. Ziotopoulou, C.S. Mantzoros, S.M. Hileman, and J.S. Flier, Differential expression of hypothalamic neuropeptides in the early phase of diet-induced obesity in mice. *Am. J. Physiol. Endocrinol. Metab.* **279**, E838-845 (2000).
110. J. Gao, L. Ghibaudi, M. van Heek, and J.J. Hwa, Characterization of diet-induced obese rats that develop persistent obesity after 6 months of high-fat followed by 1 month of low-fat diet, *Brain Res.* **936**, 87-90 (2002).
111. A. Sahu, Resistance to the satiety action of leptin following chronic central leptin infusion is associated with the development of leptin resistance in neuropeptide Y neurons, *J. Neuroendocrinol.* **14**, 796-804 (2002).
112. R. Pal, and A. Sahu, 2003 Chronic central leptin infusion results in the development of leptin resistance in proopiomelanocortin and neurotensin neurons in the hypothalamus, 85th *Annual Meeting of the Endocrine Society, June 19-22, 2003, Philadelphia, PA, Abstract# P1-255*.
113. R. Pal, and A. Sahu, Leptin signaling in the hypothalamus during chronic central leptin infusion, *Endocrinology* **144**, 3789-3798 (2003).
114. A. Sahu, and R. Pal, Phosphodiesterase 3B-cyclic AMP pathway of leptin signaling in the hypothalamus is altered during chronic central leptin infusion: implication in leptin resistance, *Program No. 231.4. 2003 Abstract Viewer/Itinerary Planner. Washington, DC: Society for Neuroscience* (2003).
115. A. Sahu, and A.R. Metlakunta, Hypothalamic phosphatidylinositol 3-Kinase (PI3K) pathway of leptin signaling is impaired in association with altered insulin receptor substrate-1 (IRS-1) phosphorylation following chronic central leptin infusion: implication in leptin resistance. 87th *Annual Meeting of the Endocrine Society, San Diego, CA; June 2005 (Abstract# OR50-2)* (2005).
116. R.S. Ahima, D. Prabakaran, C. Mantzoros, D. Qu, B. Lowell, E. Maratos-Flier, and J.S. Flier, Role of leptin in the neuroendocrine response to fasting, *Nature* **382**, 250-252 (1996).
117. J.K. Howard, G.M. Lord, G. Matarese, S. Vendetti, M.A. Ghatei, M.A. Ritter, R.I. Lechler, and S.R. Bloom, Leptin protects mice from starvation-induced lymphoid atrophy and increases thymic cellularity in ob/ob mice, *J. Clin. Invest.* **104**, 1051-1059 (1999).
118. R.S. Ahima, C.B. Saper, J.S. Flier, and J.K. Elmquist, Leptin regulation of neuroendocrine systems, *Front. Neuroendocrinol.* **21**, 263-307 (2000).
119. F.F. Chehab, M.E. Lim, and R. Lu, Correction of the sterility defect in homozygous obese female mice by treatment with the human recombinant leptin, *Nat. Genet.* **12**, 318-320 (1996).
120. F.F. Chehab, K. Mounzih, R. Lu, and M.E. Lim, Early onset of reproductive function in normal female mice treated with leptin, *Science* **275**, 88-90 (1997).
121. I.S. Farooqi, Leptin and the onset of puberty: insights from rodent and human genetics, *Semin. Reprod. Med.* **20**, 139-144 (2002).
122. I.S. Farooqi, and S. O'Rahilly, Monogenic obesity in humans. *Annu. Rev. Med.* **56**, 443-458 (2005).

123. D.R. Mann and T.M. Plant, Leptin and pubertal development in higher primates. In: Leptin and Reproduction, Edited by M. C. Hensen and V. D. Castracane, Kluwer Academic/Plenum Publishers, New York (2003).
124. E. Carro, L. Pinilla, L.M. Seoane, R.V. Considine, E. Aguilar, F.F. Casanueva, and C. Dieguez, Influence of endogenous leptin tone on the estrous cycle and luteinizing hormone pulsatility in female rats, *Neuroendocrinology* **66**, 375-377 (1997).
125. W.H. Yu, M. Kimura, A. Walczewska, S. Karanth, and S.M. McCann, Role of leptin in hypothalamic-pituitary function, *Proc. Natl. Acad. Sci. USA* **94**, 1023-1028 (1997), Erratum in: *Proc. Natl. Acad. Sci. USA* **94**, 11108 (1997).
126. E. Keen-Rhinehart, S.P. Kalra, and P.S. Kalra, AAV-mediated leptin receptor installation improves energy balance and the reproductive status of obese female Koletsky rats, *Peptides* 2005 Jul 14; [Epub ahead of print] (2005).
127. O.J. Ponzo, R. Reynoso, G. Rimoldi, D. Rondina, B. Szwarcfarb, S. Carbone, P. Scacchi, and J.A. Moguilevsky, Leptin stimulates the reproductive male axis in rats during sexual maturation by acting on hypothalamic excitatory amino acids, *Exp. Clin. Endocrinol. Diabetes* **113**, 135-138 (2005).
128. F. Elefteriou, J.D. Ahn, S. Takeda, M. Starbuck, X. Yang, X. Liu, H.Kondo, W.G. Richards, T.W. Bannon, M. Noda, K. Clement, C. Valaisse and G. Karsenty, Leptin regulation of bone resorption by the sympathetic nervous system and CART, *Nature* **434**, 514-520 (2005).
129. S.M. Appleyard, M. Hayward, J.I. Young, A.A. Butler, R.D. Cone, M. Rubinstein, and M. J. Low, A role for the endogenous opioid β-endorphin in energy homeostasis, *Endocrinology* **144**, 1753-1760 (2003).

Chapter 5

LEPTIN-INSULIN INTERRELATIONSHIPS

Asha Thomas-Geevarghese and Robert Ratner
Medstar Research Institute, Washington, DC

Abstract: The relationship of leptin to insulin is complex and our understanding of the interaction is evolving. Leptin is secreted from white adipocytes and levels correlate with adipose tissue mass. Via hypothalamic leptin receptors (ObR), it restricts food intake and increases energy expenditure in normal individuals. Leptin is implicated in decreased production and secretion of insulin by the pancreatic beta (β) cell. Insulin, conversely, stimulates leptin secretion in an adipocyte-insulin feedback loop. The studies available to date, however, have had varying results as to whether leptin is an antidiabetogenic protein. This chapter will delineate the relationships of leptin on insulin secretion and action as well as the effect of insulin on leptin secretion and action.

Key words: leptin, insulin, diabetes, pancreatic β-cells

1. INTRODUCTION

The relationship of leptin to insulin is complex and our understanding of the interaction is evolving. Obesity is associated with diabetes, and leptin is known to be elevated in most cases of obesity. Leptin is secreted from white adipocytes and levels correlate with adipose tissue mass. Via hypothalamic leptin receptors (ObR), it restricts food intake and increases energy expenditure in normal individuals. Leptin is implicated in decreased production and secretion of insulin by the pancreatic beta (β) cell. Insulin, conversely, stimulates leptin secretion in an adipocyte-insulin feedback loop. The studies available to date, however, have had varying results as to whether leptin is an antidiabetogenic protein. Leptin appears to act as both an insulin-sensitizing agent and a contributor to the insulin-resistant phenotype.[1] This chapter will delineate the relationships of leptin on insulin secretion and action as well as the effect of insulin on leptin secretion and action.

2. EFFECT OF LEPTIN ON INSULIN SECRETION AND ACTION

There is growing evidence that leptin works at the level of the pancreatic β-cell as well as centrally in the hypothalamus. The main function of the pancreatic ß-cell is the biosynthesis and appropriate secretion of insulin in response to control blood glucose levels.[2] This function is tightly regulated both by nutrients and hormonal modulators, such as enteroendocrine hormones (glucose-dependent insulinotropic polypeptide and glucagon-like peptide [GLP]-1).[2] The pathways involved in leptin signaling in pancreatic β-cells are numerous. The model of leptin deficient *ob/ob* mice has been particularly helpful in elucidating these relationships, probably secondary to the compensatory upregulation of leptin receptor signaling. As opposed to glucose and incretin-dependent insulin secretion which are short-term responders to various nutritional and hormonal inputs, leptin appears to play more of a role in the long term secretion of insulin by the β-cell. Leptin resistance at the level of the pancreatic β-cell may promote the development of hyperinsulinemia and type 2 diabetes in susceptible overweight patients.[2] In the development of type 2 diabetes in obese patients, initial hyperinsulinemia is thought to be a compensatory response of the β-cell to insulin resistance.[2,3,4] With subsequent pancreatic β-cell failure, hyperglycemia presents itself. As hyperinsulinemia may present before the onset of insulin resistance, the adipocyte-insular axis may be playing a role in the progression of Type 2 diabetes[2] (Figure 1).

Studies on the effects of leptin on insulin secretion have yielded conflicting results. The pancreatic islets of leptin-deficient *ob/ob* mice exhibit a robust reduction of insulin secretion upon leptin stimulation, likely due to higher leptin sensitivity.[2] Chronically leptin-exposed pancreatic ß-cells, however, display variable results in different experimental conditions. In pancreatic ß-cells, leptin exerts a biphasic dose response with respect to insulin secretion. In rat islets, 2 nmol/l leptin significantly and maximally suppressed insulin release, whereas high concentrations were almost ineffective.[5] Initial studies examining the effect of leptin on insulin secretion in normal rodents or cell lines has yielded varying results.[2] It has been described that under physiological conditions leptin (1–20 nmol/l) significantly reduces insulin release from pancreatic ß-cells.[2] This is also described by the majority of studies using perfused rat pancreas and isolated rat or mouse islets[2], as well as in isolated human pancreatic islets.[6] In addition, there is evidence that a physiological increase in serum leptin levels significantly reduces insulin secretion in rats in vivo.[2,7]

Whereas a number of the in vitro studies have shown an inhibitory role of leptin on glucose metabolism, the in vivo studies have demonstrated a more insulin-sensitizing role thought secondary to the central effects of leptin. The major peripheral sites of leptin action, skeletal muscle, white adipose, and liver have been shown in a number of studies to have leptin mediated insulin stimulated glucose uptake and metabolism.[1] In vivo studies infusing leptin into mouse, rat, and human soleus and epitrochlearis muscles did not alter insulin mediated glucose uptake.[8-10] These differences are likely related to the model in which these studies were conducted. In the *ob/ob* leptin deficient mice, there is a downstream upregulation of leptin receptor signaling.[11] In rodents with normal leptin and leptin receptor activity, the chronic exposure to leptin may affect the response to acute and subacute exposure to leptin. In addition, the various doses and modes of delivery of leptin, the relative long duration of action needed for leptin, and the possibility of interfering substances make the varying experimental models at times difficult to interpret.[11] Thus, the studies described here will need to be assessed with these considerations in mind.

2.1 Normal mouse studies

There is evidence that leptin directly inhibits insulin secretion from pancreatic β-cells.[11] The mode of action appears to be via the leptin receptors expressed on the β-cell and its inhibitory effect on glucose stimulated insulin secretion as well as suppressing proinsulin mRNA expression.[2] Leptin activates the ATP-sensitive potassium channels[1] with the resultant hyperpolarization preventing calcium influx and the release of insulin. Glucose-induced insulin secretion is potentiated by hormone-mediated elevation of the intracellular second messengers cAMP/protein kinase A and phospholipase C/protein kinase C.[2] The K_{ATP} channel is a molecular target of leptin in pancreatic ß-cells for inhibition of insulin secretion. Consequently, activation of K_{ATP} channels in pancreatic ß-cells by leptin reduces cytosolic calcium concentration, and this fall can be overcome by co-incubation with glucose and GLP-1.[2] The inhibitory effects of leptin on preproinsulin gene expression, however, appear to be independent of the activation of K_{ATP} channels.[2] The K_{ATP} channel opener diazoxide did not affect either leptin suppression of preproinsulin mRNA levels or inhibition of insulin promoter activity in INS-1 cells,[12] indicating that gene regulatory effects of leptin use signal transduction pathways different from those that mediate the effect on insulin secretion.

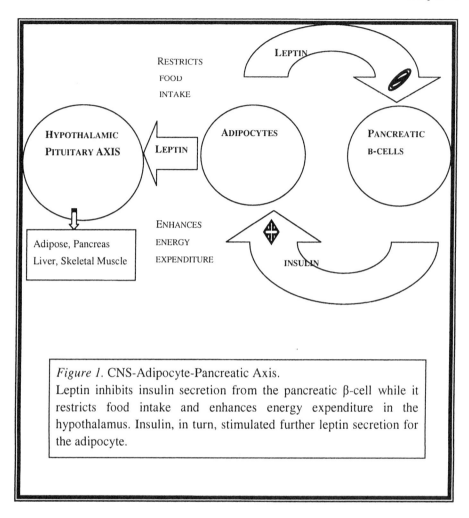

Figure 1. CNS-Adipocyte-Pancreatic Axis.
Leptin inhibits insulin secretion from the pancreatic β-cell while it restricts food intake and enhances energy expenditure in the hypothalamus. Insulin, in turn, stimulated further leptin secretion for the adipocyte.

Other proposed mechanisms include inhibition of insulin secretion by glucagon-like-peptide-1 (GLP-1), stimulation of the sympathetic nervous system[13] and reduction in protein kinase C.[1,14] By preventing triglyceride accumulation in the β-cell, however, leptin helps to maintain normal glucose stimulated insulin secretion.[15] The proinsulin gene and protein phosphatase-1 gene are leptin repressible genes and the gene for the suppressor of cytokine signaling 3 protein is a leptin-induced gene in pancreatic β-cells.[2] The molecular effects of leptin involve the restriction of insulin secretion and biosynthesis in the normal animal.[2]

To determine whether leptin has insulin sensitizing effects in normal rodents, Sivitz measured plasma glucose and insulin concentrations in male Sprague-Dawley rats treated with leptin by continuous subcutaneous infusion for 48 hours. Leptin administered 10 mcg/h, significantly reduced both plasma glucose and insulin levels and decreased circulating insulin-like growth factor-1 (IGF-1) levels. GLUT-4, the major insulin-sensitive glucose transporter expressed specifically in fat and muscle, was studied in this model.[16] The authors observed no difference in GLUT-4 content in brown and epididymal adipose tissue, suggesting that the expression of this transporter in the tissues examined is not a key factor in mediating the effects of leptin on insulin sensitivity.[17] Nonetheless, leptin could still alter glucose transport in these tissues because intrinsic transporter activity, GLUT-4 translocation, and/or transporter recycling rate can alter glucose uptake independent of transporter expression.[17] During hyperinsulinemic glucose clamps, intravenous leptin increased glucose utilization by 29% during the last 135 min of glycemia clamped at 60 mg/100 ml ($P < 0.05$) and by 30% during the last 135 min of glycemia clamped at 90 mg/dl ($P < 0.01$)[17] compared to controls. In this study, leptin increased insulin sensitivity in normal rats both under fasting conditions and in the presence of hyperinsulinemia. The 2-day leptin infused rats were of the same weight and had equal epididymal fat mass to vehicle-treated controls, suggesting that leptin has effects on insulin sensitivity independent of altered fat mass or body weight.[17] This result is likely due to increased insulin sensitivity and a leptin mediated reduction in insulin secretion. Other potential mechanisms by which leptin might enhance insulin sensitivity without directly altering glucose transport continues to be explored.

Leptin has been implicated in increasing insulin stimulated glucose uptake and inhibiting hepatic glucose production. Barzilai administered leptin vs. vehicle for 8 days to adult rats. Moderate calorie restriction resulted in similar decreases in whole body and visceral fat (20% and 21% respectively), but leptin administration led to a specific and marked decrease (by 62%) in visceral adiposity.[18] During an insulin clamp, leptin markedly enhanced insulin action on both inhibition of hepatic glucose production and stimulation of glucose uptake.[18] Hepatic gene expression of key metabolic enzymes: glucokinase (GK), glucose-6-phosphatase (Glc-6-pase), and phosphoenolpyruvate carboxykinase (*PEPCK*) were modified by leptin. Administration resulted in a marked decrease in GK mRNA and increases in both Glc-6-Pase and PEPCK mRNAs, which are likely to represent a defense against excessive storage of energy in adipose depots.[18] This study demonstrated that leptin, independent of its effect on food intake, selectively decreases visceral fat, enhances the action of insulin on peripheral glucose uptake and hepatic glucose production, modulates the gene expression of key hepatic enzymes, and determines an intrahepatic redistribution of glucose fluxes that resembles that observed with fasting.[18]

Similar results were illustrated by Kamohara who studied the in vivo effects of intravenous and intracerebroventricular (ICV) administrations of leptin on glucose metabolism. A five-hour intravenous infusion of leptin into wild-type mice increased glucose turnover and glucose uptake, but decreased hepatic glycogen content. The plasma levels of insulin and glucose did not change.[19] Similar effects were observed after intracerebroventricular infusion of leptin, suggesting that effects of leptin on glucose metabolism are mediated by the central nervous system.[19] These data indicate that leptin induces a complex metabolic response with effects on glucose as well as lipid metabolism.[19]

That leptin exerts this effect was also noted by Liu. Leptin (0.02 or 1 mcg/kg) was administered ICV for 6 hours to conscious rats, and insulin action was determined by insulin clamp. During hyperinsulinemia, the rates of glucose uptake, glycolysis and glycogen synthesis were similar in rats receiving low- and high-dose leptin versus vehicle.[20] ICV leptin resulted in a 2-3-fold increase in hepatic PEPCK mRNA levels.[20] Glycogenolysis and PEP-gluconeogenesis contributed similarly to endogenous glucose production in the vehicle-infused group. Interestingly, gluconeogenesis accounted for 80% of glucose production in both groups receiving ICV leptin, while hepatic glycogenolysis was markedly suppressed in rats receiving leptin versus vehicle.[20] This study demonstates that leptin failed to affect peripheral insulin action, but induced a striking re-distribution of intrahepatic glucose fluxes.[20]

The ventromedial hypothalamus (VMH) has been implicated as the central site of this action of leptin.[21] Minokoshi studied the effects of microinjection of leptin into the VMH and lateral hypothalamus (LH) in rats. A single VMH injection of leptin increased glucose uptake in brown adipose tissue, heart, skeletal muscle, and spleen but not in white adipose tissue or skin.[21] Injection of leptin into the LH, however, had little effect. Thus, there appears to be different leptin insulin-sensitizing effects depending on target tissue.[21,22]

The data on leptin's effect on glucose homeostasis is not altogether consistent.[20,23] Though there are a number of studies demonstrating an inhibitory effect of leptin on insulin secretion, not all have come to this conclusion. In fact, some have noted no effect or even an increase in insulin secretion. Widdowson demonstrated that acute hyperleptinemia in normal weight Wistar rats did not appear to reduce insulin sensitivity under clamp conditions.[23] Male rats received recombinant murine leptin (1 mcg/min) or vehicle. Glucose infusion rates during clamping were no different between leptin-infused and control rats, and there were no significant effects on the whole body glucose uptake or hepatic glucose production rate under basal or clamped conditions.[23]

2.2 *Ob/ob* and *db/db* mouse studies

The earliest evidence that leptin is implicated in the regulation of insulin and glucose was in *ob/ob* (leptin-deficient) and *db/db* (leptin receptor mutation) mice. Defects in the leptin pathway led to hyperinsulinemia even before the development of the diabetic, obese phenotype.[2,24,25,26] When these mice were treated with intraperitoneal leptin, improvement of the diabetic indices without significant weight loss was noted. These changes were not seen in the *db/db* leptin-resistant mice.[1,27,28,29]

Chen studied insulin secretion from islets of pre-obese, 2-week-old, *ob/ob* mice and their lean littermates.[26] The *ob/ob* mice were slightly hyperinsulinemic at 2 weeks of age. Pancreatic islet size, DNA content, and insulin content were similar in the *ob/ob* and lean mice.[26] The responsiveness of islets to glucose was unaffected. When acetylcholine and cholecystokinin (two insulin secretagogues that potentiate glucose-induced insulin secretion) were administered, they were more effective in stimulating insulin secretion from islets of *ob/ob* mice than from islets of lean mice.[26] The signal transduction pathway common to acetylcholine and cholecystokinin, and cross-talk between this pathway and the glucose-dependent insulinotropic polypeptide (GIP) signal transduction pathway are loci for early-onset defects in control of insulin secretion from islets of *ob/ob* mice.[26]

A number of initial studies used intraperitoneal leptin in *ob/ob* mice to reveal that leptin is a mediator in glucose and insulin homeostasis.[27,28,29] The administration of leptin reversed the diabetic phenotype, even in mice treated with low doe leptin without significant weight loss. This suggested a role for leptin on glucose-insulin mechanics beyond weight loss[1] Pelleymounter delivered daily intraperitoneal injections of leptin to the *ob/ob* mouse. They had decreased body weight, percent body fat, food intake, and serum concentrations of glucose and insulin. In addition, metabolic rate, body temperature, and activity levels were increased by this treatment.[29] These parameters were similar in the levels seen in the lean controls. Lean animals injected with OB protein maintained a smaller weight loss throughout the 28-day study.[29]

Adenoviral gene therapy of *ob/ob* mice with mouse leptin cDNA resulted in normalization of plasma glucose and insulin levels.[1] Muzzin showed that treatment resulted in dramatic reductions in both food intake and body weight, and the normalization of serum insulin levels and glucose tolerance.[30] The effect on serum leptin levels in treated animals, however, did not persist beyond 2-3 weeks. The subsequent decrease in leptin levels resulted in the rapid resumption of food intake and a gradual gain of body weight.[30] This correlated with the return of hyperinsulinemia and insulin resistance.[30] Several studies have suggested that the fleeting effect on the adenovirally transduced cells is due to destruction by a host immune-mediated response *in vivo*.[20,23] Recent studies have also demonstrated that cellular and humoral responses to the transgene-encoded product may play an important role in limiting the duration of transgene expression.[7,8,30]

2.3 Other models

To assess whether leptin may act independently of insulin in regulating energy metabolism in vivo, Chinookoswong studied the effects of leptin treatment alone on glucose metabolism in lean insulin-deficient streptozotocin (STZ)-induced diabetic rats.[31] Four groups of STZ-induced diabetic rats were studied: rats treated with recombinant leptin subcutaneous infusion for 12-14 days, control rats infused with vehicle, pair-fed control rats given a daily food ration, and rats treated with subcutaneous phloridzin (normalizes blood glucose via glucosuria without insulin and was used as a control for the effect of leptin in correcting hyperglycemia.) All animals were then studied with a hyperinsulinemic-euglycemic clamp. Leptin treatment in the insulin-deficient diabetic rats restored euglycemia, minimized body weight loss due to food restriction, substantially improved glucose metabolic rates during the postabsorptive state, and restored insulin sensitivities at the levels of the liver and the peripheral tissues during the glucose clamp.[31] The effects on glucose turnover appeared independent of food restriction and changes in blood glucose concentration, suggesting that the antidiabetic effects of leptin are achieved through both an insulin-independent and an insulin-sensitizing mechanism.[31]

Another model is the Otsuka Long-Evans Tokushima Fatty (OLETF) rat. This rat develops late onset hyperglycemia (at about 18 weeks of age), hyperinsulinemia and mild obesity that closely resemble non-insulin-dependent diabetes mellitus in humans. Mizuno administered leptin intravenously for 16 h to OLETF and Long-Evans Tokushima Otsuka (LETO) (lean controls) rats, followed by the measurement of insulin-stimulated glucose uptake in hindlimb muscles during hyperinsulinemic euglycemic clamp technique.[32] In the LETO rats, the administration of leptin significantly decreased plasma insulin levels, without change in plasma glucose, and led to an increase in insulin-stimulated glucose uptake in hindlimb muscles.[32] In the OLETF rats, leptin administration changed neither plasma insulin levels nor insulin-stimulated glucose uptake. The study showed that at 8 weeks of age, OLETF rats have already become resistant to high concentration of peripheral leptin.[32]

An indirect effect of leptin deficiency can also affect β-cell function. Leptin resistance in Zucker diabetic fatty (ZDF) rats has been associated with intracellular triglyceride accumulation.[15] When a certain threshold is achieved, lipotoxicity can occur resulting in a 50% loss of β-cells.[1] When the leptin receptor is overexpressed in ZDF rat pancreatic islets, the diabetic phenotype is reversed in association with the reduction of intracellular triglyceride.[1,33]

2.4 Diet Induced Obesity

Obesity is often associated with elevated leptin levels. Human obesity and high fat feeding in rats are associated with the development of insulin resistance and perturbed carbohydrate and lipid metabolism. It has been proposed that these metabolic abnormalities may be reversible by interventions that increase plasma leptin.[1] In one study, sustained increase in plasma leptin was achieved by administration of a recombinant adenovirus containing the leptin cDNA in Wistar rats fed a high-fat diet (HF) compared with standard chow-fed (SC) control animals.[34] Increasing plasma leptin levels for a period of 6 days decreased adipose mass by 40% and normalized plasma glucose and insulin levels. In addition, insulin-stimulated skeletal muscle glucose uptake was normalized in hyperleptinemic rats, an effect that correlated closely with a 60% decrease in intramuscular triglyceride (TG).[34] The moderate sustained leptin increase reversed diet-induced hyperglycemia, hyperinsulinemia, and skeletal muscle insulin resistance. These improvements appeared to be tightly linked to leptin-induced reductions in intramuscular TG.[34]

The adipo-insular axis may, however, play an important role during the development of type 2 diabetes in obese patients. During the development of type 2 diabetes, initial hyperinsulinemia is believed to represent a simple compensatory response of the pancreatic ß-cell to insulin resistance[3,4] and hyperglycemia is the consequence of pancreatic ß-cell failure. Hyperinsulinemia, however, frequently precedes the development of insulin resistance.[2] In obese animal models and in most obese patients, despite high levels of circulating leptin, leptin fails to exert its effect on the hypothalamus.[2] This observation has been termed "leptin resistance" and was attributed to several molecular alterations in postreceptor leptin signal transduction in the hypothalamus.[35] Reduced leptin sensitivity at the level of the pancreatic ß-cell leads to dysregulation of the adipo-insular axis, resulting in increased insulin release, which is then no longer under controlled repression by leptin.[2] Thus, leptin resistance at the level of the pancreatic ß-cell may promote hyperinsulinemia in obese patients prone to developing type 2 diabetes.[2] Elevated insulin concentrations promote both insulin resistance and further stimulation of leptin production and secretion from the adipose tissue, which may in turn enhance leptin resistance of the endocrine pancreas by further desensitizing leptin signal transduction pathways and constituting a vicious circle that promotes manifestation of type 2 diabetes in obese people[2] (Figure 2).

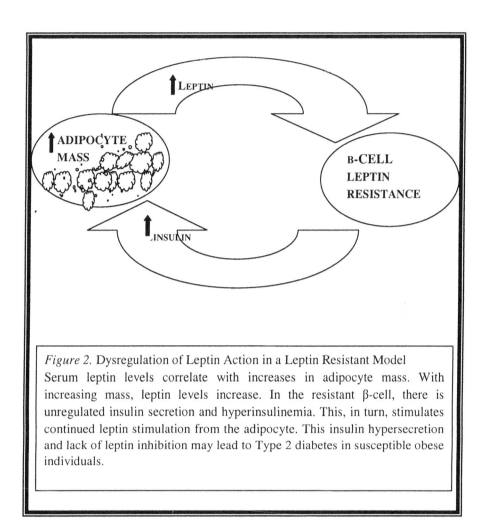

Figure 2. Dysregulation of Leptin Action in a Leptin Resistant Model
Serum leptin levels correlate with increases in adipocyte mass. With increasing mass, leptin levels increase. In the resistant β-cell, there is unregulated insulin secretion and hyperinsulinemia. This, in turn, stimulates continued leptin stimulation from the adipocyte. This insulin hypersecretion and lack of leptin inhibition may lead to Type 2 diabetes in susceptible obese individuals.

Yaspelkis, et al administered leptin to insulin-resistant rats to determine its effects on secretagogue-stimulated insulin release, whole body glucose disposal, and insulin-stimulated skeletal muscle glucose uptake and transport.[36] Male Wistar rats were fed either a normal (Con) or a high-fat (HF) diet for 3 or 6 mo. HF rats were then treated with either vehicle (HF), leptin, or food restriction (FR) for 12-15 days. Glucose tolerance and skeletal muscle glucose uptake and transport were significantly impaired in HF compared with Con. Whole body glucose tolerance and rates of insulin-stimulated skeletal muscle glucose uptake and transport in HF-Lep were similar to those of Con and greater than those of HF and HF-FR. The insulin secretory response to either glucose or tolbutamide (a pancreatic β-cell secretagogue) was not significantly diminished in HF-Lep. Total and plasma membrane skeletal muscle GLUT-4 protein concentrations were similar in Con and HF-Lep and greater than those in HF and HF-FR. The findings suggest that chronic leptin administration reversed a high-fat diet-induced insulin-resistant state, without compromising insulin secretion.[36]

To assess whether leptin can be administered in the treatment of type 2 diabetes, a mouse model of type 2 diabetes was studied. MKR mice (with transgenic overexpression of a skeletal muscle dominant-negative IGF-I receptor with a lysine-to-arginine amino acid) have normal leptin levels and are diabetic due to a primary defect in both IGF-I and insulin receptors signaling in skeletal muscle.[37] This leads to insulin resistance in liver and fat, pancreatic ß-cell dysfunction with the loss of first-phase insulin secretion, and the appearance of diabetes.[37] MKR mice have normal amounts of adipose tissue and serum leptin levels.[37] Leptin treatment increased hepatic insulin sensitivity by suppression of hepatic glucose production and increased hepatic insulin responsiveness possibly through decreasing gluconeogenesis and reducing lipid stores in liver and muscle by enhancing fatty acid oxidation and inhibiting lipogenesis.[37] Leptin also reduced gene Glc-6-pase. These findings suggest that leptin decreased glucose production through the inhibition of gluconeogenic enzymes.[37] This data suggest that leptin could be a potent antidiabetic drug in cases of type 2 diabetes that are not leptin resistant.[37] Leptin administration to the MKR mice resulted in improvement of diabetes, an effect that was independent of the reduced food intake.

Yet, other studies have shown that leptin supplementation in animals that have low plasma leptin levels in response to fat feeding may slow but may not prevent the subsequent development of diet-induced obesity.[38] Plasma leptin levels of diet- induced diabetes and obesity-prone C57BL/6J (B6) mice were increased to those seen in diabetes and obesity-resistant A/J mice and examined to see if it would prevent the development of diet-induced obesity. Four-week-old male mice were weaned onto a low-fat (11% of total kcal) diet. When the animals weighed 20 g, their diets were changed to a high-fat (HF) diet (58% of total kcal), and a continuous infusion of leptin or saline was started for 12 weeks. Chronic treatment with leptin raised plasma levels in B6 mice to that of A/J mice.[38] There were transient significant weight differences between B6 treated and B6 control groups for 2-3 weeks after pump implantation which ultimately normalized.[38] There were no differences in plasma glucose or insulin between B6 treated and control groups. This finding suggests that it is doubtful that the difference observed in leptin levels between B6 and A/J mice following the introduction of a high-fat diet is responsible for the hyperglycemia and hyperinsulinemia that subsequently develop in B6 mice. Thus, although an absolute leptin deficiency can cause diabetes, it is unlikely that relative differences in plasma leptin observed in normal individuals are related to the predisposition to develop diabetes.[38] The study demonstrated that leptin supplementation in animals that show low plasma leptin levels in response to fat feeding may slow but does not prevent the subsequent development of diet-induced obesity.[38] Further studies are ongoing to further delineate these complex relationships.

2.5 Human studies

Leptin deficiency and receptor mutations as a cause for human obesity are rare. 5-10% of obese subjects have low leptin levels relative to their adipocyte mass, a hypoleptinemic obesity.[1] Most obese subjects have high leptin levels, suggestive of a leptin resistant state. This resistance appears to be at both the level of the pancreatic β-cell and the hypothalamus. With dysregulation of the adipo-insular axis, there is increased insulin release promoting increased insulin, insulin resistance, and further stimulation of leptin from adipose tissue.[2] (Figure 2)

To assess in vivo responses to leptin, pancreatic islets were isolated from human pancreata. The presence of leptin receptors on islet β-cells was demonstrated by double fluorescence microscopy after binding of a fluorescent human leptin.[6] Leptin suppressed insulin secretion of normal islets by 20%. Intracellular calcium responses to glucose were rapidly reduced by leptin. Proinsulin m-RNA expression in islets was inhibited by leptin at higher doses of glucose. These findings demonstrate direct suppressive effects of leptin on insulin-producing β-cells in human islets at the levels of both stimulus-secretion coupling and gene expression.[6] The authors proposed that in conditions of obesity and prolonged elevated plasma leptin levels, the receptor system in pancreatic ß-cells becomes desensitize.[6] This may result in a dysregulation of the adipoinsular axis and a corresponding failure to suppress insulin secretion, resulting in chronic hyperinsulinemia and contributing to the pathogenesis of adipogenic diabetes.[6] Chronic hyperinsulinemia and failure of leptin reception set up a positive feedback loop may lead to increased adipogenesis and further increases in plasma leptin.[6]

Two cousins with severe, early-onset obesity and undetectable serum leptin concentrations were first described in 1997 to be homozygous for a frame-shift mutation in the leptin gene.[39] A trial of subcutaneous recombinant human leptin was given to the older of these children, a nine-year-old girl, for twelve months.[40] The patient had a reduction in weight (predominantly due to a loss of fat), at a rate of approximately 1 to 2 kg per month and there was a total weight loss of 16.4 kg. The patient was normoglycemic at baseline but had high fasting plasma insulin and nonesterified fatty acid (NEFA) concentrations. Her NEFA concentrations decreased, and despite a reduction in fasting insulin levels, she remained hyperinsulinemic at twelve months. The fasting insulin improved at 12 months, but remained elevated. This model of leptin deficiency is rare but illustrates the key role leptin plays in human energy balance.

Heymsfield and colleagues studied a group of lean and obese subjects after administering varying doses of recombinant human leptin daily. Lean subjects consumed a diet to maintain body weight, and obese subjects were prescribed a diet that reduced their daily energy intake by 500-kcal/d.[41] Weight changes at 24 weeks ranged from -0.7 (5.4) kg for the 0.01 mg/kg dose to -7.1 (8.5) kg for the 0.30 mg/kg dose. Fat mass declined from baseline as dose increased among all subjects at 4 weeks and among obese subjects at 24 weeks of treatment. Although baseline serum leptin concentrations were not related to weight loss, a dose-response relationship with weight and fat loss was observed with subcutaneous recombinant leptin injections in both lean and obese subjects.[41] There were no concurrent changes in glycemic control or insulin action during the course of the study.[1] The average leptin levels were 30 times higher than the placebo and baseline values, suggesting that high levels of leptin may be needed to overcome a leptin resistant state in humans.[1]

2.6 Leptin effects on pancreatic β-cell function and gene expression

The first step of insulin biosynthesis is proinsulin gene expression, with its rate-limiting step being the transcriptional regulation of the proinsulin gene promoter.[42] Many studies have reported on the suppression of preproinsulin mRNA in pancreatic ß-cells by leptin.[2] Thereby, leptin has been shown to suppress preproinsulin mRNA expression in mouse ßTC6 cells[43] in the rat pancreatic ß-cell line INS-1,[12] in isolated primary rat islets,[5,43] in ob/ob mouse islets, and in human islets.[12] In studies of human islets, human leptin (6.25 nmol/l) evokes a time-dependent decrease in preproinsulin mRNA levels in the presence of 11.1 mmol/l glucose but not 5.6 mmol/l glucose.[12] When the incretin hormone GLP-1, a known stimulator of the proinsulin gene promoter was used, leptin inhibited GLP-1–stimulated expression of preproinsulin mRNA in human islets at glucose concentrations of 5.6 and 11.1 mmol/l.[12] In contrast, in INS-1 ß-cells, leptin significantly reduced only preproinsulin mRNA expression stimulated by 25 mmol/l glucose, but not by lower glucose concentrations.[2] These observations imply that the ability of leptin to reduce preproinsulin mRNA expression in pancreatic ß-cells may depend on prior stimulation by incretin hormones or stimulatory ambient glucose concentrations. Further, the effects of leptin on steady-state preproinsulin mRNA levels in pancreatic ß-cells were only observed after 16 h of incubation and were not seen at shorter incubation periods.[12] This observation suggests that the effect of leptin on insulin biosynthesis may represent a more long-term character, and time kinetics imply that gene transcription may be necessary for this effect.

The effect of leptin on the transcriptional activity of the insulin gene promoter has also been examined. Leptin inhibited a vector expressing the luciferase gene under the control of the rat insulin I gene promoter in INS-1 cells at stimulatory glucose concentrations of 25 mmol/l but not at 5.6 mmol/l glucose.[12] In contrast, the induction of transcriptional activity of the insulin promoter by additional stimulatory concentrations of 10 nmol/l GLP-1 at 11.1 mmol/l glucose was also inhibited by leptin. These findings suggest that stimulated insulin promoter activity by either GLP-1 or high glucose represents a prerequisite for the inhibitory actions of leptin on insulin promoter activity.[12,2]

Leptin signaling through ObR is intracellularly coupled with the janus kinase (JAK)–signal transducer and activator of transcription (STAT) pathway.[2] Binding of leptin its receptor activates the receptor-associated kinase JAK2 via transphosphorylation and phosphorylates tyrosine residues on ObRb.[2] Transcription factors of the STAT family are recruited, phosphorylated, and translocate to the nucleus to regulate gene transcription. Repression of insulin promoter activity by leptin has been associated with altered binding of the isoform STAT5b to specific DNA sequences within the promoter.[12] STATs have mostly been shown to transcriptionally enhance gene expression. In contrast leptin signaling, which activates several STATs in other tissues such as the hypothalamus,[44,45] inhibits insulin biosynthesis via transcriptional repression of the proinsulin gene promoter[2,12] (Figure 3).

SOCS, suppressor of cytokine signaling molecules, inhibits JAK-STAT signal transduction by binding directly to tyrosine-phosphorylated residues on the cytokine receptor–associated kinase JAK2.[2] Expression of the SOCS proteins is induced by various cytokines and they in turn inhibit cytokine signaling via the JAK-STAT pathway in an intracellular negative feedback loop.[2] Thus, SOCS molecules may function as cytokine inducible negative regulators of cytokine signaling. In the hypothalamus, it has been demonstrated that leptin induces expression of SOCS3 mRNA in areas where ObRb is expressed.[2] Thus, the SOCS molecules may play an important role in the development of leptin resistance that is seen in obesity both in the central nervous system and the endocrine pancreatic ß-cell[2] (Figure 3).

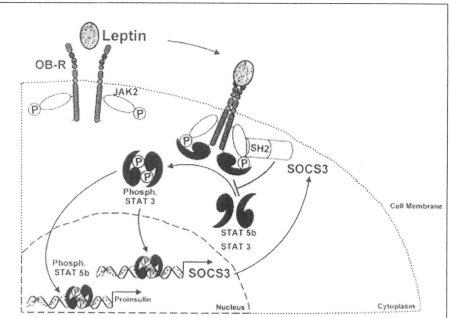

Taken with permission from: Seufert, *Diabetes* 53 (Suppl. 1): S152–S158, 2004

Figure 3. Leptin signaling and gene regulation in pancreatic ß-cells. Upon leptin stimulation, the JAK2 tyrosine kinase becomes activated via transphosphorylation and phosphorylates tyrosine residues of the leptin receptor. STAT3 and STAT5b are now recruited to the leptin receptor and are consecutively tyrosine-phosphorylated via JAK2. Phosphorylated STATs dimerize and translocate to the nucleus to regulate gene transcription. STAT5b transactivates the proinsulin gene promoter, whereas STAT3 may differentially activate the SOCS3 promoter. SOCS3 in turn inhibits the JAK-STAT signaling pathway by binding to the tyrosine-phosphorylated leptin receptor, thereby preventing recruitment of STATs to the leptin receptor. SOCS3 thereby mediates repression of leptin receptor signaling through a negative feedback loop.

3. EFFECT OF INSULIN ON LEPTIN SECRETION AND ACTION

Leptin secretion from the human white adipocyte is mediated by a number of factors. It appears to be stimulated by insulin and cortisol and inhibited by β-agonists, cAMP and thiazolidinediones.[11] Plasma insulin levels parallel levels of leptin during the fasting (decreased) and fed (increased) states. Insulin has been shown to increase leptin mRNA levels in adipocytes and increase leptin secretion and production.[46] A number of mice and rat in vitro and in vivo studies have supported this.[47,48] In the setting of acute insulin administration in fasted animals, leptin mRNA increased to levels of fed controls.[49] Insulin appears to play a chronic role in leptin gene expression and production by white adipose tissue.[11]

Numerous studies have demonstrated that hyperinsulinemia increases plasma leptin and mRNA expression in rodents and humans.[49-51,52,11] In a study of normal rats, Cusin showed that leptin mRNA is respectively up- or downregulated by a rise in insulin induced by 2-day insulin infusion while maintaining euglycemia or a decrease in insulin induced by a 3-day fast.[53] In the genetically obese fa/fa Zucker rats, white adipose tissue ob mRNA levels increase in parallel with early occurring and steadily increasing hyperinsulinemia. This results in adult obese animals having markedly higher ob mRNA levels than age-matched normoinsulinemic lean rats. Furthermore, in adult obese rats, ob mRNA escapes down-regulation as normalization of hyperinsulinemia due to fasting fails to reduce the high ob mRNA levels.[53]

To investigate the changes in leptin gene expression and production of leptin in response to insulin in vitro and in vivo, euglycemic and hyperglycemic conditions were studied in humans. Kolaczynski used three protocols: 1) a euglycemic clamp carried out for up to 5 h in 16 normal lean individuals, 30 obese individuals, and 31 patients with Type 2 DM: 2) 64-to 72-h hyperglycemic clamp performed on 5 lean individuals; and 3) long-term (96-h) primary culture of isolated abdominal adipocytes in the presence and absence of 100 nmol/l insulin.[54] Short-term (< 5 hours) hyperinsulinemia had no effect on circulating levels of leptin. During the prolonged hyperglycemic clamp, a rise in leptin was observed during the last 24 h of the study ($P < 0.001$). In the presence of insulin in vitro, OB gene expression increased at 72 h ($P < 0.01$), followed by an increase in leptin released to the medium ($P < 0.001$).[54] Insulin did not appear to stimulate leptin production acutely, but a long-term effect of insulin on leptin production could be demonstrated both in vivo and in vitro.[54] The authors suggest that insulin regulates OB gene expression and leptin production indirectly, probably through its trophic effect on adipocytes.[54]

A similar study evaluated the regulation of ob gene expression in abdominal subcutaneous adipose tissue.[55] To verify whether insulin regulates ob gene expression, six lean subjects underwent a 3-h euglycemic hyperinsulinemic (846 +/- 138 pmol/liter) clamp. Leptin and Glut 4 mRNA levels were quantified in adipose tissue biopsies taken before and at the end of the clamp. Insulin infusion produced a significant threefold increase in Glut 4 mRNA while leptin mRNA was not affected. Leptin mRNA level was highly correlated with the body mass index. Again, it was noted that ob gene expression is not acutely regulated by insulin or by metabolic factors related to fasting in human abdominal subcutaneous adipose tissue.[55]

Another study evaluated the effect of insulin on leptin in a group of diabetic patients. Plasma leptin concentrations were determined during an 8.5-h hyperinsulinaemic clamp in seven patients with non-insulin requiring diabetes versus controls. Fasting serum insulin level correlated with plasma leptin even after adjusting for the percentage of body fat.[56] During the insulin infusion, a significant increase in the plasma leptin concentration was observed after 6 h in the normal subjects and after 8.5 h in the patients with diabetes. During the saline infusion, plasma leptin concentrations decreased significantly in the normal subjects by 11 +/- 1% ($p < 0.005$) and in the patients with diabetes by 14 +/- 1% ($p < 0.01$) after 2 h. No differences were observed in plasma leptin concentrations between the normal subjects and patients with diabetes. This study revealed that prolonged exposure to insulin increases plasma leptin concentrations in humans implicating insulin in chronic but not acute regulation of plasma leptin concentrations.[56] The decrease in plasma leptin concentrations during saline infusion was greater than that expected on the basis of change in serum insulin concentrations, suggesting that factors other than insulin also contribute to regulation of plasma leptin concentrations.[56]

Insulin deficiency is associated with low levels of leptin and leptin mRNA.[11] Havel and colleagues induced diabetes in rats with streptozotocin to examine the effect of insulin-deficient diabetes and insulin treatment on circulating leptin. After 12 weeks, plasma leptin concentrations in untreated rats were all < 0.4 ng/ml versus 4.9 +/- 0.9 ng/ml in control animals ($P < 0.005$).[57] In rats treated with subcutaneous insulin implants for 12 weeks, which reduced hyperglycemia by approximately 50%, plasma leptin was 2.1 +/- 0.6 ng/ml, whereas leptin concentrations were 6.0 +/- 1.6 ng/ml in insulin-implanted rats receiving supplemental injections of insulin for 4 days to normalize plasma glucose ($P < 0.005$ vs. STZ untreated). In a second experiment, plasma leptin was monitored at biweekly intervals during 12 wk of diabetes. In rats treated with insulin implants, plasma leptin concentrations were inversely proportional to glycemia and unrelated to body weight.[57] In a third experiment, plasma leptin concentrations were examined very early after the induction of diabetes. Within 24 h after STZ injection, plasma insulin decreased from 480 +/- 30 to 130 +/- 10 pM ($P < 0.0001$), plasma glucose increased from 7.0 +/- 0.2 to 24.8 +/- 0.5 mM, and plasma leptin decreased from 3.2 +/- 0.2 to 1.2 +/- 0.1 ng/ml (delta = -63 +/- 3%, $P < 0.0001$).[57] In a subset of diabetic rats treated with insulin for 2 days, glucose decreased to 11.7 +/- 3.9 mM and leptin increased from 0.5 +/- 0.1 to 2.9 +/- 0.6 ng/ml ($P < 0.01$) without an effect on epididymal fat weight. The change of leptin was correlated with the degree of glucose lowering ($r = 0.75$, $P < 0.05$).[57] Thus insulin-deficient diabetes produces rapid and sustained decreases of leptin that are not solely dependent on weight loss, whereas insulin treatment reverses the hypoleptinemia. The authors hypothesized that decreased glucose transport into adipose tissue may contribute to decreased leptin production in insulin-deficient diabetes.[57]

To assess the short-term effects of insulin on circulating leptin levels and feeding behavior, Singh studied obesity-resistant (OR) and obesity-prone (OP) Sprague-Dawley rats. Insulin administration resulted in significant elevations of plasma leptin at 4 hours in both groups, but inhibition of the intake of chow pellets during hours 2-4 in the OR group only.[58] Thus, feeding inhibition coincides with insulin-induced elevations of plasma leptin in lean but not obese Sprague-Dawley rats suggesting that elevations of leptin within the physiological range may contribute to short-term inhibition of food intake in rats.[58] This process may be stimulated by feeding-related insulin release.[58]

Adipocyte determination differentiation dependent factor 1/sterol regulatory element binding protein 1 (ADD1/SREBP1), a candidate transcription factor, has been found to be associated with changes in insulin levels and *ob* gene expression in mice.[59] ADD1/SREBP1 expression increases upon treatment of adipocytes with insulin, and the increased ADD1/SREBP1 transactivates the leptin gene.[11] Gene expression in adipose tissue for ADD1/SREBP1 is reduced dramatically upon fasting and elevated upon refeeding. This pattern correlates with the regulation of fatty acid synthetase (FAS) and leptin, two adipose cell genes that are crucial in energy homeostasis.[11] These results indicate that ADD1/SREBP1 is a key transcription factor linking changes in nutritional status and insulin levels to the expression of certain genes that regulate systemic energy metabolism.[59] Transcription factors of the C/EBP and PPAR families, as well others to be identified, may be involved in the regulation of leptin gene expression by hormones such as insulin.[11]

4. INSULINOMA

In vivo and in vitro models of insulinoma provide an interesting clinical circumstance in which to study the leptin-insulin relationship. The dysregulated secretion of insulin produces a pathologic hyperinsulinemic state. To investigate whether leptin has a direct effect on insulin secretion in this model, isolated rat and human islets and cultured insulinoma cells were studied.[43] When mouse leptin was administered to the islet cell buffer, it inhibited insulin secretion.

To assess this relationship in humans, serum leptin concentrations were measured in five patients with insulinoma before and one month after surgery and in five control subjects.[60] The control subjects had leptin concentrations of 6.7+/-1.5 mcg/l and a BMI of 24.9+/-1.1. The mean serum leptin concentration in patients with insulinoma was 11.8+/-3.1 mcg/l (P <

0.05 vs. controls), with a BMI of 26.3+/-1.9. After surgery, a clear reduction in serum leptin concentration (5.6+/-2.4 mcg/l, P < 0.05 vs. pre surgical values and no difference vs. control subjects) occurred.[60] The area under the curve (AUC) of insulin concentration (in mU/l per 120 min) before surgery was 14421+/-4981 and after surgery was 1306-/+171 (P < 0.05).[60] This study reveals that chronic endogenous hyperinsulinemia in patients with insulinoma tumors is significantly associated with enhanced leptin secretion, an action that is reversed after successful surgery. As no changes in BMI were observed after surgery, the clear-cut reduction in leptin serum concentrations probably reflects the reduction and normalization of insulin levels.[60] This suggests that insulin has a stimulatory role in regulating serum leptin levels.

5. CONCLUSIONS

The product of the *ob* gene, leptin, plays a pivotal role in the distribution of body adiposity and exerts potent effects on insulin action and on hepatic gene expression. Leptin appears to act directly on pancreatic ß-cells in addition to its effects in the hypothalamus to reduce food intake and increase energy expenditure. (Figure 1) At the cellular level, inhibitory effects of leptin on both insulin secretion and insulin biosynthesis, mainly represented by the inhibition of preproinsulin gene expression, have been demonstrated.[2] Leptin signals the pancreas from the adipose tissue to restrict insulin secretion according to the needs that are determined by body fat stores.[2] (Figure 3) The lipogenic action of insulin has long been well established, and consequently has been demonstrated that insulin stimulates both leptin biosynthesis and secretion from white adipose tissue.[2] The effects of leptin on pancreatic ß-cells exert a physiological long-term control of insulin secretion with adaptation of insulin secretion to the degree of body fat stores.[2] This effect of leptin on insulin does not seem to interfere with the short-term stimulatory actions of nutrients and hormones, such as glucose- and incretin-dependent insulin secretion.[2]

These dramatic metabolic effects in a model of age-dependent and moderate obesity suggest that leptin action is an important factor in the pathophysiology of visceral or intraabdominal obesity and insulin resistance. Insulin resistance is associated with hyperleptinemia. As hyperinsulinemia may present before the onset of insulin resistance, the adipocyte-insular axis may be playing a role in the progression of Type 2 diabetes.[2]

REFERENCES

1. RB Ceddia, HA Koistinen, JR Zierath, G Sweeney. Analysis of paradoxical observations on the association between leptin and insulin resistance. *Faseb J*;16(10):1163-76 (2002).
2. J Seufert. Leptin effects on pancreatic beta-cell gene expression and function. *Diabetes*;53 Suppl 1:S152-8 (2004).
3. E Cerasi. Insulin deficiency and insulin resistance in the pathogenesis of NIDDM: is a divorce possible? *Diabetologia*;38(8):992-7 (1995).
4. RA DeFronzo. Pathogenesis of type 2 (non-insulin dependent) diabetes mellitus: a balanced overview. *Diabetologia*;35(4):389-97 (1992).
5. AL Pallett, NM Morton, MA Cawthorne, V Emilsson. Leptin inhibits insulin secretion and reduces insulin mRNA levels in rat isolated pancreatic islets. *Biochem Biophys Res Commun*;238(1):267-70 (1997).
6. J Seufert, TJ Kieffer, CA Leech, et al. Leptin suppression of insulin secretion and gene expression in human pancreatic islets: implications for the development of adipogenic diabetes mellitus. *J Clin Endocrinol Metab*;84(2):670-6 (1999).
7. JA Cases, I Gabriely, XH Ma, et al. Physiological increase in plasma leptin markedly inhibits insulin secretion in vivo. *Diabetes*;50(2):348-52 (2001).
8. JR Zierath, EU Frevert, JW Ryder, PO Berggren, BB Kahn. Evidence against a direct effect of leptin on glucose transport in skeletal muscle and adipocytes. *Diabetes*;47(1):1-4 (1998).
9. C Furnsinn, B Brunmair, R Furtmuller, M Roden, R Englisch, W Waldhausl. Failure of leptin to affect basal and insulin-stimulated glucose metabolism of rat skeletal muscle in vitro. *Diabetologia*;41(5):524-9 (1998).
10. S Ranganathan, TP Ciaraldi, RR Henry, S Mudaliar, PA Kern. Lack of effect of leptin on glucose transport, lipoprotein lipase, and insulin action in adipose and muscle cells. *Endocrinology*;139(5):2509-13 (1998).
11. TJ Kieffer, JF Habener. The adipoinsular axis: effects of leptin on pancreatic beta-cells. *Am J Physiol Endocrinol Metab*;278(1):E1-E14 (2000).
12. J Seufert, TJ Kieffer, JF Habener. Leptin inhibits insulin gene transcription and reverses hyperinsulinemia in leptin-deficient *ob/ob* mice. *Proc Natl Acad Sci U S A*;96(2):674-9 (1999).
13. A Mizuno, T Murakami, S Otani, M Kuwajima, K Shima. Leptin affects pancreatic endocrine functions through the sympathetic nervous system. *Endocrinology*;139(9):3863-70 (1998).
14. M Ookuma, K Ookuma, DA York. Effects of leptin on insulin secretion from isolated rat pancreatic islets. *Diabetes*;47(2):219-23 (1998).
15. RH Unger, YT Zhou, L Orci. Regulation of fatty acid homeostasis in cells: novel role of leptin. *Proc Natl Acad Sci U S A*;96(5):2327-32 (1999).
16. CF Burant, WI Sivitz, H Fukumoto, et al. Mammalian glucose transporters: structure and molecular regulation. *Recent Prog Horm Res*;47:349-87; discussion 387-8 (1991).
17. WI Sivitz, SA Walsh, DA Morgan, MJ Thomas, WG Haynes. Effects of leptin on insulin sensitivity in normal rats. *Endocrinology*;138(8):3395-401 (1997).
18. N Barzilai, J Wang, D Massilon, P Vuguin, M Hawkins, L Rossetti. Leptin selectively decreases visceral adiposity and enhances insulin action. *J Clin Invest*;100(12):3105-10 (1997).
19. S Kamohara, R Burcelin, JL Halaas, JM Friedman, MJ Charron. Acute stimulation of glucose metabolism in mice by leptin treatment. *Nature*;389(6649):374-7 (1997).

20. L Liu, GB Karkanias, JC Morales, et al. Intracerebroventricular leptin regulates hepatic but not peripheral glucose fluxes. *J Biol Chem*;273(47):31160-7 (1998).
21. Y Minokoshi, MS Haque, T Shimazu. Microinjection of leptin into the ventromedial hypothalamus increases glucose uptake in peripheral tissues in rats. *Diabetes*;48(2):287-91 (1999).
22. JL Wang, N Chinookoswong, S Scully, M Qi, ZQ Shi. Differential effects of leptin in regulation of tissue glucose utilization in vivo. *Endocrinology*;140(5):2117-24 (1999).
23. PS Widdowson, R Upton, L Pickavance, et al. Acute hyperleptinemia does not modify insulin sensitivity in vivo in the rat. *Horm Metab Res*;30(5):259-62 (1998).
24. DL Coleman. Diabetes-obesity syndromes in mice. *Diabetes*;31(Suppl 1 Pt 2):1-6 (1982).
25. DL Coleman. Obese and diabetes: two mutant genes causing diabetes-obesity syndromes in mice. *Diabetologia*;14(3):141-8 (1978).
26. NG Chen, DR Romsos. Enhanced sensitivity of pancreatic islets from preobese 2-week-old *ob/ob* mice to neurohormonal stimulation of insulin secretion. *Endocrinology*;136(2):505-11 (1995).
27. JL Halaas, KS Gajiwala, M Maffei, et al. Weight-reducing effects of the plasma protein encoded by the obese gene. *Science*;269(5223):543-6 (1995).
28. LA Campfield, FJ Smith, Y Guisez, R Devos, P Burn. Recombinant mouse OB protein: evidence for a peripheral signal linking adiposity and central neural networks. *Science*;269(5223):546-9 (1995).
29. MA Pelleymounter, MJ Cullen, MB Baker, et al. Effects of the obese gene product on body weight regulation in *ob/ob* mice. *Science*;269(5223):540-3 (1995).
30. P Muzzin, RC Eisensmith, KC Copeland, SL Woo. Correction of obesity and diabetes in genetically obese mice by leptin gene therapy. *Proc Natl Acad Sci U S A*;93(25):14804-8 (1996).
31. N Chinookoswong, JL Wang, ZQ Shi. Leptin restores euglycemia and normalizes glucose turnover in insulin-deficient diabetes in the rat. *Diabetes*;48(7):1487-92 (1999).
32. A Mizuno, T Murakami, T Doi, K Shima. Effect of leptin on insulin sensitivity in the Otsuka Long-Evans Tokushima Fatty rat. *Regul Pept*;99(1):41-4 (2001).
33. MY Wang, K Koyama, M Shimabukuro, CB Newgard, RH Unger. OB-Rb gene transfer to leptin-resistant islets reverses diabetogenic phenotype. *Proc Natl Acad Sci U S A*;95(2):714-8 (1998).
34. R Buettner, CB Newgard, CJ Rhodes, RM O'Doherty. Correction of diet-induced hyperglycemia, hyperinsulinemia, and skeletal muscle insulin resistance by moderate hyperleptinemia. *Am J Physiol Endocrinol Metab*;278(3):E563-9 (2000).
35. C Bjorbaek, JK Elmquist, JD Frantz, SE Shoelson, JS Flier. Identification of SOCS-3 as a potential mediator of central leptin resistance. *Mol Cell*;1(4):619-25 (1998).
36. BB Yaspelkis, 3rd, JR Davis, M Saberi, et al. Leptin administration improves skeletal muscle insulin responsiveness in diet-induced insulin-resistant rats. *Am J Physiol Endocrinol Metab*;280(1):E130-42 (2001).
37. Y Toyoshima, O Gavrilova, S Yakar, et al. Leptin improves insulin resistance and hyperglycemia in a mouse model of type 2 diabetes. *Endocrinology*;146(9):4024-35 (2005).
38. RS Surwit, CL Edwards, S Murthy, AE Petro. Transient effects of long-term leptin supplementation in the prevention of diet-induced obesity in mice. *Diabetes*;49(7):1203-8 (2000).
39. CT Montague, IS Farooqi, JP Whitehead, et al. Congenital leptin deficiency is associated with severe early-onset obesity in humans. *Nature*;387(6636):903-8 (1997).

40. IS Farooqi, SA Jebb, G Langmack, et al. Effects of recombinant leptin therapy in a child with congenital leptin deficiency. *N Engl J Med*;341(12):879-84 (1999).
41. SB Heymsfield, AS Greenberg, K Fujioka, et al. Recombinant leptin for weight loss in obese and lean adults: a randomized, controlled, dose-escalation trial. *Jama*;282(16):1568-75 (1999).
42. K Docherty, AR Clark, V Scott, SW Knight. Metabolic control of insulin gene expression and biosynthesis. *Proc Nutr Soc*;50(3):553-8 (1991).
43. RN Kulkarni, ZL Wang, RM Wang, et al. Leptin rapidly suppresses insulin release from insulinoma cells, rat and human islets and, in vivo, in mice. *J Clin Invest*;100(11):2729-36 (1997).
44. C Vaisse, JL Halaas, CM Horvath, JE Darnell, Jr., M Stoffel, JM Friedman. Leptin activation of Stat3 in the hypothalamus of wild-type and *ob/ob* mice but not *db/db* mice. *Nat Genet*;14(1):95-7 (1996).
45. CI Rosenblum, M Tota, D Cully, et al. Functional STAT 1 and 3 signaling by the leptin receptor (OB-R); reduced expression of the rat fatty leptin receptor in transfected cells. *Endocrinology*;137(11):5178-81 (1996).
46. N Iritani. Nutritional and insulin regulation of leptin gene expression. *Curr Opin Clin Nutr Metab Care*;3(4):275-9 (2000).
47. P Leroy, S Dessolin, P Villageois, et al. Expression of ob gene in adipose cells. Regulation by insulin. *J Biol Chem*;271(5):2365-8 (1996).
48. J Rentsch, M Chiesi. Regulation of ob gene mRNA levels in cultured adipocytes. *FEBS Lett*;379(1):55-9 (1996).
49. R Saladin, P De Vos, M Guerre-Millo, et al. Transient increase in obese gene expression after food intake or insulin administration. *Nature*;377(6549):527-9 (1995).
50. SJ Koopmans, M Frolich, EH Gribnau, RG Westendorp, RA DeFronzo. Effect of hyperinsulinemia on plasma leptin concentrations and food intake in rats. *Am J Physiol*;274(6 Pt 1):E998-E1001 (1998).
51. MF Saad, A Khan, A Sharma, et al. Physiological insulinemia acutely modulates plasma leptin. *Diabetes*;47(4):544-9 (1998).
52. T Utriainen, R Malmstrom, S Makimattila, H Yki-Jarvinen. Supraphysiological hyperinsulinemia increases plasma leptin concentrations after 4 h in normal subjects. *Diabetes*;45(10):1364-6 (1996).
53. I Cusin, A Sainsbury, P Doyle, F Rohner-Jeanrenaud, B Jeanrenaud. The ob gene and insulin. A relationship leading to clues to the understanding of obesity. *Diabetes*;44(12):1467-70 (1995).
54. JW Kolaczynski, MR Nyce, RV Considine, et al. Acute and chronic effects of insulin on leptin production in humans: Studies in vivo and in vitro. *Diabetes*;45(5):699-701 (1996).
55. H Vidal, D Auboeuf, P De Vos, et al. The expression of ob gene is not acutely regulated by insulin and fasting in human abdominal subcutaneous adipose tissue. *J Clin Invest*;98(2):251-5 (1996).
56. R Malmstrom, MR Taskinen, SL Karonen, H Yki-Jarvinen. Insulin increases plasma leptin concentrations in normal subjects and patients with NIDDM. *Diabetologia*;39(8):993-6 (1996).
57. PJ Havel, JY Uriu-Hare, T Liu, et al. Marked and rapid decreases of circulating leptin in streptozotocin diabetic rats: reversal by insulin. *Am J Physiol*;274(5 Pt 2):R1482-91 (1998).
58. KA Singh, CN Boozer, JR Vasselli. Acute insulin-induced elevations of circulating leptin and feeding inhibition in lean but not obese rats. *Am J Physiol Regul Integr Comp Physiol*;289(2):R373-R379 (2005).

59. JB Kim, P Sarraf, M Wright, et al. Nutritional and insulin regulation of fatty acid synthetase and leptin gene expression through ADD1/SREBP1. *J Clin Invest*;101(1):1-9 (1998).
60. V Popovic, D Micic, S Danjanovic, et al. Serum leptin and insulin concentrations in patients with insulinoma before and after surgery. *Eur J Endocrinol*;138(1):86-8 (1998).

Chapter 6

LEPTIN AND OTHER ENDOCRINE SYSTEMS

Robert V. Considine

Department of Medicine, Indiana University, Indianapolis, IN

Abstract: Leptin influences hypothalamic-pituitary function, particularly during the adaptation to caloric restriction and starvation. The fall in leptin with starvation is a signal to reduce energy expenditure by limiting thyroid hormone, growth hormone, and gonadal hormone secretion and by increasing cortisol release. The leptin signal is primarily mediated through receptors located within hypothalamic nuclei, although some effects may occur by leptin binding directly to cells of the anterior pituitary. Leptin may also regulate thyroid and adrenal gland function through leptin receptors located on these tissues. Finally, leptin has direct effects on adipose tissue function, which can alter secretion of various adipokines from the tissue. Thus leptin, as a signal of caloric restriction, has significant regulatory effects on many endocrine systems.

Key words: Adipose tissue; adrenal gland; anterior pituitary; catecholamines; cortisol; fasting; growth hormone; hypothalamic pituitary axis, leptin receptors; thyroid.

1. INTRODUCTION

Since the discovery of leptin[1] an ever-expanding amount of work has established that this adipocyte hormone is more than just a signal from adipose tissue to the central nervous system of the size of energy stores. In particular it has been recognized that leptin has important regulatory effects on many, if not all, other endocrine systems. Some of these systems, such as reproduction and bone metabolism, are discussed in detail in other chapters. This review will focus on the role of leptin to regulate hypothalamic pituitary function, and the thyroid, adrenal and growth hormone axes. Centrally mediated effects of leptin on these endocrine systems, as well as possible direct effects of leptin on various tissues, will be discussed. Findings in animal models and cell culture will be presented and compared/contrasted to observations in humans. Finally, the possibility that leptin may also regulate the endocrine function of adipose tissue itself will be explored.

An important conceptual model in which to understand the effect of leptin on hypothalamic pituitary function is to consider that a major effect of leptin in the central nervous system is to signal for compensation in states of energy deprivation. This model for leptin action, as well as a brief review of leptin receptor function and distribution, will be presented prior to the discussion of each endocrine system to be covered in this chapter.

2. CENTRAL AND PERIPHERAL TISSUE LEPTIN RECEPTORS

As discussed in detail in Chapter 2, there are several different leptin receptor isoforms that have been characterized. The most thoroughly studied isoform, the hypothalamic leptin receptor Ob-Rb, is a class I cytokine receptor[2]. Upon leptin binding, activation of Ob-Rb promotes janus kinase (JAK)-dependent signaling through signal transducer and activator of transcription (STAT) proteins, primarily STAT-3[3]. This leptin receptor has also been observed to activate phosphoinositol-3 kinase and phosphodiesterase 3B signaling pathways in the hypothalamus[4,5], although it is not clear that such signaling is mediated by JAK and STAT proteins.

In addition to the hypothalamic leptin receptor Ob-Rb, five other leptin receptor isoforms have been identified, all of which are encoded by alternative splicing of the same gene[6,7]. Ob-Ra (originally termed the short leptin receptor) is the best characterized of the short leptin receptor isoforms. The extracellular domain of Ob-Ra is identical to that of Ob-Rb, however the intracellular domain is truncated; thus this short leptin receptor lacks the Box 2 motif at which STAT proteins bind. Ob-Ra has been shown to activate JAK2 and MAPK in transiently transfected cell models, but the physiologic significance of this observation is not yet known[8]. Ob-Ra is most highly expressed in cerebral microvessels comprising the blood brain barrier where it functions to transport leptin from the blood to the brain[9,10].

Ob-Rb mRNA is highly expressed in the hypothalamus and most studies support the concept that this leptin receptor isoform signals for leptin action within the central nervous system. In contrast, Ob-Ra, which lacks a well-defined mechanism to signal leptin action, is found in most tissues examined and is highly expressed in white adipose tissue, adrenals and testes[9]. Although Ob-Rb mRNA can be detected in peripheral tissue, its expression is much lower than that of Ob-Ra. Therefore when considering the possibility of direct effects of leptin on peripheral tissues, it is not entirely clear which receptor isoform mediates leptin effects. However, it has been suggested, based on observations in leptin receptor transfected cells, that limited expression of Ob-Rb is sufficient to provide competent leptin signaling[11].

3. LEPTIN COORDINATES THE NEUROENDOCRINE RESPONSE TO CALORIC RESTRICTION AND STARVATION

Much work demonstrating that leptin can limit food intake and increase energy expenditure in rodents and humans support the concept that this hormone functions as the signal postulated by the lipostasis theory to regulate energy stores in the adipose tissue[12]. However, Flier has argued that from an evolutionary perspective it is difficult to conceive of a mechanism that would limit food intake and storage of fat during times of excess, as this would reduce survival during the subsequent periods of limited nutrient availability. Rather, Flier has proposed that the major function of leptin is to signal energy deficiency and integrate the neuroendocrine response to this state[13].

Energy restriction and starvation initiate a complex series of biochemical and behavioral adaptations to promote survival. Increased food seeking behavior, a switch from carbohydrate to fat metabolism, and a reduction in energy expenditure are initiated by prolonged food deprivation. Energy utilization is reduced through central mechanisms in the CNS resulting in suppression of thyroid hormone regulated thermogenesis, curtailment of reproductive function and growth, and immune suppression[13].

In the well-fed state, serum leptin is highly correlated with total body fat content in cross-sectional studies[14]. However, serum leptin falls rapidly with short-term fasting (24-72 h) in both animals[15] and humans[16,17]. The rapid fall in leptin with fasting is disproportionately greater than the small reduction in adipose tissue mass that occurs over the same time period. Thus it is reasonable to suggest that serum leptin during fasting serves as a peripheral signal to the central nervous system that caloric restriction is occurring, rather than as a signal of current energy stores in the body. Proof that leptin coordinates the neuroendocrine response to fasting was originally derived through replacement experiments in rodents[15]. In these studies recombinant leptin was administered to 48 hour fasted mice to achieve serum leptin levels similar to that observed during the fed state. Preventing the starvation-induced fall in leptin substantially blunted the change in gonadal, adrenal and thyroid axes that would occur in male mice. Leptin administration also prevented the starvation-induced delay in ovulation in female mice. More recently, Chan et al[17] have demonstrated that replacement of leptin during complete caloric restriction in men can prevent the fasting-induced reduction in testosterone and partially prevent the suppression of the hypothalamic pituitary thyroid axis. Taken together, these observations thus establish a role for leptin regulation of hypothalamic-pituitary function in both rodents and humans.

4. LEPTIN AND THE ANTERIOR PITUITARY

Studies demonstrating that leptin administration could attenuate the fasting-induced reduction in hypothalamic pituitary function suggested that leptin action was mediated through the hypothalamus via actions on NPY neurons[15]. However, leptin receptors have been found in the anterior pituitary gland, suggesting that leptin may also have direct effects on this tissue. Message for both Ob-Ra and Ob-Rb are found in normal pituitary of rodents[18,19] and in human pituitary adenomas[20,21]. Expression of Ob-Rb in normal adult pituitary is controversial with two studies[20,22] documenting Ob-Rb mRNA expression in normal human pituitary but a third finding only expression of Ob-Ra[23]. Interestingly, in the study of Shimon et al[23] Ob-Rb message was detected in normal fetal pituitary, prompting these investigators to postulate a role for leptin in pituitary development. Leptin receptor protein has been detected in corticotropes, somatropes and gonadotropes of the ovine anterior pituitary, although the antibody used in these studies does not distinguish between Ob-Ra and Ob-Rb[24].

In addition to expression of leptin receptor, it appears that cells within the anterior pituitary also synthesize leptin. Using immunoelectron microscopy to examine normal human pituitary, leptin was detected in hormone producing glandular cells but not in stellate cells[25]. Corticotrophs were most frequently labeled (70-80% of ACTH positive cells) with much lower labeling in somatotrophs (10-15%), thyrotrophs (20-25%), and gonadotrophs (25-30%). No lactotrophs stained for leptin in this study. Leptin expression is much lower in rodent pituitary with expression mainly in TSH positive cells (24% and 31% of cells in rat and mouse, respectively)[19]. Leptin secretion in vitro was observed in 16 of 47 cultured pituitary adenomas but leptin mRNA was not detected in 5 normal pituitaries obtained at autopsy in this study[22].

Direct effects of leptin to regulate anterior pituitary cell function have been observed in vitro. Yu et al[26] observed that leptin increased FSH and LH release from rat hemi-anterior pituitaries at doses of 10^{-9} to 10^{-11}M, and prolactin secretion at much higher concentrations (10^{-7}-10^{-5}M). Low concentrations of leptin stimulate GH release from human fetal pituitary cell cultures but not ACTH, prolactin or gonadotropin secretion[23]. The ability of leptin to stimulate GH release decreased as gestational age at which the pituitary was obtained increased, suggesting that leptin regulation of GH release is more important during fetal development than in adults. In one study of pituitary adenomas leptin stimulated TSH release in vitro from one tumor and FSH from a second tumor, but had no effect on six additional tumors, three of which were GH secreting adenomas[22]. In agreement Kristiansen et al[21] found no effect of leptin on GH secreting adenomas. In cultured cell lines leptin induced pancreastatin release from HP75 cells and inhibited proliferation of GH3 and TtT/GF cells[19,20].

Overall these studies suggest that leptin may have direct effects on pituitary cell function although the variability in response of various preparations suggests that leptin effects may be cell type, developmental stage and species dependent. Leptin expression in the anterior pituitary also raises the possibility of a paracrine interaction between the various cell types within the tissue, which might be independent of the prevailing serum leptin concentration. Although in vitro studies suggest that direct effects of leptin to regulate pituitary function are possible, it has not yet been established that direct effects of leptin to regulate pituitary function are significant in relation to regulation mediated by leptin action in the hypothalamus.

5. LEPTIN AND THYROID FUNCTION

5.1 Rodent studies

Thyroid hormone levels determine basal metabolic rate and are subject to significant regulation during the transition from the fed to starved state. In rodents, starvation rapidly suppresses T4 and T3 levels to reduce metabolic rate and conserve energy[27]. The reduction in thyroid hormone results from suppression of TRH synthesis in the paraventricular nucleus within the hypothalamus and the subsequent reduction in TSH production in thyrotropes of the anterior pituitary. Administration of leptin to fasted mice prevents the starvation-induced fall in thyroid hormones by maintaining TRH mRNA levels in the paraventricular nucleus[15]. This effect appears to be mediated through two hypothalamic mechanisms. The projection of leptin responsive neurons from the arcuate nucleus to TRH neurons in the paraventricular nucleus is important as ablation of the arcuate nucleus with monosodium glutamate blocks the effect of leptin administration to prevent the fasting-induced fall in thyroid hormones[28]. The effect of leptin on TRH neurons is mediated through the melanocortin system as TRH neurons within the paraventricular nucleus express melanocortin-4 receptors and central administration of α-MSH can prevent or minimize the fasting-induced fall in TRH levels[29,30]. Furthermore, central administration of AgRP can decrease plasma TSH in fed animals, and block α-MSH- and leptin-induced TRH release from hypothalamic explants[29]. As a second mechanism leptin may act directly on TRH neurons in the paraventricular nucleus. TRH neurons express Ob-Rb mRNA and leptin administration induces STAT3 phosphorylation[31] and expression of suppressor of cytokine signaling-3 mRNA[32] in TRH neurons from fasted rats, suggesting a direct binding of leptin and activation of Ob-Rb in these neurons. Leptin has also been shown to activate the TRH promoter co-transfected into 293T cells with Ob-Rb[32].

A consistent relationship between serum leptin and thyroid hormones has not been found in various states of thyroid dysfunction[33]. Serum leptin was decreased in five studies of hyperthyroid rats and increased in four studies of hypothyroid rats. In three additional studies of hypothyroidism in rats, serum leptin was unchanged. Changes in fat mass with states of hypo- and hyperthyroidism complicate studies of the relationship between thyroid hormone and leptin in these studies.

5.2   Thyroid function and leptin in humans

Evidence for leptin regulation of the hypothalamic pituitary thyroid axis has also been obtained in studies with humans. Serum leptin levels in humans are pulsatile with a nocturnal rise in the evening and nadir in the late morning[34,35]. The diurnal secretion of TSH in normal subjects is similar to that of leptin and the 24 h patterns of variability in TSH and leptin are strongly correlated[36], suggesting that leptin may regulate TSH pulsatility and circadian rhythm. Further, support for this possibility is derived from examination of four brothers of a family with leptin deficiency. In one brother homozygous for leptin deficiency (leptin is detectable but bioinactive) TSH rhythm was completely disorganized[36]. In two heterozygous brothers the 24 h leptin and TSH pattern were significantly correlated, although the strength of the correlation was less than that for TSH and leptin in the homozygous normal brother and in normal unrelated subjects.

In lean healthy men fasted for 72 h, TSH secretion is suppressed and the pulsatile pattern lost[17]. T3 levels also fall with fasting but T4 levels are unchanged over the 72 h period. Administration of recombinant leptin to replacement levels significantly blunted the fall in TSH secretion but had no effect on the reduction in T3 with fasting. These findings in humans thus confirm observations in rodent models that leptin regulates the hypothalamic pituitary thyroid response to fasting.

A 10% reduction in body weight through dieting results in decreased T3, T4 and leptin. Administration of recombinant leptin to achieve serum levels comparable to that prior to weight loss restored T3 and T4 to baseline levels[37]. There were no changes in TSH with weight reduction or leptin administration. This suggests that declines in thyroid hormones with weight loss result from decreased T3 and T4 biosynthesis in the thyroid gland through a reduction in response to TSH. There is also decreased hypothalamic pituitary sensitivity to T3 since TSH is not increased despite lower T3 in weight-reduced subjects.

In three children with congenital leptin deficiency thyroid function tests were within the normal range, as were T4 and T3 levels, prior to initiation of recombinant leptin therapy[38]. At three months of therapy T4 levels remained within the normal range but were significantly increased in all three children. T3 levels were increased in two of the three children but TSH was unchanged with leptin treatment.

An extensive amount of work has been conducted to understand the relationship between leptin and thyroid dysfunction, as recently reviewed by Zimmermann-Belsing and colleagues[33]. In humans a consistent effect of thyroid state on serum leptin levels has not been found. In hypothyroid subjects serum leptin was increased in five studies, decreased in three and unchanged in eight compared to euthyroid controls. In hyperthyroid subjects serum leptin was increased in six studies, decreased in five studies and unchanged in fourteen studies[33]. A major complicating factor in all of these studies is that changes in fat mass occur with hyper- and hypothyroidism, which makes determination of interactions between thyroid hormone and leptin difficult. The use of BMI as a surrogate measure of fat mass likely also contributed to the disparate results.

110   *Chapter 6*

5.3   Direct effects of leptin on thyroid cells

The regulation of thyroid function by leptin in vivo is mediated through effects on hypothalamic neurons. However, a recent study has suggested that leptin can inhibit TSH induced iodide uptake, thyroglobulin mRNA expression and DNA synthesis in clonal rat thyroid FRTL-5 cells[39]. The potential interaction between such direct negative effects on thyroid function and the positive effect of leptin to promote thyroid hormone synthesis and release through hypothalamic neural signaling is not readily apparent.

5.4   Regulation of leptin synthesis by TSH and thyroid hormones

The effect of TSH to regulate leptin synthesis by adipocytes in vitro has been examined in two studies with opposite results. In rat epididymal adipocytes TSH inhibited leptin release in a time- and dose-dependent manner[40]. In contrast TSH dose-dependently stimulated leptin secretion from cultured omental adipose tissue pieces derived from normal to overweight humans over a 48 h period[41]. A major difference between these two studies is the use of adipose tissue pieces, which maintains the structural framework and interaction of various cells within the tissue, and does not expose the adipocytes to collagenase. Treatment of both cultured human adipose tissue pieces[42] and isolated rat adipocytes[43] with T3 results in inhibition of leptin mRNA and secretion. As TSH and T3 appear to have opposite effects on leptin release from human adipocytes experiments to assess the effects of these two hormones in the presence of each other need to be done. Further, the lack of a relationship between thyroid hormone status and serum leptin in vivo raise the question whether the in vitro effects of thyroid hormone on leptin synthesis are relevant in vivo. The fact that TSH may stimulate leptin release from human adipocytes could explain the highly synchronized diurnal and ultradian rhythms of these two hormones.

6.   ADRENAL FUNCTION AND LEPTIN

6.1   Animal studies

Several studies in rodents support a role for leptin in regulating hypothalamic pituitary adrenal function. Starvation activates the hypothalamic pituitary adrenal axis. Leptin administration to starved mice prevents the starvation-induced increase in ACTH and corticosterone levels[15]. Leptin treatment also blunts the rise in ACTH and cortiosterone that occurs in response to restraint stress in mice[44] or exposure to a new environment in rats[45]. In obese leptin deficient *ob/ob* mice glucocorticoid levels are 85% higher than that in 8 week old lean control mice. Injection of recombinant leptin acutely reduced serum corticosterone (24 h following initiation of treatment) prior to significant changes in body weight[46]. Chronic leptin infusion also attenuated the increase in plasma cortisol and ACTH in female rhesus monkeys that occurs in response to an unpredictable situation[47]. Taken together these findings support a role for leptin in inhibiting hypothalamic pituitary adrenal activation in response to stress.

The effect of leptin to prevent activation of the hypothalamic pituitary adrenal function appears to be mediated by inhibition of corticotropin releasing hormone (CRH) synthesis. In isolated rat hypothalmi leptin dose-dependently prevented the increase in CRH release induced by low glucose, but had no effect on ACTH release from cultured primary rat pituitary cells[44]. In a second study leptin infusion in starved mice reduced CRH mRNA in cells of the paraventricular nucleus and activation of these neurons[48]. However, other studies suggest that intracerebroventricular administration of leptin acutely increases CRH message and protein in the hypothalamus, a response in line with the function of CRH to inhibit food intake and increase energy expenditure[49,50,51]. The discrepancies between these observations may due to different model systems used. Alternatively, it has been hypothesized that there may be subsets of CRH neurons in the paraventricular nucleus that respond differently to leptin to regulate food intake and stress response[52].

6.2   Human studies

Frequent blood sampling techniques have been used to demonstrate that serum leptin levels are pulsatile and inversely related to the rapid fluctuations in ACTH and cortisol[35]. This observation prompted speculation that leptin may regulate hypothalamic pituitary adrenal function in humans as observed in rodents. However, in contrast to observations in animals, humans with leptin deficiency or leptin receptor mutations have normal levels of ACTH and cortisol[53,54]. Treatment with recombinant leptin to achieve significant weight loss had no effect on urinary cortisol concentrations in leptin deficient subjects[38]. Fasting in healthy men for 72 h had no effect on urine free cortisol or serum cortisol concentrations but did significantly increase the 24 h mean cortisol concentration, indicating a mild activation of the HPA axis[17]. Recombinant leptin had no effect on serum or urinary cortisol parameters in this study. Recombinant leptin treatment also had no effect on cortisol or ACTH in women with hypothalamic amenorrhea, despite increasing T3 and T4 within the normal range, and increasing markers of bone formation[55]. Leptin therapy, which improved reproductive hormone function, in lipodystrophic women also had no effect on ACTH or cortisol, which were normal prior to treatment[56]. Taken together, these results suggest that if leptin regulates hypothalamic pituitary adrenal function in humans, the extent of this regulation may not be as great as observed in rodents.

6.3 Direct leptin effects on adrenal function

Leptin receptors are present on adrenal cortical and medullary cells [57,58,59]. Leptin inhibits cortisol secretion from adrenocortical cells obtained from bovine, human and rodents in a dose-dependent manner[58,59,60]. In bovine or porcine adrenal medullary chromaffin cells leptin stimulates catecholamine synthesis and secretion[61,62]. These findings are in keeping with observations that leptin activates the sympathetic nervous system. Interestingly, in the only study to use human adrenal chromaffin cells, leptin was without effect on basal catecholamine secretion[59], possibly suggesting species differences in leptin effects on adrenomedullary function.

6.4 Regulation of leptin synthesis by cortisol and catecholamines

Cortisol is a potent simulus for leptin synthesis and secretion from adipocytes in vivo and in vitro[63,64,others]. Local synthesis of cortisol from inactive metabolites by 11β-hydroxysteroid dehydrogenase is likely an important source of cortisol regulating leptin synthesis in adipose tissue[65]. The mechanism through which glucocorticoids regulate leptin synthesis in adipocytes is not completely understood as the glucocorticoid response element on the Lep gene promoter is not needed for dexamethasone to stimulate promoter activity[66].

Activation of the sympathetic nervous system is postulated to be a negative feedback loop to inhibit leptin synthesis and release from adipose tissue. Support for this postulate is derived from different experimental paradigms including administration of catecholamines to human subjects, which acutely reduces serum leptin[67]. In vitro, catecholamines and cAMP reduce *LEP* mRNA and leptin synthesis in human adipose tissue pieces, human adipocytes differentiated in vitro, 3T3-L1 cells and rodent adipocytes[68,69].

7. LEPTIN AND GROWTH HORMONE

7.1 Animal studies

Growth hormone in rats is markedly suppressed in nutritionally deprived states and several studies support a role for leptin in signaling for this response to food restriction. In 48 h food restricted rats intracerebroventricular leptin reversed the inhibitory effect of caloric restriction on growth hormone secretion[70,71]. In contrast intracerebroventricular administration of leptin antiserum to fed rats results in a significant decrease in mean growth hormone amplitude and area under the curve for growth hormone secretion compared to animals receiving normal rabbit serum[70]. Finally, chronic peripheral infusion of leptin results in a dramatic increase in growth hormone pulse height despite its effects to reduce food intake[72].

Growth hormone release is stimulated by growth hormone releasing hormone and inhibited by somatostatin. A role for both factors in the regulation of growth hormone secretion by leptin has been established. Leptin inhibited somatostatin release from cultured fetal hypothalamic neurons[73] and increased growth hormone secretion in response to growth hormone releasing hormone in fasted rats[74], suggesting that leptin also inhibited somatostatin release in vivo. Leptin attenuated the fasting-induced fall in growth hormone releasing hormone mRNA in the hypothalamus in one study[75] and increased growth hormone releasing hormone mRNA in freely moving fed rats during a three day intracerebroventricular administration[76]. More recently it has been shown using an in vivo hypothalamic perfusion technique that intracerebroventricular leptin both increases hypothalamic growth hormone releasing hormone secretion and decreases somatostatin secretion[77]. Leptin receptors and STAT3 have been colocalized with growth hormone releasing hormone-containing neurons in rat hypothalamus[78], suggesting that leptin directly acts on these neurons to regulate growth hormone releasing hormone secretion.

As discussed above leptin may also directly regulate growth hormone release from somatotropes in the anterior pituitary[23,79], although the in vivo relevance of this effect is not established.

7.2 Human studies

Growth hormone levels are reduced in obese humans and leptin levels are significantly increased. Observations that leptin could regulate growth hormone secretion in rodents therefore led to the hypothesis that the elevated leptin levels in obese humans might inhibit growth hormone release. To test this hypothesis Ozata et al[80] compared basal and stimulated growth hormone secretion in subjects either homozygous or heterozygous for mutations in the leptin gene, to adiposity and gender-matched controls. Subjects with leptin gene mutations would be obese without elevated leptin. Therefore, if leptin inhibits growth hormone secretion subjects deficient in leptin should have higher basal and./or stimulated growth hormone levels compared to obese subjects with elevated leptin levels. In both controls and subjects with leptin deficiency obesity was associated with lower basal and stimulated growth hormone release, but there was no additional effect of leptin to reduce growth hormone secretion in subjects without leptin gene mutations. These findings thus rule out the possibility that elevated serum leptin inhibits growth hormone secretion in obese humans.

In leptin deficient children linear growth was not stunted in the untreated state or altered by recombinant leptin administration[38]. Plasma IGF-1 levels were normal before treatment and increased with age. Whole body bone mineral content and density were age and gender appropriate in these children, although skeletal maturation was increased by a mean of 2.1 years. These findings demonstrate that leptin deficiency in humans does not result in impaired linear growth as observed in *ob/ob* mice.

In contrast to rodents, fasting in humans results in increased growth hormone secretion. Administration of recombinant leptin to healthy men fasted for 72 h had no effect on fasting-induced changes in growth hormone secretion[17]. However leptin therapy for 3 months in women with hypothalamic amenorrhea did result in an increase in IGF-1 and IGF binding protein 3[55].

In growth hormone deficient subjects leptin levels are elevated due to increased fat mass. Growth hormone therapy results in lower serum leptin due to its effects to reduce fat mass and increase lean mass in treated patients[81,82,others]. Thus these studies have not found that growth hormone regulates leptin levels independently of its effects on body fat content. However in two separate studies a single supraphysiologic dose of growth hormone elicited a significant increase in serum leptin 24 h following hormone administration[83,84]. Both studies suggest that this effect of growth hormone was not mediated by an increase in insulin, suggesting that growth hormone at very high doses either acts directly on adipocytes or induces another factor that acts on adipocytes to increase serum leptin.

Overall observations in humans from several different studies have not provided strong evidence that leptin regulates growth hormone to the extent seen for other hypothalamic pituitary axis hormones such as thyroid hormone.

8. LEPTIN REGULATION OF ADIPOSE TISSUE FUNCTION

Adipose tissue is an endocrine organ that secretes a large number of different hormones and cytokines in addition to leptin[85,86]. The serum concentration of many of these adipose tissue secretory products, with the exception of adiponectin, are increased in obesity and have been linked to the development of insulin resistance, diabetes and cardiovascular disease. Leptin effects mediated through the hypothalamus to reduce adipose tissue mass should therefore result in reduced expression of many these adipose tissue factors, including leptin itself. However, leptin also has direct effects on tissues that are not mediated through the central nervous system[87]. Of particular relevance to this chapter, work from several different laboratories has established that leptin can induce lipolysis in isolated rodent adipocytes[88,89,90]. This effect is mediated by leptin receptors as leptin has no lipolytic effect on adipocytes with defective leptin receptors obtained from *db/db* mice or *fa/fa* rats. Further evidence for leptin signaling through Ob-Rb on adipocytes is provided by the observations that STAT-3 in adipose tissue is phosphorylated three minutes after intravenous injection, but not intracerebroventricular administration, of leptin[91]. Leptin also activated STAT-3 and MAPK in adipose tissue ex vivo. These findings thus support the hypothesis that leptin has direct effects on adipose tissue and may therefore directly influence the release of hormones and cytokines from the tissue. In support of such an effect Wang et al[90] observed that leptin inhibited expression of *Lep* mRNA in isolated adipocytes. More recently it has been observed that TNFα, and leptin expression are increased in adipocytes of mice with a selective ablation of leptin receptors in adipose tissue[92]. Adiponectin expression in this model is reduced. As these mice are more obese than wild-type controls, it remains to be determined if these changes in adipokine synthesis result from an inability of leptin to directly signal in adipocytes or are secondary changes in response to increased adiposity. However, these intriguing observations indicate that additional work is necessary to fully appreciate the possibility that leptin may directly regulate the endocrine function of adipose tissue.

9. SUMMARY

Nutritional status has profound effects on all physiologic processes in the body and ultimately determines survival of the organism. Endocrine networks have thus developed to coordinate the function of various tissues in response to periods of caloric deprivation and excess. As illustrated in Figure

1, leptin has important regulatory effects on hypothalamic pituitary function that become readily apparent during periods of caloric deprivation, although differences exist in the extent to which leptin regulates these systems in rodents and humans. Leptin, as a signal of both energy stores within the adipose tissue, and acute reductions in caloric intake during fasting, thus appears to be a master coordinator of the central nervous system response to changes in nutritional status. The extent to which leptin regulates other endocrine systems may differ in times of nutrient excess, or in various disease states such as diabetes and obesity.

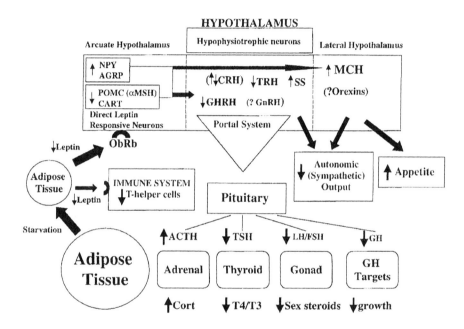

Figure 1. Role of leptin in the adaptation to starvation. The fall in leptin with starvation results in an increase in neuropeptide Y (NPY) and agouti-related peptide (AGRP) levels, and a decrease in proopiomelanocortin (POMC) and cocaine- and amphetamine-regulated transcript (CART) levels in the arcuate hypothalamic nucleus. NPY, POMC, AGRP, and CART neurons are directly responsive to leptin. NPY and AGRP stimulate feeding, whereas melanocyte stimulating hormone (a product of POMC) and CART inhibit feeding. These neurons also project to the lateral hypothalamus and regulate the expression of melanin-concentrating hormone (MCH), a major stimulator of feeding. In addition, leptin targets in the arcuate hypothalamic nucleus respond to low leptin levels by regulating the neuroendocrine axis and decreasing sympathetic nervous output. The metabolic and neuroendocrine adaptations to fasting mediated by leptin are likely to be of greater survival value in rodents since short-term starvation has more severe consequences in this species. CRH (corticotropin-releasing hormone), TRH (thyrotropin-releasing hormone), GHRH (growth hormone-releasing hormone), SS (somatostatin), GnRH (gonadotropin-releasing hormone), GH (growth hormone). From Ahima and Flier[93]. Reprinted, with permission, from the *Annual Review of Physiology,* Volume 62 ©2000 by Annual Reviews   www.annualreviews.org.

REFERENCES

1. Y. Zhang, R. Proenca, M. Maffei, M. Barone, L. Leopold and J.M. Friedman, Positional cloning of the mouse obese gene and its human homologue. *Nature,* 372:425-432 (1994).
2. L.A. Tartaglia, The leptin receptor. *J Biol Chem,* 272:6093-6096 (1997).
3. C. Vaisse, J.L. Halaas, C.M. Horvath, J.E. Darnell Jr, M. Stoffel and J.M. Friedman, Leptin activation of STAT3 in the hypothalamus of wild-type and *ob/ob* mice but not *db/db* mice. *Nature-Genetics* 14:95-97 (1996).
4. K.D. Niswender, G.J. Morton, W.H. Stearns, C.J. Rhodes, M.G. Myers Jr and M.W. Schwartz, Intracellular signalling. Key enzyme in leptin-induced anorexia. *Nature,* 413:794-795 (2001).
5. A.Z. Zhao, J.N. Huan, S. Gupta, R. Pal and A. Sahu, A phosphatidylinositol 3-kinase phosphodiesterase 3B-cyclic AMP pathway in hypothalamic action of leptin on feeding. *Nature Neurosci,* 5:727-728 (2002).
6. G.H. Lee, R. Proenca, J.M. Montez, K.M. Carroll, J.G. Darvishzadeh, J.I Lee and J.M. Friedman, Abnormal splicing of the leptin receptor in *diabetic* mice. *Nature* 379:632-635 (1996).
7. M.-Y.Wang, Y.T. Zhou, C.B. Newgard and R.H. Unger, A novel leptin receptor isoform in rat. *FEBS Lett,* 392:87-90 (1996).
8. C. Bjorbaek, S. Uotani, B. da Silva and J.S. Flier, Divergent signaling capacites of the long and short isoforms of the leptin receptor. *J Biol Chem,* 272:32686-32695 (1997).
9. L.A. Tartaglia, M. Dembski, X. WengN. Deng, J. Culpepper, R. Devos, G.J. Richards, L.A. Campfield, F.T. Clark, J. Deeds, C. Muir, S. Sanker, A. Moriarty, K.J. Moore, J.S. Smutko, G.G. Mays, E.A. Woolf, C. Selent-Munro and R.I. Tepper, Identification and expression cloning of the a leptin receptor, OB-R. *Cell* 83:1263-1271 (1995).
10. S.M. Hileman, D.D. Pierroz, H. Masuzaki, C. Bjorbaek, K. El-Haschimi, W.A. Banks and J.S. Flier, Characterizaton of short isoforms of the leptin receptor in rat cerebral microvessels and of brain uptake of leptin in mouse models of obesity. *Endocrinology* 143:775-783 (2002).
11. C. Bjorbaek and B.B. Kahn, Leptin signaling in the central nervous system and the periphery. *Recent Prog Horm Res,* 59:305-331 (2004).
12. J.F. Caro and R.V. Considine, Leptin: From laboratory to clinic. In. *Handbook of Obesity,* G.A Bray GA and C. Bouchard Eds., 2nd Ed. Marcel Dekker, Inc, New York, pp. 275-295 (2004).
13. J.S. Flier, What's in a name? In search of leptin's physiologic role. *J Clin Endocrinol Metab,* 83:1407-1413 (1998).
14. R.V. Considine, M.K. Sinha, M.L. Heiman, A. Kriauciunas, T.W. Stephens, M.R. Nyce, J.P. Ohannesian, C.C. Marco, L.M. McKee, T.L. Bauer and J.F. Caro, Serum immunoreactive-leptin concentrations in normal weight and obese humans. *N Eng J Med,* 334:292-5 (1996).
15. R.S. Ahima, D. Prabakaran, C. Mantzoros, D. Qu, B. Lowell, E. Maratos-Flier and J.S. Flier, Role of leptin in the neuroendocrine response to fasting. *Nature,* 382:250-252 (1996).
16. J.W. Kolaczynski, R.V. Considine, J. Ohannesian, C. Marco, I. Opentanova, M.R. Nyce, M. Myint and J.F. Caro, Responses of leptin to short-term fasting and

refeeding in humans: A link with ketogenesis but not ketones themselves. *Diabetes*, **45**:1511-1515 (1996).
17. J.L. Chan, K. Heist, A.M. DePaoli, J.D. Veldhuis and C.S. Mantzoros, The role of falling leptin levels in the neuroendocrine and metabolic adaptation to short-term starvation in healthy men. *J Clin Invest*, **111**:1409-1421 (2003).
18. P.L. Zamorano, V.B. Mahesh, L.M. De Sevilla, L.P. Chorich, G.K. Bhat and D.W. Brann, Expression and localization of the leptin receptor in endocrine and neuroendocrine tissues of the rat. *Neuroendocrinology*, **65**:223-228 (1997).
19. L. Jin, S. Zhang, B.G. Burguera, M.E. Couce, R.Y. Osamura, E. Kulig and R.V. Lloyd, Leptin and leptin receptor expression in rat and mouse pituitary cells. *Endocrinology*, **141**:333-339 (2000).
20. L. Jin, B.G. Burguera, M.E. Couce, B.W. Scheithauer, J. Lamsan, N.L. Eberhardt, E. Kulig and R.V. Lloyd, Leptin and leptin receptor expression in normal and neoplastic human pituitary: evidence of a regulatory role for leptin on pituitary cell proliferation. *J Clin Endocrinol Metab*, **84**:2903-2911 (1999).
21. M.T. Kristiansen, L.R. Clausen, S. Nielsen, O. Blaabjerg, T. Ledet, L.M. Rasmussen and J.O. Jorgensen, Expression of leptin receptor isoforms and effects of leptin on the proliferation and hormonal secretion in human pituitary adenomas. *Horm Res*, **62**:129-136 (2004).
22. M. Korbonits, M.M. Chitnis, M. Gueorguiev, D. Norman, N. Rosenfelder, M. Suliman, T.H. Jones, K. Noonan, A. Fabbri, G.M. Besser, J.M. Burrin and A.B. Grossman, The release of leptin and its effect on hormone release from human pituitary adenomas. *Clin Endocrinol (Oxf)*, **54**:781-789 (2001).
23. I. Shimon, X. Yan, D.A. Magoffin, T.C. Friedman and S. Melmed, Intact leptin receptor is selectively expressed in human fetal pituitary and pituitary adenomas and signals human fetal pituitary growth hormone secretion. *J Clin Endocrinol Metab*, **83**:4059-4064 (1998).
24. J. Iqbal, S. Pompolo, R.V. Considine and I.J. Clarke, Localization of leptin receptor-like immunoreactivity in the corticotropes, somatotropes, and gonadotropes in the ovine anterior pituitary. *Endocrinology*, **141**:1515-1520 (2000).
25. S. Vidal, S.M. Cohen, E. Horvath, K. Kovacs, B.W. Scheithauer, B.G. Burguera and R.V. Lloyd, Subcellular localization of leptin in non-tumorous and adenomatous human pituitaries: an immuno-ultrastructural study. *J Histochem Cytochem*, **48**:1147-1152 (2000).
26. W.H. Yu, M. Kimura, A. Walczewska, S. Karanth and S.M. McCann, Role of leptin in hypothalamic-pituitary function. *Proc Natl Acad Sci USA*, **94**:1023-1028 (1997).
27. N.G. Blake, D.J. Eckland, O.J. Foster and S.L. Lightman, Inhibition of hypothalamic thyrotropin-releasing hormone messenger ribonucleic acid during food deprivation. *Endocrinology*, **129**:2714-2718 (1991).
28. G. Legradi, C.H. Emerson, R.S. Ahima, W.M. Rand, J.S. Flier and R.M. Lechan, Arcuate nucleus ablation prevents fasting-induced suppression of ProTRH mRNA in the hypothalamic paraventricular nucleus. *Neuroendocrinology*, **68**:89-97 (1998).
29. M.S. Kim, C.J. Small, S.A. Stanley, D.G. Morgan, L.J. Seal, W.M. Kong, C.M. Edwards, S. Abusnana, D. Sunter, M.A. Ghatei and S.R. Bloom, The central melanocortin system affects the hypothalamo-pituitary thyroid axis and may mediate the effect of leptin. *J Clin Invest*, **105**:1005-1011 (2000).

30. C. Fekete, G. Legradi, E. Mihaly, J.B. Tatro, W.M. Rand and R.M. Lechan, alpha-Melanocyte stimulating hormone prevents fasting-induced suppression of corticotropin-releasing hormone gene expression in the rat hypothalamic paraventricular nucleus. *Neurosci Lett,* **289**:152-156 (2000).
31. L. Huo, H. Munzberg, E.A. Nillni and C. Bjorbaek, Role of signal transducer and activator of transcription 3 in regulation of hypothalamic trh gene expression by leptin. *Endocrinology,* **145**:2516-2523 (2004).
32. M. Harris, C. Aschkenasi, C.F. Elias, A. Chandrankunnel, E.A. Nillni, C. Bjoorbaek, J.K. Elmquist, J.S. Flier and A.N. Hollenberg, Transcriptional regulation of the thyrotropin-releasing hormone gene by leptin and melanocortin signaling. *J Clin Invest,* **107**:111-120 (2001).
33. T. Zimmermann-Belsing, G. Brabant, J.J. Holst and U. Feldt-Rasmussen, Circulating leptin and thyroid dysfunction. *Eur J Endocrinol,* **149**:257-271 (2003).
34. M.K. Sinha, J.P. Ohannesian, M.L. Heiman, A. Kriauciunas, T.W. Stephens, S. Magosin, C. Marco and J.F. Caro, Nocturnal rise of leptin in lean, obese, and non-insulin dependent diabetes mellitus subjects. *J Clin Invest,* **97**:1344-1347 (1996).
35. J. Licinio, C. Mantzoros, A.B. Negrao, G. Cizza, M.L. Wong, P.B. Bongiorno, G.P. Chrousos, B. Karp, C. Allen, J.S. Flier and P.W. Gold, Human leptin levels are pulsatile and inversely related to pituitary-adrenal function. *Nature Med,* **3**:575-579 (1997).
36. C.S. Mantzoros, M. Ozata, A.B. Negrao, M.A. Suchard, M. Ziotopoulou, S. Caglayan, R.M. Elashoff, R.J. Cogswell, P. Negro, V. Liberty, M.L. Wong, J. Veldhuis, I.C. Ozdemir, P.W. Gold, J.S. Flier and J. Licinio, Synchronicity of frequently sampled thyrotropin (TSH) and leptin concentrations in healthy adults and leptin-deficient subjects: evidence for possible partial TSH regulation by leptin in humans. *J Clin Endocrinol Metab,* **86**:3284-3291 (2001).
37. M. Rosenbaum, E.M. Murphy, S.B. Heymsfield, D.E. Matthews and R.L. Leibel, Low dose leptin administration reverses effects of sustained weight-reduction on energy expenditure and circulating concentrations of thyroid hormones. *J Clin Endocrinol Metab,* **87**:2391-2394 (2002).
38. I.S. Farooqi, G. Matarese, G.M. Lord, J.M. Keogh, E. Lawrence, C. Agwu, V. Sanna, S.A. Jebb, F. Perna, S. Fontana, R.I. Lechler, A.M. DePaoli and S. O'Rahilly, Beneficial effects of leptin on obesity, T cell hyporesponsiveness, and neuroendocrine/metabolic dysfunction of human congenital leptin deficiency. *J Clin Invest,* **110**:1093-1103 (2002).
39. O. Isozaki, T. Tsushima, Y. Nozoe, M. Miyakawa and K. Takano, Leptin regulation of the thyroids: negative regulation on thyroid hormone levels in euthyroid subjects and inhibitory effects on iodide uptake and Na+/I- symporter mRNA expression in rat FRTL-5 cells. *Endocr J,* **51**:415-423 (2004).
40. M. Shintani, H. Nishimura, T. Akamizu, S. Yonemitsu, H. Masuzaki, Y. Ogawa, K. Hosoda, G. Inoue, Y. Yoshimasa and K. Nakao, Thyrotropin decreases leptin production in rat adipocytes. *Metabolism,* **48**:1570-1574 (1999).
41. C. Menendez, R. Baldelli, J.P. Camina, B. Escudero, R. Peino, C. Dieguez and F.F. Casanueva, TSH stimulates leptin secretion by a direct effect on adipocytes. *J Endocrinol,* **176**:7-12 (2003).
42. K. Kristensen, S.B. Pedersen, B.L. Langdahl and B. Richelsen, Regulation of leptin by thyroid hormone in humans: studies in vivo and in vitro. *Metabolism,* **48**:1603-1607 (1999).

43. G. Medina-Gomez, R.M. Calvo and M.J. Obregon, T3 and Triac inhibit leptin secretion and expression in brown and white rat adipocytes. *Biochim Biophys Acta,* **1682**:38-47 (2004).
44. M.L. Heiman, R.S. Ahima, L.S. Craft, B. Schoner, T.W. Stephens and J.S. Flier, Leptin inhibition of the hypothalamic-pituitary-adrenal axis in response to stress. *Endocrinology,* **138**:3859-3863 (1997).
45. K.W. Nowak, K. Pierzchala-Koziec, C. Tortorella, G.G. Nussdorfer and L.K. Malendowicz, Effects of prolonged leptin infusion on rat pituitary-adrenocortical function. *Int J Mol Med,* **9**:61-64 (2002).
46. R.S. Ahima, D. Prabakaran and J.S. Flier, Postnatal leptin surge and regulation of circadian rhythm of leptin by feeding. Implications for energy homeostasis and neuroendocrine function. *J Clin Invest,* **101**:1020-1027 (1998)
47. M.E. Wilson, J. Fisher and J. Brown, Chronic subcutaneous leptin infusion diminishes the responsiveness of the hypothalamic-pituitary-adrenal (HPA) axis in female rhesus monkeys. *Physiol Behav,* **84**:449-458 (2005).
48. Q. Huang, R. Rivest and D. Richard, Effects of leptin on corticotropin-releasing factor (CRF) synthesis and CRF neuron activation in the paraventricular hypothalamic nucleus of obese (ob/ob) mice. *Endocrinology,* **139**:1524-1532 (1998).
49. M.W. Schwartz, R.J. Seeley, L.A. Campfield, P. Burn and D.G. Baskin, Identification of targets of leptin action in rat hypothalamus. *J Clin Invest,* **98**:1101-1106 (1996).
50. Y. Uehara, H. Shimizu, K. Ohtani, N. Sato and M. Mori, Hypothalamic corticotropin-releasing hormone is a mediator of the anorexigenic effect of leptin. *Diabetes* **47**:890-893 (1998).
51. M. Jang, A. Mistry, A.G. Swick and D.R. Romsos, Leptin rapidly inhibits hypothalamic neuropeptide Y secretion and stimulates corticotropin-releasing hormone secretion in adrenalectomized mice. *J Nutr,* **130**:2813-2820 (2000).
52. R.S. Ahima and S.Y. Osei, Leptin signaling. *Physiol Behav,* **81**:223-241 (2004).
53. C.T. Montague, I.S. Farooqi, J.P. Whitehead, M.A. Soos, H. Rau, N.J. Wareham, C.P. Sewter, J.E. Digby, S.N. Mohammed, J.A. Hurst, C.H. Cheetham, A.R. Earley, A.H. Barnett, J.B. Prins and S. O'Rahilly, Congenital leptin deficiency is associated with severe early-onset obesity in humans. *Nature,* **387**:903-908 (1997).
54. K. Clement, C. Vaisse, N. Lahlou, S. Cabrol, V. Pelloux, D. Cassuto, M. Gourmelen, C. Dina, J. Chambaz, J.M. Lacorte, A. Basdevant, P. Bougneres, Y. Lebouc, P. Froguel and B. Guy-Grand, A mutation in the human leptin receptor gene causes obesity and pituitary dysfunction. *Nature,* **392**:398-401 (1998).
55. C.K. Welt, J.L. Chan, J. Bullen, R. Murphy, P. Smith, A.M. DePaoli, A. Karalis and C.S. Mantzoros, Recombinant human leptin in women with hypothalamic amenorrhea. *N Engl J Med,* **351**:987-997 (2004).
56. E.A.Oral, E. Ruiz, A. Andewelt, N. Sebring, A.J. Wagner, A.M. Depaoli and P. Gorden, Effect of leptin replacement on pituitary hormone regulation in patients with severe lipodystrophy. *J Clin Endocrinol Metab,* **87**:3110-3117 (2002).
57. G.Y. Cao, R.V. Considine and R.B. Lynn RB, Leptin receptors in the adrenal medulla of the rat. *Am J Physiol,* **273**:E448-E452 (1997).
58. S.R. Bornstein, K. Uhlmann, A. Haidan, M. Ehrhart-Bornstein and W.A. Scherbaum, Evidence for a novel peripheral action of leptin as a metabolic signal to

the adrenal gland: leptin inhibits cortisol release directly. *Diabetes,* **46**:1235-1238 (1997).
59. A. Glasow, A. Haidan, U. Hilbers, M. Breidert, J. Gillespie, W.A. Scherbaum, G.P. Chrousos and S.R. Bornstein, Expression of Ob receptor in normal human adrenals: differential regulation of adrenocortical and adrenomedullary function by leptin. *J Clin Endocrinol Metab,* **83**:4459-4466 (1998).
60. F.P. Pralong, R. Roduit, G. Waeber, E. Castillo, F. Mosimann, B. Thorens and R.C. Gaillard, Leptin inhibits directly glucocorticoid secretion by normal human and rat adrenal gland. *Endocrinology,* **139**:4264-4268 (1998).
61. K. Takekoshi, M. Motooka, K. Isobe, F. Nomura, T. Manmoku, K. Ishii and T. Nakai, Leptin directly stimulates catecholamine secretion and synthesis in cultured porcine adrenal medullary chromaffin cells. *Biochem Biophys Res Commun,* **261**:426-431 (1999).
62. I. Shibuya, K. Utsunomiya, Y. Toyohira, S. Ueno, M. Tsutsui, T.B. Cheah, Y. Ueta, F. Izumi and N. Yanagihara, Regulation of catecholamine synthesis by leptin. *Ann N Y Acad Sci,* **971**:522-527 (2002).
63. H. Larsson and B. Ahren, Short-term dexamethasone treatment increases plasma leptin independently of changes in insulin sensitivity in healthy women. *J Clin Endocrinol Metab,* **81**:4428-4432 (1996).
64. L.B. Williams, R.L. Fawcett, A.S. Waechter, P. Zhang, B.E. Kogon, R. Jones, M. Inman, J. Huse and R.V. Considine, Leptin production in adipocytes from morbidly obese subjects: stimulation by dexamethasone, inhibition with troglitazone, and influence of gender. *J Clin Endocrinol Metab,* **85**:2678-2684 (2000).
65. D.J. Wake and B.R. Walker, 11 beta-hydroxysteroid dehydrogenase type 1 in obesity and the metabolic syndrome. *Mol Cell Endocrinol,* **215**:45-54 (2004).
66. P. De Vos, A.M. Lefebvre, I. Shrivo, J.C. Fruchart and J. Auwerx, J Glucocorticoids induce the expression of the leptin gene through a non-classical mechanism of transcriptional activation. *Eur J Biochem,* **253**:619-626 (1998).
67. A.L.Mark, K. Rahmouni, M. Correia and W.G. Haynes, A leptin-sympathetic-leptin feedback loop: potential implications for regulation of arterial pressure and body fat. *Acta Physiol Scand,* **177**:345-349 (2003).
68. R.V. Considine, Regulation of leptin production. *Rev Endocr Metab Disord,* **2**:357-363 (2001).
69. D.V. Rayner and P. Trayhurn, Regulation of leptin production: sympathetic nervous system interactions. *J Mol Med,* **79**:8-20 (2001).
70. E. Carro, R. Senaris, R.V. Considine, F.F. Casanueva and C. Dieguez, Regulation of in vivo growth hormone secretion by leptin. *Endocrinology,* **138**:2203-2206 (1997).
71. E. Carro, L.M. Seoane, R. Senaris, R.V. Considine, F.F. Casanueva and C. Dieguez, Interaction between leptin and neuropeptide Y on in vivo growth hormone secretion. *Neuroendocrinology,* **68**:187-191 (1998).
72. G.S. Tannenbaum, W. Gurd and M. Lapointe, Leptin is a potent stimulator of spontaneous pulsatile growth hormone (GH) secretion and the GH response to GH-releasing hormone. *Endocrinology,* **139**:3871-3875 (1998).
73. M. Quintela, R. Senaris, M.L. Heiman, F.F. Casanueva and C. Dieguez, Leptin inhibits in vitro hypothalamic somatostatin secretion and somatostatin mRNA levels. *Endocrinology,* **138**:5641-5644 (1997).

74. E. Carro, L.M. Seoane, R. Senaris, F.F. Casanueva and C. Dieguez, Leptin increases in vivo GH responses to GHRH and GH-releasing peptide-6 in food-deprived rats. *Eur J Endocrinol*, **142**:66-70 (2000).
75. N, LaPaglia, J. Steiner, L. Kirsteins, M. Emanuele and N. Emanuele, Leptin alters the response of the growth hormone releasing factor- growth hormone--insulin-like growth factor-I axis to fasting. *J Endocrinol*, **159**:79-83 (1998).
76. D. Cocchi, V. De Gennaro Colonna, M. Bagnasco, D. Bonacci and E.E. Muller, Leptin regulates GH secretion in the rat by acting on GHRH and somatostatinergic functions. *J Endocrinol*, **162**:95-99 (1999).
77. H. Watanobe and S Habu, Leptin regulates growth hormone-releasing factor, somatostatin, and alpha-melanocyte-stimulating hormone but not neuropeptide Y release in rat hypothalamus in vivo: relation with growth hormone secretion. *J Neurosci*, **22**:6265-6271 (2002).
78. M.L. Hakansson, H. Brown, N. Ghilardi, R.C. Skoda and B. Meister, Leptin receptor immunoreactivity in chemically defined target neurons of the hypothalamus. *J Neurosci*, **18**:559-572 (1998).
79. S.G. Roh, G.Y. Nie, K. Loneragan, A. Gertler and C. Chen, Direct modification of somatotrope function by long-term leptin treatment of primary cultured ovine pituitary cells. *Endocrinology*, **142**:5167-5171 (2001).
80. M. Ozata, C. Dieguez and F.F. Casanueva, The inhibition of growth hormone secretion presented in obesity is not mediated by the high leptin levels: a study in human leptin deficiency patients. *J Clin Endocrinol Metab*, **88**:312-316 (2003).
81. Y.J. Janssen, M. Frolich, P. Deurenberg and F. Roelfsema, Serum leptin levels during recombinant human GH therapy in adults with GH deficiency. *Eur J Endocrinol*, **137**:650-654 (2003).
82. H.S. Randeva, R.D. Murray, K.C. Lewandowski, C.J. O'Callaghan, R. Horn, P. O'Hare, G. Brabant, E.W. Hillhouse and S.M. Shalet, Differential effects of GH replacement on the components of the leptin system in GH-deficient individuals. *J Clin Endocrinol Metab*, **87**:798-804 (2002).
83. M.S. Gill, A.A. Toogood, J. Jones, P.E. Clayton and S.M. Shalet, Serum leptin response to the acute and chronic administration of growth hormone (GH) to elderly subjects with GH deficiency. *J Clin Endocrinol Metab*, **84**:1288-1295 (1999).
84. C.A. Lissett, P.E. Clayton and S.M. Shalet, The acute leptin response to GH. *J Clin Endocrinol Metab*, **86**:4412-4415 (2001).
85. P.J. Havel, Update on adipocyte hormones: regulation of energy balance and carbohydrate/lipid metabolism. *Diabetes*, **53 Suppl 1**:S143-S151 (2004).
86. H. Hauner, Secretory factors from human adipose tissue and their functional role. *Proc Nutr Soc*, **64**:163-169 (2005).
87. R.V. Considine and J.F. Caro, Pleotropic Cellular Effects of Leptin. *Curr Opin Endocrinol Diabetes*, **6**:163-169 (1999).
88. G. Fruhbeck, M. Aguado and J.A. Martinez, In vitro lipolytic effect of leptin on mouse adipocytes: evidence for a possible autocrine/paracrine role of leptin. *Biochem Biophys Res Commun*, **240**:590-594 (1997).
89. C.A. Siegrist-Kaiser, V. Pauli, C.E. Juge-Aubry, O. Boss, A. Pernin, W.W. Chin, I. Cusin, F. Rohner-Jeanrenaud, A.G. Burger, J. Zapf and C.A. Meier, Direct effects of leptin on brown and white adipose tissue. *J Clin Invest*, **100**:2858-2864 (1997).
90. M.Y. Wang, Y. Lee and R.H. Unger, Novel form of lipolysis induced by leptin. *J Biol Chem*, **274**:17541-17544 (1999).

91. Y.B. Kim, S. Uotani, D.D. Pierroz, J.S. Flier and B.B. Kahn, In vivo administration of leptin activates signal transduction directly in insulin-sensitive tissues: overlapping but distinct pathways from insulin. *Endocrinology,* **141**:2328-2339 (2000).
92. J.N. Huan, J. Li, Y. Han, K. Chen, N. Wu and A.Z. Zhao, Adipocyte-selective reduction of the leptin receptors induced by antisense RNA leads to increased adiposity, dyslipidemia, and insulin resistance. *J Biol Chem,* **278**:45638-45650 (2003).
93. R.S. Ahima and J.S. Flier, Leptin. *Annu Rev Phyisol,* **62**:413-437 (2000).

Chapter 7

LEPTIN AND IMMUNE FUNCTION, INFLAMMATION AND ANGIOGENESIS

Giuseppe Matarese, Claudio Procaccini and Veronica De Rosa
Gruppo di ImmunoEndocrinologia, Istituto di Endocrinologia e Oncologia Sperimentale, Consiglio Nazionale delle Ricerche c/o Laboratorio di Immunologia, Dipartimento di Biologia e Patologia Cellulare e Molecolare, Università di Napoli "Federico II", Napoli, Italy

Abstract: Over the last few years the intricate interaction between immunity and metabolism has been recognized. Indeed, it has been suggested that adipose tissue is not merely the site of energy storage, but can be considered as an "immune-related" organ producing a series of molecules named "adipocytokines." Among these, leptin seems to play a pivotal role in the regulation of several neuroendocrine and immune functions. In this chapter, we describe the effects of leptin on innate/adaptive immunity and angiogenesis and speculate on the possible modulation of the leptin axis in novel therapeutic settings.

Key words: Leptin, T cells, endothelial cells, inflammation, immunity, autoimmunity

1. INTRODUCTION

Leptin, a hormone mainly secreted by adipocytes, belongs to the helical cytokine family; its plasma concentrations correlate with fat mass and respond to changes in energy balance. This molecule, that is encoded by the *obese* (*ob*) gene localized on human and mouse 7 and 6 chromosomes, respectively, is a 16-kDa non-glycosylated protein[1]. Structurally, leptin belongs to the type I cytokine family and is characterized by a long-chain four-helical bundle structure, such as growth hormone (GH), prolactin (PRL), erythropoietin (EPO), interleukin (IL)-3, IL-11, leukemia inhibitory factor

(LIF), ciliary neurotrophic factor (CNTF), IL-12, oncostatin M (OSM) and granulocyte-colony stimulating factor (G-CSF)[2]. Initially, leptin was considered as an anti-obesity hormone, but experimental evidence has also shown pleiotropic effects of this molecule on hematopoiesis[3], angiogenesis, lymphoid organs homeostasis and T lymphocyte functions[4]. More specifically, leptin links the pro-inflammatory T helper (Th1) immune response to nutritional status and energy balance. Indeed, decreased leptin concentrations during conditions of food deprivation lead to impaired immune capabilities. This chapter focuses on the potential therapeutic utilities for agents that manipulate the leptin-adipocyte axis and discusses the role of leptin on inflammation, immunity and angiogenesis.

2. DISTRIBUTION AND INTRACELLULAR SIGNALING OF THE LEPTIN RECEPTOR ON IMMUNE CELLS

The leptin receptor (Ob-R) is encoded by the *diabetes* (*db*) gene, that was first cloned from mouse choroid plexus[5]. The Ob-R mRNA is alternatively spliced giving rise to six different spliced forms of the receptor known as Ob-Ra, Ob-Rb, Ob-Rc, Ob-Rd, Ob-Re and Ob-Rf. Ob-R is a member of the class I cytokine receptor family, which includes receptor for IL-6, LIF, G-CSF and gp120 with predominantly hematopoietic expression. The different mRNA spliced forms encode for ObR with different length cytoplasmic domains: Ob-Rb, also known as the long receptor isoform, has 302 cytoplasmic residues containing the activation and the signal transduction motifs; the other forms with a 34-amino acid residue cytoplasmic domain and the soluble one (Ob-Re) lack some or all of these motifs[6]. The short forms of the leptin receptor are expressed in several tissues, where presumably they mediate leptin transport into the brain and its degradation. Ob-Rb is primarily expressed at high levels in hypothalamus, especially in the arcuate, dorsomedial, ventromedial and lateral hypothalamic nuclei, that secrete neuropeptides and neurotransmitters involved in the regulation of appetite and body weight. Furthermore, the long isoform is expressed in murine and human fetal liver, jejunal epithelium, pancreatic ß cells, ovarian follicular cells, vascular endothelial cells, CD34 hematopoietic bone marrow precursors and T lymphocytes.

Lord and colleagues[4] demonstrated that leptin may amplify CD4 T cell responses and Ob-Rb RNA expression has been detected in human CD4 T lymphocytes; in addition, human monocytes, which have been shown to be activated by high-dose leptin, also express Ob-Rb. Martin-Romero *et al.*[7] demonstrated Ob-Rb expression not only on CD4 but also on CD8 human T cells. More recently, in a mouse model of colitis, Siegmund et al.[8] demonstrated the expression of Ob-Rb on T cells which mediate the regulation of immune responses. Finally, Zhao and colleagues[9] reported constitutive expression of both long and short Ob-R forms on human natural killer (NK) cells, which mediate regulation of NK cytotoxicity.

In lymphoid cells, leptin binding to Ob-Rb activates JAK (Janus kinases) and STAT (signal transducers and activators of transcription) proteins as the other members of the class I cytokine receptor family. All the four membrane-bound leptin receptors contain in the cytoplasmic tail a box 1 motif, strongly conserved within most members of this receptor family, whereas a box 2 motif is found only in the long isoform. These two domains are involved in the interaction and activation of JAK2 tyrosine kinase, that phosphorylates and activates members of STAT family, as STAT1, STAT5 and STAT3. Activated JAK2 then phosphorylates phosphotyrosine residues in the intracellular domain of Ob-Rb, providing binding motifs for SHP-2 and STAT proteins. The latter, after tyrosine-phosphorylation in response to JAK activation, translocate to the nucleus where they activate gene transcription. In particular, leptin modulates the expression of STAT3-dependent target genes, which include c-fos, c-jun, suppressor of cytokine signaling (SOCS-3)[10]. Furthermore, *in vitro* and *in vivo* studies show that Ob-Rb can stimulate SH protein tyrosine phosphatase-2 (SHP-2)-dependent ERK1/2 activation, tyrosine phosphorylation of Insulin Receptor Substrate-1 (IRS-1) and Phosphatidylinositol 3-Kinase (PI3-kinase) activity[11].

3. LEPTIN IN IMMUNE RESPONSE AND INFLAMMATION: INFECTION SUSCEPTIBILITY *VERSUS* AUTOIMMUNITY

Over the last few years experimental evidence has shown the effect of leptin not only on neuroendocrine and metabolic functions, but also on several systems such as the acute phase response, bone marrow function, and the natural and adaptive immune response (Figure 1). Recent reports have shown that deficiency of leptin is responsible for the immunosuppression and thymic atrophy observed during acute starvation and undernutrition. As previously mentioned, leptin has great structural similarities with molecules produced by the immune system such as cytokines. Following nutritional deprivation, leptin blood levels fall due to reduction in body fat, causing impairment of the immune function. Therefore, leptin seems to be one of the major players in the immunoendocrine *scenario* regulating the correlation among nutritional status, basal metabolism and immune function.

On innate immunity, leptin modulates the activity and the function of neutrophils by increasing chemotaxis and the secretion of oxygen radicals (such as hydrogen peroxide, H_2O_2, and superoxide, O_2^-), through direct and indirect mechanisms[12]. In mice, leptin seems to activate neutrophils directly, while in humans (Figure1) the action of leptin seems to be mediated by Tumour Necrosis Factor (TNF) secreted by monocytes[13]. Moreover, leptin increases phagocytosis by monocytes/macrophages, enhances the secretion of pro-inflammatory mediators of the acute-phase response and the expression of adhesion molecules[14]. On NK cells, leptin increases cytotoxic ability through the secretion of perforin and IL-2[15] (Figure 1).

The effects of leptin on adaptive immune responses have been extensively investigated on human CD4 T cells (Figure 1). Addition of physiological concentrations of leptin to a Mixed Lymphocyte Reaction (MLR) induces a dose-dependent increase in CD4 T-cell proliferation[4]. However, leptin has different effects on proliferation and cytokine production by human naive (CD45RA) and memory (CD45RO) CD4 T cells (both of which express Ob-Rb). Leptin promotes proliferation and IL-2 secretion by naive T cells, through the activation of mitogen-activated protein kinase (MAPK) and PI3-K pathways. On memory T cells, instead, leptin promotes the switch towards Th1-cell immune responses by increasing interferon-γ (IFN-γ) and TNF secretion, IgG2a production by B cells and promoting delayed-type hypersensitivity (DTH) responses. This process is then sustained by an autocrine loop of leptin secretion by Th1 cells. Furthermore, leptin increases the expression of adhesion molecules, such as intercellular adhesion molecule1 (ICAM1, CD54) and very late antigen 2 (VLA2, CD49B), by CD4 T cells, possibly through the induction of pro-inflammatory cytokines such as IFNγ[4]. Increased expression of adhesion molecules could then be responsible for the induction of clustering, activation and migration of immune cells to sites of inflammation. Recent evidences indicate that leptin also affects the generation, maturation and survival of thymic T cells by reducing their rate of apoptosis[16,17].

Another important role of leptin in adaptive immunity is highlighted by the observation that leptin deficiency in *ob/ob* mice is associated with immunosuppression and thymic atrophy, a finding similar to that observed in acute starvation[4]. Furthermore, *ob/ob* and *db/db* (leptin receptor deficient) animals have long been described as models of obesity, hyperphagia and hyperinsulinemia. Interestingly, naturally leptin-deficient obese *ob/ob* mice display many abnormalities similar to those observed in starved animals and malnourished humans, including impaired CD4 T lymphocyte functions. More specifically, chronic leptin deficiency in these animals determined reduced secretion, upon antigen specific stimulation, of the classical Th1-type pro-inflammatory cytokines such as IL-2, IFN-γ, IL-18, TNF-α and an increased production of IL-4, typical of the Th2 regulatory phenotype[4]. Usually, Th1 and Th2 CD4 helper T lymphocytes cross-regulate one another because their respective cytokines act antagonistically. IFNγ and IL-18 are typically secreted during inflammation and cell-mediated immunity. They determine Th1 differentiation of CD4 naive T cells; conversely, IL-4 causes Th2 differentiation and inhibits the generation of IFNγ-secreting cells.

Regarding the effect of leptin on lymphoid tissue homeostasis, it has been shown that it participates in the mainteinance of thymic maturation of double-positive CD4 CD8 cells and in the prevention of glucocorticoid-induced apoptosis of thymocytes. Indeed, leptin deficient *ob/ob* or wild type starved mice show reduction in thymic size particularly affecting the cortex of this organ where the majority of double positive cells are present. Leptin replacement in *ob/ob* and starved wild type animals restores a normal thymic fuctionality increasing the number on double positive T cells and reducing the thymic apoptosis rate[16]. *Ob/ob* mice display also reduced numbers of mature CD4 and not of CD8 T cells in the periphery mainly for the altered anatomical structure of lymph nodes (adipose-metaplasia) together with reduced thymic output.

4. LEPTIN AND AUTOIMMUNITY

Current evidence from the literature suggests that leptin is involved in autoimmune disease susceptibility. As mentioned earlier, *ob/ob* mice have several abnormalities that are common to starved animals[18]. However, *ob/ob* (and *db/db*) mice also have additional endocrine and metabolic disturbances that could affect the immune system[18].

More importantly, *ob/ob* mice have reduced secretion of IL-2, IFNγ, TNF and IL-18 and increased production of Th2-type cytokines, such as IL-4 and IL-10, after mitogenic stimulation[4,19,20]. As a result, they are resistant to the induction of several experimentally induced autoimmune diseases. For example, in Antigen-Induced Arthritis (AIA)[20], *ob/ob* mice have less severe joint inflammation, reduced T cell proliferation, lower concentrations of antibodies specific for the inducing antigen methylated bovine serum albumin, reduced expression of Th1-type cytokines and a bias towards the production of Th2-type cytokines.

Ob/ob mice are also protected from Experimental Autoimmune Encephalomyelitis (EAE)[21,22], whereas administration of leptin to susceptible wild-type mice worsens EAE by increasing the secretion of pro-inflammatory cytokines and directly correlates with pathogenic T cell autoreactivity[21,22]. Notably, leptin is expressed by T cells and macrophages in both the lymph nodes and active inflammatory lesions of the CNS during acute and relapsing EAE, but not during remission[22]. Finally, increased leptin expression has recently been described in active inflammatory lesions of the CNS in patients with multiple sclerosis (MS)[23] and in the serum of patients with MS before relapses after treatment with IFNβ[24].

Protection of *ob/ob* mice from autoimmune damage is also observed in Experimentally Induced Hepatitis (EIH)[19], in which leptin deficiency protects against the T-cell-mediated liver damage induced by administration of concanavalin A (ConA) or *Pseudomonas aeruginosa* exotoxin A. Also in this case, leptin administration restores responsiveness of these mice to ConA. Of note, the liver of *ob/ob* mice with EIH shows reduced production of TNF, IFNγ and IL-18.

Finally, *ob/ob* mice are resistant to acute and chronic intestinal inflammation induced by dextran sodium sulphate and to colitis induced by trinitrobenzene sulphonic acid (Experimentally Induced Colitis, EIC)[25]. In acute EIC, these mice do not develop intestinal inflammation and show decreased secretion of pro-inflammatory cytokines and chemokines. As expected, leptin replacement increases cytokine production to the levels observed in control mice[25]. Similarly, in chronic colitis, *ob/ob* mice have decreased secretion of pro-inflammatory cytokines, such as TNF, IFNγ, IL-1β, IL-6 and IL-18, and reduced production of chemokines, such as CXC-chemokine ligand 2 (CXCL2; macrophage inflammatory protein 2, MIP2) and CC-chemokine ligand 3 (CCL3; macrophage inflammatory protein 1α, MIP1α)[25]. Of interest, recent reports have shown that leptin secreted by the gastric mucosa is not completely degraded by proteolysis and can therefore reach the intestine in an active form, where it can control the expression of sodium/glucose and peptide transporters on intestinal epithelial cells. As a result, leptin might have a dual nature: on the one hand, leptin could function as a growth factor for the intestine, because of its involvement in the absorption of carbohydrates and proteins; on the other hand, leptin could function as a mediator of intestinal inflammation[25].

Most recently, protection from autoimmunity in *ob/ob* mice has been observed in experimentally induced glomerulonephritis[26]. In this immune-complex-mediated inflammatory disease, induced by the injection of sheep antibodies specific for mouse glomerular basement membrane into mice pre-immunized against sheep IgG, Tarzi *et al.*[26] have observed renal protection of *ob/ob* mice associated with reduced glomerular-crescent formation and reduced macrophage infiltration. These protective effects were associated with concomitant defects of both adaptive and innate immune responses (testified by reduced *in vitro* proliferation of splenic T cells and reduced humoral responses to sheep IgG, respectively). In spite of this trend, in one experiment, *ob/ob* mice showed normal humoral responses (compared to wild-type mice) and one out of six mice developed histological injury. Tarzi *et al.* hypothesized that defective innate effector responses were present in *ob/ob* mice, in line with *in vitro* experiments that have indicated defective phagocytosis and cytokine production in *ob/ob* mice[26].

All these studies concern a role for leptin in experimentally induced autoimmunity. However, leptin is also important in spontaneous autoimmune diabetes in non-obese diabetic (NOD) mice[27]. Female NOD mice have increased levels of serum leptin before the development of disease, and administration of exogenous leptin accelerates the onset and progression of disease by promoting insulitis and local production of IFNγ[27]. Of interest, IL-2-deficient mice, which develop spontaneous Inflammatory Bowel Disease (IBD), have increased levels of pro-inflammatory cytokines, including leptin, after food deprivation. Incidentally, in this case, the increase in leptin concentration seems to depend on the secretion of TNF[28]. Taken together, the data in NOD mice and IL-2-deficient mice indicate that the production of leptin can be favoured and/or sustained by ongoing inflammation[28].

Another indication that leptin could be involved in autoimmunity is the sexual dimorphism of serum leptin concentration (higher in females than in males matched for age and body mass index). In this sense, leptin could add to the list of hormones, such as oestradiol and prolactin, that have long been known to have a role in favouring the predisposition of females to the development of autoimmunity[29]. In particular, only hyperleptinaemic female mice develop autoimmunity, whereas hypoleptinaemic mice are protected, and treatment of EAE-resistant SJL/J males with recombinant leptin renders them susceptible to EAE[29].

All this evidence indicates that alterations in leptin levels and in its responsiveness are important issues to be taken in account in the study of the pathogenesis of a number of autoimmune diseases. These close interactions among leptin, cytokines, lymphocytes, and nutritional status may help to better understand the regulation of the immune and inflammatory response and to promote novel and safe therapeutic immune interventions.

5. LEPTIN AND ANGIOGENESIS: A NOVEL LINK AMONG INFLAMMATION, ENDOTHELIAL CELLS AND CANCER?

Angiogenesis is a process involving several cell types and mediators, which interact to establish a specific microenvironment suitable for the formation of new blood vessels by capillary sprouting from pre-existing vessels. It occurs in several physiological and pathological conditions, such as embryo development and wound healing, diabetic retinopathy and tumours[30]. Inflammatory cells fully participate in the angiogenic process by secreting cytokines that may affect endothelial cell (EC) functions, including EC proliferation, migration and activation.

Angiogenesis is the result of a net balance between the activities exerted by positive regulators, including Vascular Endothelial Growth Factor (VEGF), fibroblast growth factor (FGF), and negative antiangiogenic factors such as endostatin and angiostatin[31]. With regard to inflammatory cells and endothelium cross-talk, such balance is conceptually very similar to that of pro-inflammatory and anti-inflammatory mediators that modulate an appropriate inflammatory response.

Obesity is characterized by an excess of fat mass as a consequence of adipocyte hypertrophy and hyperplasia. The excessive growth of adipose tissue requires the formation of new capillaries for proper function. Because the development of the vascular bed in adipose tissue is tightly connected to both number and size of adipocytes and adipose tissue serves as an important conduit for growing blood vessels, it is conceivable that adipocytes may modulate the growth of the vasculature in a paracrine manner.

Several reports have shown that adipocytes are not only sites of energy storage but also are important sources of cytokines such as IL-1 and TNFα, growth factors such as VEGF, and hormones such as leptin. The expression and the plasma concentration of leptin were found to be markedly increased in human obesity and positively correlated to body fat mass[4]. Because leptin is secreted into the plasma, endothelial cells could be exposed to much higher concentrations of this hormone than other cell types; so, it is tempting to speculate that the leptin-mediated cross-talk between adipocytes and endothelial cells promotes angiogenesis, which in turn participates in the additional increment of the adipose mass[34].

Proliferation of endothelial cells constitutes one key event in the complex angiogenic process[31]. Angiogenesis starts by cell-mediated degradation of the basement membrane, followed by the migration and the proliferation of endothelial cells[34]. The morphogenesis of the cells into capillary tubes finishes this process. Using two different *in vitro* models of angiogenesis (ie, endothelial cell–coated microcarrier-induced and monolayer-induced formation of capillary-like tubes in fibrin gels), Bouloumié *et al.*[34] demonstrated that leptin promotes endothelial cell survival and proliferation *in vitro* (Figure 1). Moreover, *in vivo* angiogenic assay using chicken chorioallantoic membrane assay (CAMs) showed clearly that leptin enhanced the formation of new blood vessels. Uckaya *et al.*[35] also found that patients suffering from diabetic retinopathy (an angiogenic disease) had higher plasma leptin levels the more advanced the retinopathy[35].

The angiogenic process does not occur only in physiological conditions but plays a key role for tumor growth and progression. Today it is widely accepted that vessel growth, induced by tumor cells through the release of angiogenic factors (basic-fibroblast growth factor and vascular endothelial growt factor), leads to hypervascularization of tumor tissue[36]. On the other hand, it has been demonstrated that tumors also induce angiogenesis through the down regulation or inhibition of endogenous angiogenic inhibitors (thrombospondin-1)[37].

Leptin, as an angiogenic factor, is not well investigated in tumor angiogenesis. However, Bertolini *et al.*[38] had shown no significant differences of circulating leptin levels between patients with non-Hodgkin's lymphoma and the ones that had complete remission of the disease. Moreover, Tessitore et al.[39] found high plasma leptin levels in breast cancer patients, while in other cancers as colorectal and lung cancer, this correlation could not be seen. However, the interaction of leptin expression and tumor growth are not perfectly understood, but it is important to consider that stimulation and/or inhibition of angiogenesis is a local process not necessarily associated with elevated leptin serum levels.

Thus, this experimental evidence demonstrates that leptin could be a potent modulator of the angiogenic process. This opens a promising perspective concerning future investigations of leptin-dependent angiogenesis modulation both in physiological and pathological conditions.

6. POSSIBLE THERAPEUTIC RELEVANCE OF LEPTIN

Leptin-based therapies are currently applied to only a few cases of genetically leptin-deficient individuals or in extremely obese non-leptin-deficient patients. These treatments are effective in reducing food intake and obesity and in restoring some of the impaired neuroendocrine functions of genetically leptin-deficient individuals such as the reproductive function. While leptin-deficient patients display great peripheral and central sensitivity to leptin (due to Ob-Rb upregulation on the cell surface), non-leptin-deficient obese patients only benefit of modest effects from leptin administration probably secondary to Ob-Rb desensitization caused by the high circulating leptin levels.

Despite the limited use of leptin, new clinical applications can be envisaged particularly because of the immunoregulatory properties of leptin on the CD4 T cells. For example, in HIV-1 infection, serum leptin is dramatically reduced. Leptin administration could enhance immunoreconstitution of CD4 T cell numbers and functions in these patients because of its effects on thymic output of T cells and cell-mediated Th1 responses. Indeed, immunization of experimental animals in the absence of leptin or in the presence of reduced leptin concentration leads to decreased DTH response and to a switch towards a Th2-cytokine profile; as a consequence, administration of leptin restores DTH as well as Th1 response. For the same reasons, the potentiation of this response could also be useful in the treatment of resistant tuberculosis (TB) in immunocompromised hosts and/or as an adjuvant also in vaccination protocols of normal individuals.

Proinflammatory cytokines such as IL-1, IL-6, IL-12, IFNγ and TNFα play an important role in the pathogenesis of several animal and human autoimmune diseases; *in vivo* neutralization of these cytokines often ameliorates clinical score and delays progression of the disease. For example, administration of anti-IL-12 blocking monoclonal antibodies to mice reduced clinical score, demyelinization and paralysis in EAE and pancreatic β-cell damage in IDDM in NOD mice. A similar approach has also been used successfully with anti-TNFα antibodies in experimental autoimmune arthritis and it has in recent times become the gold-standard therapy for RA patients.

Modulation of circulating leptin levels may as well be suggested as a strategy to dampen pro-inflammatory responses. This approach could be attained *via* nutritional intervention such as caloric restriction, and/or immune intervention through the use of blocking anti-leptin antibodies, thus overcoming drug-related side effects. Interestingly, clinical trials involving starvation to modulate proinflammatory responses in human autoimmune diseases have already been reported to successfully improve disease activity and delay its progression. For example, in RA patients a week after caloric restriction, which associates with loss of body weight and reduced leptin levels, showed significant decrease of joint count, erythrocyte sedimentation rate, C-reactive protein level, lower CD4 and CD8 counts and decreased T cell activation accompanied by increased IL-4 secretion.

Reduced caloric restriction, alone or together with coadministration of soluble recombinant leptin-receptor (which reduces circulating levels of leptin upon binding), could well complement the treatment of certain autoimmune diseases. Thus, patients affected by autoimmune diseases could be treated with combined therapies considering nutritional regime, administration of n-3 PUFA and/or zinc free diets and eventual use of blocking anti-leptin antibodies, soluble leptin receptor or leptin receptor antagonists.

7. CONCLUDING REMARKS

Despite a series of important studies carried out recently, many cellular and molecular aspects of the role of leptin in immune homeostasis remain elusive. Nonetheless, particularly because of its dual role in nutrition and autoimmunity and its modulation by food intake, leptin could be a new immunotherapeutic target in conditions where leptin is thought to promote disease. For example, Steinman and colleagues[40] have suggested that the stress responses of acute starvation could prove beneficial in certain autoimmune conditions in which leptin promotes chronic inflammation. However, acute starvation and subsequent hypoleptinaemia would be detrimental during infection as they might result in suppression of immune responses.

Another unresolved issue is whether modulation of leptin might sufficiently impact immune processes alone or whether it would be necessary to complement it with other approaches to attain beneficial effects. Moreover, new studies will need to address the role of leptin in other aspects of the immune response that have not yet been investigated, such as immune regulation and tolerance, survival of autoreactive T cells and antigen-presenting cell function.

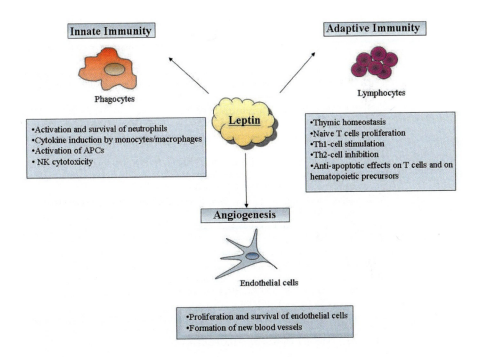

Figure 1. Immune and angiogenic actions of leptin

ACKNOWLEDGMENTS

The authors are supported by grants from Fondazione Italiana Sclerosi Multipla (n. 2002/R/55) and JDRF-Telethon (n. GJT04008).

REFERENCES

1. Y. Zhang, R. Proenca, M. Maffei, M. Barone, L. Leopold, and J. M. Friedman, Positional cloning of the mouse obese gene and its human homologue, *Nature* **372**(6505), 425-432 (1994).
2. F. Zhang, M. B. Basinski, J. M. Beals, S. L. Briggs, L. M. Churgay, D. K. Clawson, R. D. DiMarchi, T. C. Furman, J. E. Hale, H. M. Hsiung, B. E. Schoner, D. P. Smith, X. Y. Zhang, J. P. Wery, and R. W. Schevitz, Crystal structure of the obese protein leptin-E100, *Nature* **387**(6629), 206-209 (1997).
3. B. D. Bennett, G. P. Solar, J. Q. Yuan, J. Mathias, G. R. Thomas, and W. Matthews, A role for leptin and its cognate receptor in hematopoiesis, *Curr. Biol.* **6**(9), 1170-1180 (1996).
4. G. M. Lord, G. Matarese, J. K. Howard, R. J. Baker, S. R. Bloom, and R. I. Lechler, Leptin modulates the T-cell immune response and reverses starvation-induced immunosuppression, *Nature* **394**(6696), 897-901 (1998).
5. L. A. Tartaglia, The leptin receptor, *J. Biol. Chem.* **272**(10), 6093-6100 (1997).
6. L. A. Tartaglia, M. Dembski, X. Weng, N. Deng, J. Culpepper, R. Devos, G. J. Richards, L. A. Campfield, F. T. Clark, J. Deeds, C. Muir, S. Sanker, A. Moriarty, K. J. Moore, J. S. Smutko, G. G. Mays, E. A. Wool, C. A. Monroe, and R. I. Tepper, Identification and expression cloning of a leptin receptor, OB-R, *Cell.* **83**(7), 1263-1271 (1995).
7. C. Martin-Romero, J. Santos-Alvarez, R. Goberna, and V. Sanchez-Margalet, Human leptin enhances activation and proliferation of human circulating T lymphocytes, *Cell. Immunol.* **199**(1), 15-24 (2000).
8. B. Siegmund, J. A. Sennello, J. Jones-Carson, F. Gamboni-Robertson, H. A. Lehr, A. Batra, I. Fedke, M. Zeitz, and G. Fantuzzi, Leptin receptor expression on T lymphocytes modulates chronic intestinal inflammation in mice, *Gut* **53**(7), 965-972 (2004).
9. Y. Zhao, R. Sun, L. You, C. Gao, and Z. Tian, Expression of leptin receptors and response to leptin stimulation of human natural killer cell lines, *Biochem. Biophys. Res. Commun.* **300**(2), 247-252 (2003).
10. A. S. Banks, S. M. Davis, S. H. Bates, and M. G. Jr Myers, Activation of downstream signals by the long form of the leptin receptor, *J. Biol. Chem.* **275**(19), 14563-14572 (2000).
11. C. Bjorbaek, R. M. Buchholz, S. M. Davis, S. H. Bates, D. D. Pierroz, H. Gu, B. G. Neel, M. G. Jr Myers, and J. S. Flier, Divergent roles of SHP-2 in ERK activation by leptin receptors, *J. Biol. Chem.* **276**(7), 4747-4755 (2001).
12. F. Caldefie-Chezet, A. Poulin, and M. P. Vasson, Leptin regulates functional capacities of polymorphonuclear neutrophils, *Free Radic. Res.* **37**(8), 809-814 (2003).
13. H. Zarkesh-Esfahani, A. G. Pockley, Z. Wu, P. G. Hellewell, A. P. Weetman, and R. J. Ross, Leptin indirectly activates human neutrophils via induction of TNF-alpha, *J. Immunol.* **172**(3), 1809-1814 (2004).
14. H. Zarkesh-Esfahani, G. Pockley, R. A. Metcalfe, M. Bidlingmaier, Z. Wu, A. Ajami, A. P. Weetman, C. J. Strasburger, and R. J. Ross, High-dose leptin activates human leukocytes via receptor expression on monocytes, *J. Immunol.* **167**(8), 4593-4599 (2001).
15. Y. Zhao, R. Sun, L. You, C. Gao, and Z. Tian, Expression of leptin receptors and response to leptin stimulation of human natural killer cell lines, *Biochem. Biophys. Res. Commun.* **300**(2), 247-252 (2003).

16. J. K. Howard, G. M. Lord, G. Matarese, S. Vendetti, M. A. Ghatei, M. A. Ritter, R. I. Lechler, and S. R. Bloom, Leptin protects mice from starvation-induced lymphoid atrophy and increases thymic cellularity in ob/ob mice, *J. Clin. Invest.* **104**(8), 1051-1059 (1999).
17. G. M. Lord, G. Matarese, J. K. Howard, and R. I. Lechler, The bioenergetics of the immune system, *Science* **292**(5518), 855-856 (2001).
18. J. M. Friedman, and J. L. Halaas, Leptin and the regulation of body weight in mammals, *Nature*, **395**(6704), 763-770 (1998).
19. R. Faggioni, J. Jones-Carson, D. A. Reed, C. A. Dinarello, K. R. Feingold, C. Grunfeld, and G. Fantuzzi, Leptin-deficient (ob/ob) mice are protected from T cell-mediated hepatotoxicity: role of tumor necrosis factor alpha and IL-18, *Proc. Natl. Acad. Sci. U S A* **97**(5), 2367-2372 (2000).
20. N. Busso, A. So, V. Chobaz-Peclat, C. Morard, E. Martinez-Soria, D. Talabot-Ayer, and C. Gabay, Leptin signaling deficiency impairs humoral and cellular immune responses and attenuates experimental arthritis, *J. Immunol.* **168**(2), 875-882 (2002).
21. G. Matarese, A. Di Giacomo, V. Sanna, G. M. Lord, J. K. Howard, A. Di Tuoro, S. R. Bloom, R. I. Lechler, S. Zappacosta, and S. Fontana, Requirement for leptin in the induction and progression of autoimmune encephalomyelitis, *J. Immunol.* **166**(10), 5909-5916 (2001).
22. V. Sanna, A. Di Giacomo, A. La Cava, R. I. Lechler, S. Fontana, S. Zappacosta, and G. Matarese, Leptin surge precedes onset of autoimmune encephalomyelitis and correlates with development of pathogenic T cell responses, *J. Clin. Invest.* **111**(2), 241-250 (2003).
23. G. Matarese, P. B. Carrieri, A. La Cava, F. Perna, V. Sanna, V. De Rosa, D. Aufiero, S. Fontana, and S. Zappacosta, Leptin increase in multiple sclerosis associates with reduced number of CD4(+)CD25+ regulatory T cells, *Proc. Natl. Acad. Sci. U S A* **102**(14), 5150-5155 (2005).
24. A. P. Batocchi, M. Rotondi, M. Caggiula, G. Frisullo, F. Odoardi, V. Nociti, C. Carella, P. A. Tonali, and M. Mirabella, Leptin as a marker of multiple sclerosis activity in patients treated with interferon-beta, *J. Neuroimmunol.* **139**(1-2), 150-154 (2003).
25. B. Siegmund, H. A. Lehr, and G. Fantuzzi, Leptin: a pivotal mediator of intestinal inflammation in mice, *Gastroenterology* **122**(7), 2011-2025 (2002).
26. R. M. Tarzi, H. T. Cook, I. Jackson, C. D. Pusey, and G. M. Lord, Leptin-deficient mice are protected from accelerated nephrotoxic nephritis, *Am. J. Pathol.* **164**(2), 385-390 (2004).
27. G. Matarese, V. Sanna, R. I. Lechler, N. Sarvetnick, S. Fontana, S. Zappacosta, and A. La Cava, Leptin accelerates autoimmune diabetes in female NOD mice, *Diabetes* **51**(5), 1356-1361 (2002).
28. L. M. Gaetke, H. S. Oz, R. C. Frederich, and C. J. McClain, Anti-TNF-alpha antibody normalizes serum leptin in IL-2 deficient mice, *J. Am. Coll. Nutr.* **22**(5), 415-420 (2003).
29. G. Matarese, V. Sanna, A. Di Giacomo, G. M. Lord, J. K. Howard, S. R. Bloom, R. I. Lechler, S. Fontana, and S. Zappacosta, Leptin potentiates experimental autoimmune encephalomyelitis in SJL female mice and confers susceptibility to males, *Eur. J. Immunol.* **31**(5), 1324-1332 (2001).
30. M. Klagsbrun, and P. A. D'Amore, Regulators of angiogenesis, *Annu. Rev. Physiol.* **53**, 217-239 (1991).
31. J. Folkman, Angiogenesis and angiogenesis inhibition: an overview, *EXS.* **79**, 1-8 (1997)
32. P. Bjorntorp, Adipose tissue distribution and function, *Int. J. Obes.* **2**, 67-81 (1991).

33. Q. X. Zhang, C. J. Magovern, C. A. Mack, K. T. Budenbender, W. Ko, and T. K. Rosengart, Vascular endothelial growth factor is the major angiogenic factor in omentum: mechanism of the omentum-mediated angiogenesis, *J. Surg. Res.* **67**(2), 147-154 (1997).
34. A. Bouloumie, H. C. Drexler, M. Lafontan, and R. Busse R, Leptin, the product of Ob gene, promotes angiogenesis, *Circ. Res.* **83**(10), 1059-1066 (1998).
35. G. Uckaya, M. Ozata, Z. Bayraktar, V. Erten, N. Bingol, and I. C. Ozdemir, Is leptin associated with diabetic retinopathy? *Diabetes Care.* **23**(3), 371-376 (2000).
36. D. Hanahan, and R. A., Weinberg, The hallmarks of cancer, *Cell.* **100**(1), 57-70 (2000).
37. S. C. Campbell, O. V. Volpert, M. Ivanovich, and N. P. Bouck, Molecular mediators of angiogenesis in bladder cancer, *Cancer Res.* **58**(6), 1298-1304 (1998).
38. F. Bertolini, M. Paolucci, F. Peccatori, S. Cinieri, A. Agazzi, P. F. Ferrucci, E. Cocorocchio, A. Goldhirsch, and G. Martinelli, Angiogenic growth factors and endostatin in non-Hodgkin's lymphoma, *Br. J. Haematol.* **106**(2), 504-509 (1999).
39. L. Tessitore, B. Vizio, O. Jenkins, I. De Stefano, C. Ritossa, J. M. Argiles, C. Benedetto, and A. Mussa, Leptin expression in colorectal and breast cancer patients, *Int. J. Mol. Med.* **5**(4), 421-426 (2000).
40. L. Steinman, P. Conlon, R. Maki,, and A. Foster, The intricate interplay among body weight, stress, and the immune response to friend or foe, *J. Clin. Invest.* **111**(2), 183-185 (2003).

Chapter 8

LEPTIN AND BONE
Central control of bone metabolism by leptin

Shu Takeda
Department of Orthopedics and 21COE, Tokyo Medical and Dental University, Tokyo, Japan

Abstract: Leptin, following the binding to ObRb in the hypothalamus, affects bone formation and resorption through multiple pathways. Through the sympathetic nervous system, leptin inhibits bone formation via CREB, AP-1 and the molecular clock, while stimulates bone resorption via ATF4. Moreover, leptin also inhibits bone resorption via CART through an unidentified mechanism.

Key words: bone formation, bone resorption, hypothalamus, sympathetic nervous system, β blocker, cocaine- and amphetamine-regulated transcript

1. INTRODUCTION

With the increase in longevity, osteoporosis is now emerging as a major concern for public health, since it is the most common degenerative bone disease in the developed world[1]. Osteoporosis is caused by an imbalance between bone formation and bone resorption[2]. Clinically, the most frequent cause for osteoporosis is menopause, on the other hand, obese individuals are relatively protected from the development of osteoporosis[2]. These observations suggest that there may be a link between fat mass and bone mass. Furthermore, as osteoblasts and adipocytes originate from the same mesenchymal progenitor cells[3], many investigators searched for molecules linking fat and bone biology. Recently, our laboratory discovered the existence of hypothalamic control of bone remodeling[4], a discovery that was confirmed subsequently by others. Leptin regulates bone formation and resorption via the hypothalamus and sympathetic nervous system[5]. Considering that most of leptin's physiological actions are mediated by the hypothalamus[6], the notion that central control of bone metabolism by leptin seems to be quite reasonable. However, leptin has been shown to directly affect cells localized in bone in some reports. Before discussing the central nature of leptin in bone metabolism, I would like to summarize leptin's local effect on bone.

2. LOCAL ACTION OF LEPTIN ON BONE CELL

Leptin is not only produced by visceral or subcutaneous adipocytes, but from bone marrow adipocytes[7]. Several reports indicate that leptin affects bone cells locally. Leptin functional receptors *ObRb* are expressed in osteoblasts[8,9], osteoclasts and chondrocytes[10,11], cells indispensable for bone modeling and remodeling. Interestingly, osteoblasts produce and secrete leptin[8], suggesting the autocrine nature of leptin in bone remodeling. Moreover, exogenous leptin increased osteoblastic differentiation or mineralization[8,9,12] in vitro, thus demonstrating an anabolic action on bone metabolism. On the contrary, others reported that leptin induced apoptosis of bone marrow stromal cells [13]. Those direct effects of leptin were not confined to osteoblasts. Namely, leptin inhibited osteoclast differentiation[14] or stimulated chondrocyte proliferation[11]. In vivo, intraperitoneal treatment of leptin stimulated bone growth of *ob/ob* mice[15] and reduced ovariectomy-induced bone loss[16]. These results suggest that leptin affects bone cells in local microenvironment. However, leptin overexpression in bone using bone-specific a1(I) collagen promoter does not affect bone metabolism in vivo[5]. The reason for this discrepancy can be partly explained by the fact that most in vitro studies were performed using supraphysiological amounts of leptin. Taken together, it is indicated that the primary action of leptin in vivo is not mediated by direct action on bone cells.

3. EFFECT OF LEPTIN ON BONE FORMATION THROUGH CENTRAL NERVOUS SYSTEM

Since most of the physiological condition are under control of the central nervous system, especially hypothalamus, one may hypothesize that bone remodeling does not escape this rule. As a molecule explaining the bone sparing effect of obesity, we focused on leptin, which many known actions result following its binding to specific receptors on hypothalamic neurons and whose deficiency causes morbid obesity. Mouse models of leptin deficiency (*ob/ob*) and leptin receptor-deficiency (*db/db*) demonstrated a marked high bone mass phenotype[4]. This was quite unexpected, since there is no other mouse model in which hypogonadism and high bone mass phenotypes co-exist. Subsequent studies of the ob/ob mice showed an increased bone formation and resorption, suggesting that high bone mass is due to enhanced bone formation. Intracerebroventricular infusion of leptin results in bone loss in ob/ob mice and wild-type mice without raising serum concentration of leptin, thus established antiosteogenic function of leptin via the hypothalamus[4] (Figure 1).

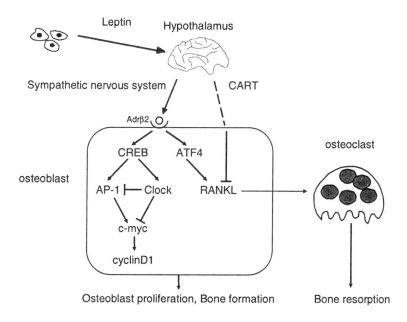

Figure 1. Model of central control of bone metabolism by leptin.

Leptin inhibits osteoblast proliferation via sympathetic nervous system. CREB, AP-1 and Clock are involved in this regulation. Leptin also affects bone resorption through osteoclast differentiation factor RANKL.

The melanocortin pathway has a crucial role in leptin's regulation of food intake[6]. However, genetic (Agouti yellow mice and melanocortin 4 receptor-deficient mice) or pharmacological (MC4R agonist) manipulation of melanocortin pathway did not affect the antiosteogenic i.e. inhibition of bone formation action of leptin[5], suggesting that pathways regulating antiosteogenic and anorexigenic function of leptin are different. In the diverse phenotypic abnormality observed in ob/ob mice, low tonus of sympathetic abnormality caught our attention. Namely, we tested if leptin's antiosteogenic function is mediated via sympathetic nervous system. Indeed, dopamine-β-hydroxylase (DBH)-deficient mice, which are unable to synthesize catecholamines and mice treated with non-selective β blocker (propranolol) displayed the same high bone mass phenotype than ob/ob mice, Moreover, the fact that icv infusion of leptin decreased body weight in DBH-deficient mice or propranolol-treated mice, but not their bone mass, demonstrated the essential role of sympathetic nervous system in antiosteogenic action of leptin[5] not in its control of body weight (Figure 1). This observation raises the prospect that blockade of the sympathetic nervous system could be potentially a novel therapy for osteoporosis.

Subsequent analysis of mice lacking the adrenergic β2receptor, the only adrenergic receptor expressed in osteoblasts, revealed high bone mass phenotype accompanied by an increase in bone formation[17], as expected. More recently, circadian genes were discovered to act as downstream signaling molecules of sympathetic signaling in osteoblasts[18]. Indeed, mice lacking molecular clock components displayed high bone mass and showed a paradoxical increase in bone formation following leptin icv infusion. In osteoblasts, leptin and sympathetic nervous system induced clock genes expression, which antagonizes AP-1 family-mediated osteoblast proliferation. Thus, the molecular mechanism of leptin's antiosteogenic action partly, if not all, is now being clarified[18](ure 1).

4. CENTRAL EFFECT ON OSTEOCLASTS BY LEPTIN AND SNS

Surprisingly, adrb2-deficient mice developed another bone phenotype, which is a decrease in bone resorption[17]. Leptin icv infusion caused an increase in bone resorption in wild-type mice, but not in adrb2-deficient mice, demonstrating that leptin increases bone resorption via the sympathetic nervous system. Isoproterenol, a β receptor agonist, favored osteoclastic bone resorption by inducing the expression of the osteoclast differentiation factor RANKL in osteoblasts while no effect of sympathetic signaling on osteoclasts could be found. This effect of sympathetic signaling on RANKL expression required the osteoblast specific transcription factor ATF4 phosphorylation by PKA. Importantly, adrb2-deficent mice are protected from gonadectomy-induced bone loss, indicating that sympathetic nervous system is indispensable for the development of postmenopausal osteoporosis. These results demonstrated that leptin regulates both axis of bone remodeling centrally[17] and gave further importance to this regulation since very few molecules regulate both aspects of bone remodeling (Fig. 1).

5. CENTRAL EFFECT ON OSTEOCLASTS BY CART

The increase in bone resorption observed in ob/ob mice was interpreted to be secondary to hypogonadism initially. However, the dissociation of bone resorption status in ovariectomized-b2adr-deficient mice and ob/ob mice argued against that. Namely, though both mutant mouse strains display a hypogonadism and a decrease in sympathetic tone, the former model displayed normal bone resorption, while the latter showed increased bone resorption. These results suggested that the action of leptin on bone resorption is not solely dependent on sympathetic nervous system and led to the identification of CART as another molecule implicated in leptin's action on bone resorption[17]. CART is a gene whose expression is regulated by leptin and is nearly absent in ob/ob mice that was thought to be anorectic[19]. However, CART-deficient mice have a normal food intake, are lean on normal diet[20]. In contrast, CART-deficient mice are osteopenic due to an isolated increase in osteoclastic resorption[17]. Leptin icv caused a further reduction of bone loss compared to wild type animal, suggesting that CART mediates leptin's action modulating bone resorption. In addition, high bone mass phenotype observed in MC4R-deficient mice and human patients can be explained by their increase in CART expression. Taken together these data establish that, leptin regulates bone resorption centrally, through two different pathways, sympathetic nervous system-ATF4-RANKL and CART[17].

6. LEPTIN, β BLOCKERS AND OSTEOPOROSIS IN CLINICAL MEDICINE

Clinically, the association of serum leptin concentration and bone mass or bone metabolic markers are under intensive investigation. However, results of various studies are conflicting. Some reports showing no correlation between serum leptin level and bone metabolic markers in postmenopausal women[21,22], while positive correlation was observed between serum leptin level and bone mass in women[23-25]. On the contrary, studies including adult men show that serum leptin level was inversely correlated with bone formation markers and bone mineral density[26] or bone mineral density[27]. These results might suggest a gender specific effect of leptin in bone metabolism. However, more importantly, the association of leptin and other parameters are lost or diminished after adjusting body weight in most studies. It is well accepted that obesity leads to leptin-resistance, as hyperinsulinemia does in type2 diabetes patients. This is best demonstrated by the fact that serum leptin concentration and body weight is positively correlated[28]. Given the fact that a clinical marker reflecting leptin's action in vivo is not available, studies exploring leptin and bone mineral density in human beings need to be carefully interpreted.

A few studies were conducted to address if leptin treatment affects bone mass in human patients. Farroqi et. al. reported the decrease of bone mineral density after leptin replacement therapy to a single leptin-deficient patient[29]. It has also been shown that leptin supplementation to 2 lipodystrophic patients did not affect bone mass[30]. Clearly, larger clinical trials are necessary to address the role of leptin on bone metabolism in human beings. Although the most interesting aspect of this regulation is the involvement of a sympathetic tone which is more amenable to therapeutic manipulations.

Since blockade of sympathetic regulation of bone remodeling increases bone mass in mouse, clinical researchers examined if a β blocker, a most commonly prescribed drug, may be beneficial for bone metabolism in human. Some prospective studies reported the lack of association between β blocker usage and bone density[31,32], while two large cohort studies found almost 30% reduction of bone fracture by propranolol[33,34]. Recently, a randomized trial assessing the effect of propranolol on bone metabolic markers reported no beneficial effect of a β blocker. However, considering that this study was conducted in a relatively short period with a small number of patients a larger randomized study is warranted.

7. CONCLUSION

Leptin has become, in relatively few years, a major regulator of bone metabolism, whose mode of action has been largely elucidated[35]. Recently, various neuropeptides and their receptors, such as NPY[36], MCH[37] and cannabinoid [38], were identified as regulator of bone metabolism, thus our understanding of central control of bone metabolism is expanding. However, several questions remain to be elucidated. One is obviously the molecular mechanism how CART affects bone resorption. In addition, there may be some other molecules mediating leptin-dependent sympathetic regulation of bone formation. From the clinical point of view, modulating leptin and its downstream pathway, especially bone-specific β blockers, is a potential therapeutic target for the treatment of osteoporosis.

ACKNOWLEDGEMENTS

I thank Gerard Karsenty for critical reading of the manuscript. This work was supported in part by grants from Ministry of Education, Culture, Sports, Science, Japan, grants from Center of Excellence Program for Frontier Research on Molecular Destruction and Reconstruction of Tooth and Bone, Japan Society for Promotion of Science, Tokyo, grants from Ono Medical Research Foundation, and grants from Kanae Foundation for Life and Socio-Medical Science.

REFERENCES

1. C. Cooper & L. J. I. Melton. in *Osteoporosis* (eds. R. Marcus, D. Feldman & J. Kelsey) 419-434 (Academic Press, San Diego, 1996).
2. B. L. Riggs, S. Khosla & L. J. Melton, 3rd. A unitary model for involutional osteoporosis: estrogen deficiency causes both type I and type II osteoporosis in postmenopausal women and contributes to bone loss in aging men. *J Bone Miner Res*, **13**, (5), 763-773. (1998).
3. D. J. Prockop. Marrow stromal cells as stem cells for nonhematopoietic tissues. *Science*, **276**, (5309), 71-4 (1997).
4. P. Ducy, M. Amling, S. Takeda, M. Priemel, A. F. Schilling, T. Beil, J. Shen, C. Vincon, J. M. Rueger & G. Karsenty. Leptin inhibits bone formation through a hypothalamic relay: A central control of bone mass. *Cell*, **100**, 197-207 (2000).
5. S. Takeda, F. Elefteriou, R. Levasseur, X. Liu, L. Zhao, K. L. Parker, D. Armstrong, P. Ducy & G. Karsenty. Leptin regulates bone formation via the sympathetic nervous system. *Cell*, **111**, (3), 305-17 (2002).
6. R. S. Ahima & J. S. Flier. Leptin. *Annu Rev Physiol*, **62**, 413-437 (2000).
7. P. Laharrague, D. Larrouy, A. M. Fontanilles, N. Truel, A. Campfield, R. Tenenbaum, J. Galitzky, J. X. Corberand, L. Penicaud & L. Casteilla. High expression of leptin by human bone marrow adipocytes in primary culture. *Faseb J*, **12**, (9), 747-52 (1998).
8. J. E. Reseland, U. Syversen, I. Bakke, G. Qvigstad, L. G. Eide, O. Hjertner, J. O. Gordeladze & C. A. Drevon. Leptin is expressed in and secreted from primary cultures of human osteoblasts and promotes bone mineralization. *J Bone Miner Res*, **16**, (8), 1426-33 (2001).
9. T. Thomas, F. Gori, S. Khosla, M. D. Jensen, B. Burguera & B. L. Riggs. Leptin acts on human marrow stromal cells to enhance differentiation to osteoblasts and to inhibit differentiation to adipocytes. *Endocrinology*, **140**, (4), 1630-8 (1999).
10. K. Kume, K. Satomura, S. Nishisho, E. Kitaoka, K. Yamanouchi, S. Tobiume & M. Nagayama. Potential Role of Leptin in Endochondral Ossification. *J. Histochem. Cytochem.*, **50**, (2), 159-170 (2002).
11. G. Maor, M. Rochwerger, Y. Segev & M. Phillip. Leptin acts as a growth factor on the chondrocytes of skeletal growth centers. *J Bone Miner Res*, **17**, (6), 1034-43 (2002).
12. Y. J. Lee, J. H. Park, S. K. Ju, K. H. You, J. S. Ko & H. M. Kim. Leptin receptor isoform expression in rat osteoblasts and their functional analysis. *FEBS Lett*, **528**, (1-3), 43-7 (2002).

13. G. S. Kim, J. S. Hong, S. W. Kim, J. M. Koh, C. S. An, J. Y. Choi & S. L. Cheng. Leptin induces apoptosis via ERK/cPLA2/cytochrome c pathway in human bone marrow stromal cells. *J Biol Chem*, **278,** (24), 21920-9 (2003).
14. W. R. Holloway, F. M. Collier, C. J. Aitken, D. E. Myers, J. M. Hodge, M. Malakellis, T. J. Gough, G. R. Collier & G. C. Nicholson. Leptin inhibits osteoclast generation. *J Bone Miner Res*, **17,** (2), 200-9 (2002).
15. C. Steppan, D. Crawford, K. Chidsey-Frink, H. Ke & A. Swick. Leptin is a potent stimulator of bone growth in ob/ob mice. *Regulatory Peptides*, **92,** (1-3), 73-78 (2000).
16. B. Burguera, L. C. Hofbauer, T. Thomas, F. Gori, G. L. Evans, S. Khosla, B. L. Riggs & R. T. Turner. Leptin reduces ovariectomy-induced bone loss in rats. *Endocrinology*, **142,** (8), 3546-53 (2001).
17. F. Elefteriou, J. D. Ahn, S. Takeda, M. Starbuck, X. Yang, X. Liu, H. Kondo, W. G. Richards, T. W. Bannon, M. Noda, K. Clement, C. Vaisse & G. Karsenty. Leptin regulation of bone resorption by the sympathetic nervous system and CART. *Nature*, **434,** (7032), 514-20 (2005).
18. L. Fu, M. S. Patel, A. Bradley, E. F. Wagner & G. Karsenty. The molecular clock mediates leptin-regulated bone formation. *Cell*, **122,** (5), 803-15 (2005).
19. J. K. Elmquist. Hypothalamic pathways underlying the endocrine, autonomic, and behavioral effects of leptin. *Int J Obes Relat Metab Disord*, **25 Suppl 5**, S78-82 (2001).
20. M. A. Asnicar, D. P. Smith, D. D. Yang, M. L. Heiman, N. Fox, Y. F. Chen, H. M. Hsiung & A. Koster. Absence of cocaine- and amphetamine-regulated transcript results in obesity in mice fed a high caloric diet. *Endocrinology*, **142,** (10), 4394-4400. (2001).
21. A. Goulding & R. W. Taylor. Plasma leptin values in relation to bone mass and density and to dynamic biochemical markers of bone resorption and formation in postmenopausal women. *Calcif Tissue Int*, **63,** (6), 456-8 (1998).
22. G. Martini, R. Valenti, S. Giovani, B. Franci, S. Campagna & R. Nuti. Influence of insulin-like growth factor-1 and leptin on bone mass in healthy postmenopausal women. *Bone*, **28,** (1), 113-7 (2001).
23. J. A. Pasco, M. J. Henry, M. A. Kotowicz, G. R. Collier, M. J. Ball, A. M. Ugoni & G. C. Nicholson. Serum Leptin Levels Are Associated with Bone Mass in Nonobese Women. *J Clin Endocrinol Metab*, **86,** (5), 1884-1887 (2001).
24. H. Blain, A. Vuillemin, F. Guillemin, R. Durant, B. Hanesse, N. de Talance, B. Doucet & C. Jeandel. Serum Leptin Level Is a Predictor of Bone Mineral Density in Postmenopausal Women. *J Clin Endocrinol Metab*, **87,** (3), 1030-1035 (2002).
25. T. Thomas, B. Burguera, L. J. Melton, 3rd, E. J. Atkinson, W. M. O'Fallon, B. L. Riggs & S. Khosla. Role of serum leptin, insulin, and estrogen levels as potential mediators of the relationship between fat mass and bone mineral density in men versus women. *Bone*, **29,** (2), 114-20 (2001).
26. M. Sato, N. Takeda, H. Sarui, R. Takami, K. Takami, M. Hayashi, A. Sasaki, S. Kawachi, K. Yoshino & K. Yasuda. Association between Serum Leptin Concentrations and Bone Mineral Density, and Biochemical Markers of Bone Turnover in Adult Men. *J Clin Endocrinol Metab*, **86,** (11), 5273-5276 (2001).
27. C. E. Ruhl & J. E. Everhart. Relationship of serum leptin concentration with bone mineral density in the United States population. *Journal of Bone and Mineral Research*, **17,** (10), 1896-903 (2002).
28. J. S. Flier. Clinical review 94: What's in a name? In search of leptin's physiologic role. *Journal Of Clinical Endocrinology And Metabolism*, **83,** (5), 1407-13 (1998).
29. I. S. Farooqi, S. A. Jebb, G. Langmack, E. Lawrence, C. H. Cheetham, A. M. Prentice, I. A. Hughes, M. A. McCamish & S. O'Rahilly. Effects of recombinant leptin therapy in a child with congenital leptin deficiency. *N Engl J Med*, **341,** (12), 879-84 (1999).
30. V. Simha, J. E. Zerwekh, K. Sakhaee & A. Garg. Effect of subcutaneous leptin replacement therapy on bone metabolism in patients with generalized lipodystrophy. *J Clin Endocrinol Metab*, **87,** (11), 4942-5 (2002).

31. L. Rejnmark, P. Vestergaard, M. Kassem, B. R. Christoffersen, N. Kolthoff, K. Brixen & L. Mosekilde. Fracture risk in perimenopausal women treated with beta-blockers. *Calcif Tissue Int*, **75**, (5), 365-72 (2004).
32. I. R. Reid, G. D. Gamble, A. B. Grey, D. M. Black, K. E. Ensrud, W. S. Browner & D. C. Bauer. beta-Blocker Use, BMD, and Fractures in the Study of Osteoporotic Fractures. *J Bone Miner Res*, **20**, (4), 613-8 (2005).
33. J. A. Pasco, M. J. Henry, K. M. Sanders, M. A. Kotowicz, E. Seeman & G. C. Nicholson. Beta-adrenergic blockers reduce the risk of fracture partly by increasing bone mineral density: Geelong Osteoporosis Study. *J Bone Miner Res*, **19**, (1), 19-24 (2004).
34. R. G. Schlienger, M. E. Kraenzlin, S. S. Jick & C. R. Meier. Use of beta-blockers and risk of fractures. *Jama*, **292**, (11), 1326-32 (2004).
35. S. Harada & G. A. Rodan. Control of osteoblast function and regulation of bone mass. *Nature*, **423**, (6937), 349-55 (2003).
36. P. A. Baldock, A. Sainsbury, M. Couzens, R. F. Enriquez, G. P. Thomas, E. M. Gardiner & H. Herzog. Hypothalamic Y2 receptors regulate bone formation. *J Clin Invest*, **109**, (7), 915-921. (2002).
37. Y. M. Bohlooly, M. Mahlapuu, H. Andersen, A. Astrand, S. Hjorth, L. Svensson, J. Tornell, M. R. Snaith, D. G. Morgan & C. Ohlsson. Osteoporosis in MCHR1-deficient mice. *Biochem Biophys Res Commun*, **318**, (4), 964-9 (2004).
38. A. I. Idris, R. J. van 't Hof, I. R. Greig, S. A. Ridge, D. Baker, R. A. Ross & S. H. Ralston. Regulation of bone mass, bone loss and osteoclast activity by cannabinoid receptors. *Nat Med*, **11**, (7), 774-9 (2005).

Chapter 9

ROLES AND REGULATION OF LEPTIN IN REPRODUCTION

Michael C. Henson[1] and V. Daniel Castracane[2]

[1]*Department of Biological Sciences, Purdue University Calumet, Hammond, IN*
[2]*Texas Tech University School of Medicine, Lubbock, TX*

Abstract: Leptin is the endocrine product of the *LEP* gene, which in addition to influencing satiety and energy metabolism, is associated with puberty onset, fertility, and pregnancy. Therefore, second only to its association with obesity, leptin's role as a reproductive regulator represents the primary research focus of the scientific community to date. A correlation with adipose mass is at least partly responsible for serum leptin concentrations being higher in females than in males, but as maternal levels in pregnancy are greater still, regulatory mechanisms linked to the steroid hormones are strongly suggested. In this regard, leptin levels may directly influence testicular steroidogenesis and be linked to testis development. These mechanisms are further evidenced by animal and in vitro studies that demonstrate a stimulatory influence of estrogen on leptin synthesis, as well as an inhibitory influence of androgens. An association with gonadotropins demonstrates a role for leptin at the hypothalamic level in controlling menstrual cyclicity and ovarian function. Results of clinical reports in humans, in vitro experiments employing human tissues, and interventional studies utilizing rodent and nonhuman primate models, have demonstrated a number of roles for the polypeptide, acting through both membrane-bound and soluble forms of its receptor, with respect to implantation, placental function, conceptus growth, and fetal development. Further associations with intrauterine growth restriction, preeclampsia, pregnancy-associated diabetes, and the fetal origin of adult diseases help to place leptin in the forefront of research in reproductive biology.

Key words: puberty, menstrual cycle, fertility, pregnancy, fetal origin of adult diseases

1. INTRODUCTION

Following the discovery of leptin in 1994 by Friedman's group[1], studies rapidly followed to determine the physiologic role(s) of this new protein that was expressed abundantly in adipose tissues in normal rodents. Leptin was defined in the rodent as the product of the *ob* (now *Lep*) gene and was not present in the $Lep^{ob}Lep^{ob}$ obese mouse, while its specific receptor was not present in obese $Lepr^{db}Lepr^{db}$ mice. It had been known for many years that both of these genetic models, in addition to being afflicted with hyperglycemia, hyperinsulinemia and other metabolic dysfunctions, were infertile. While food restriction would restore normal body weight in the $Lep^{ob}Lep^{ob}$ mouse, it would not restore fertility. However, the administration of leptin would decrease obesity to normal body weight and restore fertility[2]. These were the first definitive indications that leptin was associated with reproduction. Early studies also demonstrated a relationship with the onset of puberty, as administration of leptin to normal prepubertal mice would advance the timing for the initiation of pubertal development[3,4]. Soon, it was demonstrated that the leptin message was expressed not only in adipose tissue, but also in the placenta[5], and extended the polypeptide's interactions with reproductive biology to include pregnancy.

Subsequent studies expanded these associations to interactions with virtually every aspect of reproductive function in females, as well as in males. Leptin functions via a specific receptor that is a member of the class I cytokine receptor super family and is manifested in alternatively spliced isoforms that are distinguished by the relative lengths of their cytoplasmic regions. These include a long form ($LEPR_L$) that predominates in the hypothalamus, and a short form ($LEPR_S$) that is found in many organs and tissues. $LEPR_L$ exhibits consensus amino acid sequences involved in binding to Janus tyrosine kinases (JAK/STAT); while $LEPR_S$ has distinct signaling capabilities involving mitogen activated protein kinase (MAPK)[6]. A soluble, circulating leptin receptor (solLEPR) is generated in humans by the proteolytic cleavage of membrane bound receptors[7]. Mice[8] and rats[9] manifest their own version of the circulating receptor ($LEPR_E$), which is highly expressed in the placenta.

In little more than a decade since leptin's discovery and its initial association with satiety and energy balance, it is now evident that the "fat hormone" plays important roles in reproduction. Therefore, a thorough review of reproductive endocrinology is no longer complete without its inclusion. The pleiotropic actions of leptin are well represented in this volume, but the association of leptin with reproduction may represent the area of greatest research activity outside of those directly addressing obesity itself. Therefore, in this chapter, we will review the roles and regulation of leptin that touch the many areas of reproductive physiology.

2. GENDER DIFFERENCES

The rapid development of leptin radioimmunoassays allowed the measurement of serum leptin levels in humans as one of the first possible studies, long before the administration of leptin was considered appropriate for our species. These first studies provided several important findings. First, that a positive correlation exists for increases in serum leptin with increases in measures of body fat mass no matter how this was measured (percent body fat, body mass index [BMI], or fat cell mass)[10,11]. Interestingly, obese individuals of either sex did not exhibit a decrease in serum leptin with increasing adiposity and gave rise to the concept of leptin resistance[12,13]. Of greater interest, with regard to leptin's role in reproduction, was the observation that females always had higher leptin levels than males[14-16].

There are two general observations that must be considered with respect to this gender difference. The first is that although females generally have a greater percentage body fat than males of similar body weight or BMI, leptin levels are greater in females over males of equivalent fat mass[17]. Differences in relative amounts of subcutaneous versus visceral adipose tissues may be important, with females having greater subcutaneous adipose tissue than males. Leptin secretion has been reported to be greater in subcutaneous than omental adipocytes for the same subject[18-20]. The second important factor in this gender difference is the endogenous hormonal milieu, with estrogens generally reported to increase leptin production[21] and testosterone or androgens to suppress leptin levels[22-24]. In addition to in vivo studies, these same steroid effects have been observed in adipocytes in vitro, as well[25-27].

3. LEPTIN AND GONADOTROPINS

A component of the lipostat theory years ago was the hypothesis that some biochemical signal from adipose tissue serves as the feedback regulator to tell the brain the status of peripheral body nutrition. This signal is now understood to be leptin, which feeds back to the arcuate nucleus in the regulation of neuropeptide Y (NPY), as the most important molecule involved in appetite regulation. The arcuate nucleus is also the site of key reproductive control as the origin of GnRH. Early studies tested the hypothesis that leptin may be involved in both hypothalamic and pituitary gonadotropin regulation. McCann and his colleagues[28] incubated hemi-anterior pituitaries of adult male rats with increasing concentrations of leptin for 3 hours and observed a dose dependent stimulation of FSH and LH release. Prolactin secretion was also increased in a dose dependent manner, but only at higher leptin concentrations. These studies were the first to demonstrate a direct in vitro effect of leptin on pituitary LH, FSH and prolactin secretion.

These same investigators[28] also examined the action of leptin on median eminence-arcuate nucleus transplants from the same animals. They found a stimulation of GnRH release only at the lowest leptin concentrations and a suppression of GnRH release at higher leptin levels. As a third study, using estradiol benzoate-treated ovariectomized female rats, they administered leptin through a third ventricle cannula 72 hours after estrogen treatment. Leptin treatment resulted in a highly significant increase in plasma LH, 10-50 minutes after the initiation of leptin administration. There was no effect on FSH. Dearth and co-workers[29] were able to demonstrate the effectiveness of leptin administered into the third ventricle to stimulate LH release in late juvenile rats and that immunoneutralization of GnRH would block this action, confirming the results from the earlier studies of McCann's group. Other studies demonstrated that leptin plays a role in stimulating NOS and increasing NO release from the hypothalamus and anterior pituitary. The NOS inhibitor, NMMA, can block the action of leptin at both hypothalamus and pituitary and indicates that leptin may affect GnRH and LH release through the stimulation of NOS[30].

Galanin is a peptide found throughout the hypothalamus and has been implicated in the regulation of food intake and body weight and in the neuroendocrine control of reproduction[31,32]. Ohtaki and colleagues[33] have identified a novel galanin-like peptide (GALP) from porcine hypothalamus. GALP is a 60 amino acid peptide that, unlike galanin, has a non-amidated C-terminus, but residues 9-21 are identical to the biologically active C-terminus (1-13) portion of galanin. There are at least three galanin receptor subtypes and rat GALP selectively recognizes GALPR2 with high affinity and GALPR1 with lower affinity, while galanin is relatively non-selective for these receptors. The distribution of GALP neurons in the hypothalamus is predominately in the arcuate nucleus but also in the caudal dorsomedial nucleus, median eminence and the pituitary in the rodent[34-37]. Similar distribution has been reported for the nonhuman primate hypothalamus[38]. GALP neurons in the hypothalamus are colocalized with leptin receptor in several species[38,39]. GALP neurons respond to leptin treatment with an increase in the expression of *GALP* mRNA. Central administration of GALP activates GnRH immunoreactive neurons and increases plasma LH levels. Leptin serves to link the body adiposity with the hypothalamic regulation of reproduction[37,40]. A reduction in the level of hypothalamic GALP mRNA was found in the Lep^{ob}/Lep^{ob} and Lep^{db}/Lep^{db} mice[36,39] and intracerebral ventricle administration of leptin to Lep^{ob}/Lep^{ob} mice increased both the number of GALP mRNA expressing neurons and their content of GALP mRNA[36].

For many years, fasting has been known to result in a decrease in serum LH and testosterone in male primates as well as rodents and heifers[41-44]. Similarly, Cameron and Nosbeich[41] fasted young male monkeys for 48 hours and observed a decrease in LH surges. Fasting even for as short as 24-48 hours is also known to decrease serum leptin levels[45,46]. Finn and collaborators[47] were able to demonstrate the cessation of LH pulses in monkeys within 48 hours of fasting and that 2 days of leptin infusion would restore LH pulses. This is presumably the action of leptin at hypothalamic-pituitary sites as discussed earlier. Conversely, Lado-Abeal and others[48] using a similar animal preparation, the peripubertal male rhesus monkey, could not restore the LH pulses after fasting with infusion of recombinant rhesus leptin, nor were increases in cortisol or the frequency of GH pulses corrected with treatment. The relationship of stress changes to this effect on LH surges, separate from leptin involvement, has been discussed by Lado-Abeal and Norman[49]. Ages in these two studies were similar but the differences have not been resolved but may involve the source and dose of the leptin preparation used in each study.

4. LEPTIN AND STEROID HORMONES

Ovariectomy diminished leptin gene expression in white adipose tissue and caused a decline in serum leptin levels in rats[50-52], while administration of estradiol (E_2) reversed all the effects of ovariectomy. Ovariectomy also reduced serum leptin levels in humans[53]. Although leptin and E_2 demonstrate similar profiles during the human menstrual cycle[54], leptin levels were unaffected by the relatively small increases in estrogen associated with normal menstrual cyclicity, but were up-regulated by the large increases that typically result from ovulation induction, effects that may identify estrogen as a dose-dependent regulator[16, 55-57]. Estrogens may regulate leptin expression by acting on a portion of the estrogen response element in the leptin promoter[58], with leptin production by cultured first trimester human cytotrophoblast cells being dose-responsively potentiated by E_2[59]. The presence of estrogen receptor in primate trophoblast[60] suggests that, as in adipose tissue[61], this is an estrogen receptor-mediated phenomenon. Because commensurate administration of E_2 and progesterone to normally cycling women resulted in increased serum leptin concentrations, cooperative mechanisms mediated by the two steroids might also be implied during the luteal phase of the menstrual cycle[62]. However, in late pregnancy when placental progesterone production is at its height, progesterone has been reported to inhibit leptin secretion by human placental cells in culture[63].

Estrogen administration was also reported to elicit an increase in hypothalamic expression of the long form of the leptin receptor in rats[64]. This potential was elucidated by Lindell et al[65] who reported that a putative estrogen response element, close to the most frequently used transcriptional start sites of the leptin receptor gene in the rat hypothalamus, might be a mechanism by which estrogen regulates the leptin receptor.

5. PUBERTY

With the first availability of the ob (now Lep) protein (leptin), several studies demonstrated that leptin administration to the prepubertal mouse would advance the time of puberty[3, 4]. Furthermore, in the $Lep^{ob}Lep^{ob}$ mouse, without leptin, which never enters puberty, administration of leptin would result in a normal pubertal process[66]. These early studies stimulated investigations into the role of leptin and puberty in many species, including the human. In the rat, mild food restriction was found to result in a delay of sexual maturation, which could be overcome with leptin administration. When the food restriction was more severe, leptin was not able to overcome this effect. Cheung et al[67] concluded that leptin has a permissive role, but that leptin is not the major metabolic factor that initiates pubertal development in the rat. Similarly, Gruaz, et al[68] administered leptin into the cerebral ventricle of the rat and was able to initiate early pubertal onset, indicating an action for leptin in the central nervous system. Presumably, the action of leptin on the hypothalamus or pituitary may mediate this stimulatory effect on pubertal development.

In both the mouse and the rat, a rise in serum leptin levels that precedes pubertal development has been noted. In the mouse, a clear prepubertal surge has been reported[69,] while in the rat a gradual increase occurs, although the frequency of sampling precluded the detection of a true surge[68]. In other species, an increase in serum leptin has been reported prior to pubertal development, and would include the pig and the sheep[70, 71]. Exogenous leptin has even been reported to advance puberty in the domestic hen[72].

Most importantly, studies in the human also demonstrated a role for leptin during the pubertal process. Serum leptin levels were reported to rise during the years preceding pubertal development and reach high levels around the time of puberty onset. In females, the leptin levels continue to rise, while in males, the leptin levels decline, probably related to the testosterone effect[73]. In an early study, Mantzoros et al[22] were able to demonstrate, in an elegant set of serial samples obtaining over several years in young boys approaching the normal age of puberty, that a surge in leptin was clearly evident before any significant increases in serum testosterone were observed, suggesting a role for leptin in the initiation of this process. Unfortunately, the leptin levels are markedly different among the individual boys, with some levels quite low, although clearly increased above baseline levels. The role of leptin is also seen in other conditions, for example, an earlier age for puberty has been observed in obese girls, presumably related to the higher leptin levels in this group[74]. In girls with premature pubarche were found to have elevated leptin levels, independent of insulin or androgen levels, and these girls may be considered at risk for metabolic syndrome[75]. It has been reported many times that young girls in serious gymnastic or ballet programs have a delay in pubertal development and serum leptin levels in both of these groups are noted to be decreased[76]. Perhaps the most revealing clinical situation on the role of leptin in pubertal development is seen in those children with the rare mutation which results in the absence of leptin. In these children, no sign of pubertal development is typically observed, but when treatment with leptin is initiated, the first signs of endocrine changes characteristic of puberty are noted[66].

Whether or not leptin binding protein in the serum plays a role in pubertal development has also been studied. There are several reports to demonstrate that leptin binding protein declines during the prepubertal years in both males and females. These decreased levels of the circulating binding protein would allow a greater amount of free leptin, with greater biological activity that could result in a greater effective action for serum leptin[77-79]. The literature reporting studies in humans clearly demonstrates a relationship between increasing leptin and pubertal development but whether or not this role is permissive or the primary factor that initiates the sequence of endocrine changes resulting in puberty remains to be determined.

The use of nonhuman primates has served as a valuable experimental model and presents a close nonhuman surrogate for the human. In the rhesus monkey, several studies report that no observable increase in serum leptin is observed prior to the initiation of puberty and suggest that leptin may not be involved in the pubertal process in this species[80-82]. More recently, however, Suter et al[83] observed that nocturnal increases in leptin may be important. Therefore, it is well known that the initiating endocrine events of pubertal development are nocturnal events and this hypothesis would fit well with the known changes in gonadotropins and gonadal steroids described for primates. This area remains controversial[84-85] and whether or not leptin plays a role in rhesus pubertal development adequate serum levels of leptin may still play a permissive role and cannot be discounted.

6. MENSTRUAL CYCLE

Earlier in this chapter we described those studies that described the roles for leptin in the hypothalamus and pituitary resulting in the stimulation of GnRH and LH, respectively. Similarly, the action of leptin on steroid hormone synthesis is well documented and the effects of steroid hormones on leptin synthesis have been described. These actions are part of the intricate interactions by which leptin exerts its influence on the menstrual cycle. Several studies, using infrequent blood sampling during the menstrual cycle have reported inconsistent results. When blood samples were collected on the 7th, 14th and 21st day of the cycle, there was no quantitative change in serum leptin noted[86]. In some studies, no changes in serum leptin were observed, but the timing of blood sampling resulted in an inability to observe any luteal phase increase[92]. In another study, samples at four different windows during the cycle were not sufficient to denote any changes in serum leptin levels that could be correlated with specific ovarian and endocrine changes[88]. However, a similar study with five sampling windows, observed a peak in serum leptin in the late luteal phase with a drop in the early follicular phase and a return to higher levels in the next luteal phase[89]. Similar results were also reported by others[90]. When samples were obtained every 1-2 days throughout the menstrual cycle, plasma leptin was seen to increase from the early follicular phase to peak levels at the midluteal phase, returning to baseline by menses[91]. Clearly, a greater sampling frequency results in a better descriptive picture of leptin changes during the cycle. Despite minor differences, the luteal phase, either mid or late, is reported to be the period of peak serum leptin concentrations, with some studies also noting an increase during the late follicular phase. Tataranni et al[92] did not find serum leptin changes over the course of the menstrual cycle and suggested that body fat content may be a more important determinant of serum leptin levels than cycle stage.

In our own studies, which featured daily sampling, we demonstrated changes in serum leptin that were related to the stage of the cycle in normal weight women, with leptin levels increasing during follicular development and a secondary increase in the luteal phase. In obese women who continued to experience ovulatory cycles, at best an infrequent occurrence, there was no pattern of leptin associated with cycle stage, but rather leptin levels were markedly elevated above those in normal ovulatory cycles. In this group of obese women, luteal phase progesterone levels were significantly reduced in comparison to those during control cycles, and may represent an action of elevated leptin on luteal steroidogenesis[93].

Several reports have demonstrated the regulation of leptin production and its relationship to progesterone and may account for the generally reported increase in serum leptin during the luteal phase. In one such study, following ovariectomy, women received either no treatment, treatment with E_2, or treatment with E_2 plus progesterone. In both untreated and E_2-treated women, a decline in serum leptin concentrations over four days was observed, but following treatment with E_2 plus progesterone, leptin levels were significantly increased[94]. In a similar study, cycling women were either untreated or treated with E_2 or E_2 plus progesterone during the early follicular phase. In the untreated and E_2-treated women there was no increase in serum leptin, but those that received E_2 plus progesterone demonstrated enhanced leptin concentrations over the three days of treatment, with levels declining after cessation of treatment[95]. This relationship might account for the previously noted luteal phase increase in serum leptin levels and probably represents the action of ovarian steroids on production of the polypeptide in adipose tissue. The increase seen in the late follicular phase of the menstrual cycle may be due to E_2 increases at that phase of the cycle, since there are multiple reports that suggest or demonstrate a stimulatory effect of estrogens on serum leptin levels[17, 21]. The small increase in progesterone, which begins in the late follicular phase, may also contribute to this effect.

7. INFERTILITY, OVULATION INDUCTION AND IN VITRO FERTILIZATION

The changes in serum leptin concentrations during the menstrual cycle suggest a strong relationship with the ovarian cycle and the logical extension would be to situations of infertility, especially ovulation induction and the resulting in vitro fertilization (IVF) following controlled ovarian hyperstimulation (COH). It is well known that obesity has a deleterious effect on fertility, affecting many parameters, ranging from poor ovulation to the cessation of menstrual cycles, and ultimately the development of polycystic ovarian syndrome (PCOS). It has been reported that obese hyperandrogenic, amennorheic women were less likely to ovulate after clomiphene citrate (CC) medication, which is the first line of treatment for these anovulatory patients. Typically, peripheral leptin levels in these obese women are markedly elevated and leptin concentrations are generally more reliable than BMI or waist to hip ratio to predict which of those patients will remain anovulatory after CC medication. These investigators suggested that leptin is more involved in ovarian dysfunction in these patients than are other endocrine events and that this may be a direct action of leptin on ovarian dysfunction[96].

A number of reports have indicated that leptin levels are markedly increased during COH, specifically treatment with FSH to increase the number of ovulated oocytes for IVF. Interestingly, in most studies, the increase in leptin is rarely observed in 100% of subjects, but rather about 20% of patients do not show the leptin increases that seem to parallel E_2 increases and follicular development in the remaining 80% of these women In PCOS patients, those women who became pregnant following assisted reproduction treatment, tended to have lower mean follicular fluid leptin concentrations than women with PCOS who did not become pregnant with the same treatment[97]. Fedorcsak et al[98] was able to show that specific leptin binding activity was higher in the plasma than in the follicular fluid and that follicular fluid to plasma leptin ratio was independently associated with the FSH dose used to stimulate ovulation. These authors inferred that intrafollicular fluid leptin levels resulting from obesity affects ovarian function in PCOS patients and may induce a relative resistance to gonadotropic stimulation. This effect might even be heightened because of the low leptin binding activity within the preovulatory follicle of obese patients.

Butzow et al[99] were able to demonstrate that leptin production following FSH stimulation was influenced by the ovarian functional state. The high relative leptin increases associated with adiposity was associated with a reduced ovarian response. The results suggested that high leptin levels may reduce ovarian responsiveness to gonadotropins and may be the reason that obese patients require greater amounts of gonadotropins than lean subjects to achieve a successful stimulation and ovulation. Zhao et al[100] was able to demonstrate the increase in leptin associated with FSH treatment and that this correlated with increasing E_2 concentrations across all days of stimulation, in contrast to other studies which did not report this correlation. Brannian et al[101] compared pregnancy rate in IVF patients with the leptin concentration:BMI ratio. This comparison demonstrated that with a higher leptin concentration per BMI, the success rate declines significantly in a stepwise manner. These results suggest that the greater the leptin production the less successful is the IVF procedure to result in a pregnancy. This approach has not been adopted by infertility practitioners and indeed, some reports suggest that there is no relationship between leptin levels and pregnancy success rate[102, 103]. Therefore, further study in this area is warranted.

The use of leptin in conditions of low levels of this hormone, have been reported to have beneficial effects. A group of women (n=8) with hypothalamic amenorrhea and low leptin levels, were studied by Welt et al[104] for one control month before receiving recombinant human leptin for up to three months and a separate control group (n=6) received no treatment. Controls were essentially unchanged over the course of the study. Conversely, recombinant human leptin increased LH levels and LH pulse frequency after two weeks, with an increase in maximum follicular diameter and the number of dominant follicles, ovarian volume and E_2 levels over three months. Ovulatory menstrual cycles were reported in three subjects and two other women had preovulatory follicular development with withdrawal bleeding during treatment. These studies suggest that leptin may be required for normal reproductive and neuroendocrine function and may be of clinical utility in the treatment of leptin deficiency in women with hypothalamic amenorrhea. Collectively, the studies discussed above indicate an association of leptin with the normal physiology of the menstrual cycle and a potential role for the polypeptide in the treatment of women undergoing controlled ovarian hyperstimulation. Further work will be needed to fully understand this association and the potential clinical use of leptin in the infertility patient.

8. PREGNANCY

Ontogeny and species specificity - Leptin is produced by adipose tissues and the placental trophoblast, with maternal hyperleptinemia common to many species. Serum leptin concentrations are elevated in human pregnancy, rise along with estrogen and are correlated in the first trimester with hCG[105-110]. Fetal adipose tissue produces leptin[111], although the decline in neonatal levels following birth suggests a placental contribution to the fetus[112]. The presence of *LEP* mRNA transcripts in the trophoblast prompted the contention that maternal hyperleptinemia is exclusively placental[113], although two other observations contributed to this assumption. The first is the postpartum decline in leptin levels observed after placental delivery; a decrease that is relatively prolonged for a hormone with such a short half-life and the second results from the outcome of placental perfusions[114]. We examined the role of placental mass in the pregnant rat by adjusting the number of fetal-placental units shortly after implantation, so that rats had either 1-2, 4-5, or greater than 10 implantation sites. Maternal serum leptin levels were highest in those animals with fewer implantations and conversely, were least in those with the greatest number of implantations[115]. We then compared maternal serum leptin concentrations in women (15-20 weeks of gestation) with singleton or twin pregnancies. Mean leptin levels and leptin levels plotted against BMI were virtually identical for both groups. In addition, serial samples from singleton, twin and triplet pregnancies revealed that placental number was not related to maternal serum leptin levels but rather, that maternal adiposity was the controlling factor[116]. These studies, in different species, suggested that increases in maternal leptin levels were not related to increased placental mass, but that the hormonal milieu of pregnancy upregulates leptin synthesis in maternal adipose tissue.

Leptin/leptin receptor regulation and function in rodent pregnancy[117-119] differ from that during pregnancy in both humans[120] and nonhuman primates[121, 122]. Thus, although maternal peripheral leptin concentrations increase with gestational age in the human, *LEP* mRNA in placental villous tissue is greater in the first trimester than at term[120]. In contrast, Amico et al[123] reported that placental leptin mRNA increased 4- to 5-fold over the final one-third of rat pregnancy, while Garcia et al[124] observed that *LEP* mRNA in placenta increased throughout gestation. Although leptin transcripts may be expressed in both the placenta and fetus[125], there is some disagreement as to whether the mouse placenta produces leptin at all[126]. To better understand regulatory mechanisms in human pregnancy we employed a well-characterized nonhuman primate model, the baboon (Papio sp.), an old world primate[127-129] that differs in some respects from other monkeys[122, 130] with regard to leptin production. Leptin concentrations in pregnant baboons are much higher than in either cycling or postpartum animals and increase about 2.5-fold between days 60 and 160 of gestation[121]. Term is approximately 184 days. As in humans, leptin transcripts in placental villous tissue decline with advancing gestation, but maternal serum leptin levels increase almost 3-fold with pregnancy and are correlated with gestational age. Because the presence of both leptin and its receptor in the placenta, amnion, chorion, and umbilical vasculature[105,-107, 131] suggest important roles in human pregnancy, we assessed these tissues and omental and subcutaneous fat at early (day 60), mid (day 100) and late (day 160) baboon pregnancy[132]. A resurgent corpus luteum and decidual tissue were also collected on day 160, as was fetal hypothalamus. *LEPR$_L$* and *LEPR$_S$* mRNA transcripts were detected in all tissues and were constitutively expressed throughout gestation in placenta and fat, with *LEPR$_S$* expressed in greater abundance than *LEPR$_L$* in all tissues. As in humans[120], in situ hybridization localized transcripts for leptin and its receptor in baboon trophoblast. Expression intensity for leptin was highest in early pregnancy, reflecting the greater abundance of leptin transcripts at that time[121].

In pregnancy, as in some forms of obesity, "leptin resistance" may result from inhibited transport across the blood-brain barrier[133] or sequestration of bioactive leptin in the circulation by solLEPR[134, 135]. Correspondingly, we have reported that transcripts for $LEPR_L$ and $LEPR_S$ were expressed in human trophoblast both early (7-14 weeks) in gestation and at term[120]. Although there is some disagreement as to whether soluble leptin receptor concentrations increase[136] or remain unchanged[137] with pregnancy in women, we have suggested that an increase in solLEPR and hence, the level of bound leptin in the maternal circulation, increases with advancing gestation[105-107]. In the human, at least two soluble leptin receptor isoforms bind leptin and perhaps potentiate leptin resistance[138, 139], as in the mouse[140], with an increase in receptor protein proposed to explain the enhancement in maternal leptin typical of pregnancy. Schulz et al[141] identified two isoforms of the receptor in human placenta that are similar in size to two we have identified in the baboon[142]. A 50 kDa solLEPR was recently identified in baboon decidua that was down regulated by chorionic gonadotropin[143]; perhaps further suggesting that increasing receptor concentrations play a role in regulating leptin availability.

Roles of leptin in pregnancy - Many physiological roles have been suggested for leptin in human pregnancy[105-110]. Thus, the presence of placental leptin/leptin receptors suggests the potential for autocrine and paracrine mechanisms in that tissue[127, 144]. The addition of recombinant leptin enhanced hCG release by cultured cytotrophoblast cells[145] and stimulated hCG secretion by human placental explants, while inducing and stimulating the amplitude of hCG pulses[146] and release of pro-inflammatory cytokines and prostaglandins[147]. The expression of leptin and leptin receptor in human placenta[148] and uterine endometrium[149] and the observation that endometrial leptin secretion is enhanced by a viable blastocyst also link the polypeptide to early conceptus development[150, 151] and suggest its place among the hormones that regulate implantation[152-154]. Leptin may also augment the conceptus' ability to sustain embryonic development, as it potentiates a down-regulation of apoptosis in the early blastocyst[155]. Because leptin receptor is expressed in maternal decidua and the uterine endometrium is identified as a target for leptin action, a definitive role is suggested in the blastocyst-endometrial dialogue[156-158]. Specifically with respect to primate pregnancy, in vitro investigations in the baboon revealed that decidual leptin secretion was enhanced by chorionic gonadotropin[159]. The obligatory nature of leptin signaling in mammalian implantation[160] was illustrated by experiments in the mouse that demonstrated that endometrial leptin receptor expression was pregnancy-dependent and that intrauterine injection of a leptin peptide antagonist or a leptin antibody impaired implantation. To this end, leptin enhances the invasiveness of mouse trophoblast cells via up-regulation of matrix metalloproteinases[161].

Leptin has also been linked to fetal development, in that administration restored the depressed brain weights of leptin-deficient $Lep^{ob}Lep^{ob}$ neonates[162] and concentrations in umbilical cord blood were highly correlated with birth and placental weights[163, 164], infant length[165, 166], and head circumference[166]. In addition, decreases in placental leptin mRNA are linked with decreased leptin concentrations in umbilical vein blood in intrauterine growth restriction (IUGR)[167], suggesting that leptin influences fetal growth in response to a fetal demand that is relative to placental supply[114]. Study of a twin pregnancy found that a growth-restricted twin had markedly lower placental leptin than its normal size sibling[168] and that cord blood leptin levels directly reflected placental concentrations. Subsequent observations of monochorionic twin pregnancies revealed that fetal and cord leptin levels were at least two-fold higher in normal size fetuses than in their growth restricted twins[168, 169], indicating a pivotal role in regulating growth[175]. Decreased leptin levels in cord and placenta of growth-restricted twins may be indirectly reflected by high levels in amniotic fluid and an increased rate of premature delivery that investigators postulated was attributable to hypoxia and poor cytrophoblastic invasion[171]. IUGR babies maintain depressed leptin levels as adults, suggesting permanently altered adipocyte function[172]. Leptin has also been proposed to directly stimulate bone growth[173] via changes in the rates of osteoblast/osteoclast growth and differentiation[174, 175] or by the inhibition of bone resorption that results in a net increase in bone mass[176]. It has also been suggested that leptin influences endochondral ossification by regulating angiogenesis[177], a process illustrated in various developmental models[178, 179]. With respect to the means by which it could facilitate angiogenesis in pregnancy, the polypeptide was reported to enhance vascular endothelial growth factor synthesis in cultured human cytotrophoblast cells[180]. Leptin is also associated with fetal pulmonary development, as it is expressed by fibroblasts and its receptor expressed by type II cells in fetal rat lung[181], with leptin directly enhancing surfactant synthesis[182]. We reported that in late baboon pregnancy the abundances of $LEPR_S$ and $LEPR_L$ mRNA transcripts in fetal lung were 8- to 10-fold greater than in early pregnancy[183]. Receptor protein, undetectable in fetal lungs at early and mid gestation, was detected by western blotting in late gestation and localized immunohistochemically in distal pulmonary epithelial cells, including type II cells.

Leptin regulation in pregnancy - Increases in maternal serum leptin levels in early pregnancy may be owed to the stimulation of maternal adipose tissue by gestational steroids[184, 185]. Placental estrogens increase with advancing gestation[127] and E_2 administration enhances leptin mRNA transcript expression and protein secretion by adipocytes, both in vitro[184-186] and in vivo[187]. Like the human, the baboon relies on androgen precursors from the fetal adrenal gland for placental estrogen synthesis[127]. Thus, the surgical removal of the fetus, but not the placenta (fetectomy), inhibits estrogen production by the syncytiotrophoblast and dramatically reduces maternal serum E_2. Therefore, we collected placental villous tissue, and subcutaneous adipose tissue from baboons in late (day 160) pregnancy[188]. In another group of pregnant baboons, estrogen production was inhibited at day 100 by fetectomy. Placentae were left in situ until day 160 of gestation, when they were surgically retrieved. Maternal adipose tissues were collected at both days 100 and 160 of pregnancy. Although fetectomy did not result in a decline in maternal E_2 to a level that would approximate levels in nonpregnant baboons, it did elicit an 87% decrease in maternal serum E_2 concentrations. Leptin levels were unaltered by fetectomy, although in maternal fat the abundance of *LEP* mRNA transcripts declined about five-fold as a consequence of fetectomy, while transcripts increased almost 3-fold in placenta. In fat, leptin levels in fetectomized baboons were about one-half that of controls, while placental levels were 3-fold higher in fetectomized animals than in those with intact pregnancies. Therefore, although adipose leptin expression declined, increased placental expression suggested a compensatory mechanism and tissue-specific regulation by estrogen (stimulatory in fat, inhibitory in placenta). A divergence in transcriptional regulation in placenta and adipose tissue might be suspected due to a functional enhancer for the leptin gene that exists only in placental cells[189, 190].

We further hypothesized that pregnancy-induced increases in estrogen would prompt commensurate increases in leptin transcripts in leptin-producing tissues. Thus, when venous blood and adipose tissues were collected from nonpregnant baboons in the mid luteal phase of the menstrual cycle and from pregnant animals throughout gestation, E_2 concentrations were lowest in cycling animals (0.06 ± 0.02 ng/ml) and increased with pregnancy and advancing gestation (4.17 ± 0.87 ng/ml on day 160), as expected. However, although the abundance of *LEP* mRNA transcripts in adipose tissue was unchanged with regard to pregnancy or advancing gestation, tissue leptin concentrations in subcutaneous fat were significantly higher in pregnancy, and with advancing gestation. In addition, soluble receptor levels in maternal serum increased approximately 60% between early and late normal pregnancy, with levels in fetectomized (estrogen deprived) baboons being less than one-half that in pregnancy-intact controls[142]. The 3-fold increase in soluble receptor over that of nonpregnant baboons approximated that observed in human pregnancy[136]. Soluble receptor was only minimally detectable following cesarean delivery. One 130 kDa isoform of the leptin receptor was identified in decidua and amniochorion. In decidua this receptor increased 4-fold and in amniochorion increased 10-fold from early to late gestation. Two isoforms (130 kDa, 150 kDa) of the leptin receptor were present in placenta, with levels of the 130 kDa isoform increasing 3-fold from early to late gestation. Following fetectomy, abundance of the 150 kDa isoform declined 50%. Intriguingly, a soluble form of the leptin receptor has been proposed to serve as the physiological vehicle for the transplacental movement of leptin into the fetal circulation for modulating fetal development in rats[191]. The results of later experiments in choriocarcinoma cells strongly suggested a potential for maternal-fetal leptin exchange across the human placenta as well[192].

Glucocorticoids also enhance leptin synthesis and secretion in adipose tissues[193-195]. In ovine pregnancy, treatment with corticosteroids increased fetal leptin concentrations, while adrenalectomy suppressed them[194]. Leptin infusion just prior to delivery suppressed fetal cortisol concentrations by 40%, evidencing a negative feedback loop between leptin and the fetal HPA axis[196]. Indeed, recombinant leptin infused into the fetal circulation inhibited activation of the HPA axis in late ovine pregnancy, suggesting that mechanisms controlling the initiation of labor might be fine-tuned by a metabolic cue that is related to fetal growth and originates in the placenta or fetal adipocytes[197]. In this regard, leptin levels in women suffering spontaneous first trimester abortions were abnormally low, implying a direct role in pregnancy maintenance[198]. With respect to the leptin receptor, maternal treatment with dexamethasone reduced leptin receptor mRNA in porcine adipose tissue[199] and rat placenta[200, 201], an interruption in leptin signaling that could be exacerbated by direct inhibition of the JAK/STAT pathway[202]. Collectively, these effects suggest that glucocorticoid-induced IUGR could be mediated, at least in part, by leptin/leptin receptor regulation in conceptus tissues.

Leptin and pregnancy-specific pathologies - Perhaps related to leptin's role in implantation, preeclampsia is associated with shallow endometrial invasion, maternal hypertension, and maternal/fetal leptin concentrations that are enhanced over the level of hyperleptinemia characteristic of human pregnancy[203-210]. Placental "susceptibility genes" most likely to be associated with onset of the condition were evaluated by microarray and leptin was up-regulated 44-fold, an elevation reflected by commensurate protein levels. Even in preeclamptic women that had not yet evidenced elevated peripheral leptin levels, enhanced amniotic fluid leptin levels identified the earliest stages of the condition[211]. It has been suggested that this exaggerated hyperleptinemia is a compensatory response to increase nutrient delivery to an under-perfused placenta[212] and may be linked to both maternal adiposity and changes in bioavailable estrogen levels[213]. Although preeclampsia-associated hyperleptinemia has also been linked to enhanced solLEPR levels[214], conflicting reports[215, 216] call for further study. Pregnancy-associated diabetes is also characterized by increased placental leptin contributions to enhanced maternal leptin levels[217, 218]. Cord leptin levels in diabetic pregnancies were strongly correlated with conceptus growth[219, 220], and among the offspring of gestational diabetics serum levels were enhanced over population norms until at least nine years of age[221]. Recently, Lappas and colleagues reported that a dysregulation of placental leptin metabolism and/or function may be directly linked to the pathogenesis of gestational diabetes[222]. Interestingly, both preeclampsia[223] and pregnancy-associated diabetes[224] are associated with fetal hypoxia. Thus, Grosfeld et al[225] reported that decreased oxygen tension up-regulated leptin gene expression in trophoblast-derived BeWo choriocarcinoma cells, an effect proposed to be mediated by activation of distinct cis-acting sequences of the leptin promoter[226].

Leptin and the fetal origin of adult health and disease - Since Barker[227, 228] originally observed the relationship between low birthweight and the adult onset of diseases such as diabetes mellitus, hypertension, and coronary heart disease, much interest has been generated in the "fetal programming" paradigm. In this capacity, Bouret and colleagues[229, 230] suggested that alterations in leptin levels in utero prompt substantive hypothalamic changes in fetuses that eventually result in altered nutritional intake, energy metabolism, and adiposity in children and adults. In addition to studies in rodents, observations in sheep mimic those in women subjected to famine, which suggest that cardiovascular physiology and phenotypic predisposition to obesity are programmed as a natural component of fetal development[231]. Recently, Lecklin et al reported that female rats injected with a recombinant adeno-associated virus vector that encoded the Lep gene, evidenced decreased food intake and commensurate loss of body weight, traits that were maintained throughout their subsequent breeding, pregnancies, and deliveries[232]. Although these primary results illustrated the investigators' main goal of demonstrating the efficacy of leptin gene therapy to elicit weight loss, later observations confirmed that first generation offspring of leptin-transgene expressing females also weighed significantly less than peer controls from birth into adulthood.

9. LEPTIN AND MALE PHYSIOLOGY

Gender differences have been described earlier in this chapter, but we should take the opportunity to present, in greater detail, the situation in males and females from fetal life to adulthood. Numerous studies have demonstrated the gender difference in neonatal samples (cord blood) with female leptin levels always significantly greater than male neonates[233-236]. Generally, E_2 and testosterone levels were not different between males and females in term deliveries[233, 235] and an apparent fall in leptin levels was evident by the fifth postnatal day[239]. In all cases, fetal leptin concentrations correlated with fetal weight. Gender differences between boys and girls between three and 90 days of life were not observed, despite increasing leptin levels during this time period[237]. During pubertal development, leptin levels in boys and girls are similar until activation of gonadal steroidogenesis In girls, leptin levels increase with the initial increases in gonadal estrogen production, conversely, as the testes becomes active in testosterone production, a clear decline in serum leptin is evident[22, 73]. In adults, the classic gender differences described by many investigators are present in normal adults and demonstrate a clear correlation with indices of body fat[14-16]. Levels in normal males are always less than levels in normal females of the same BMI. Considerations of the reasons for this gender difference have been discussed earlier in this chapter.

Perhaps of greater significance are the leptin mediated events within the testes. Tena-Sempere et al[238] identified the leptin receptor in the rat testis. While all splice variants of the leptin receptor were recognized, the long form ($Lepr_b$ isoform) was highest in pubertal testes (15 to 30 day old rats) and declined in adulthood. Testicular *Lepr* mRNA expression was sensitive to neonatal endocrine influence, since neonatal treatment with estradiol benzoate (E_2B) resulted in a permanent increase in the relative expression of *Lepr* mRNA. E_2B treatment had a differential effect on the different isoforms of the leptin receptor. These studies were the first to indicate a direct role for leptin in testicular regulation in the rat.

Caprio et al[239] report a different pattern of leptin receptor in the rat testes. Using an immunohistochemical approach, they demonstrated that Lepr is absent in early embryonic stages (14.5 days) and only appears in late embryonic testes (19.5 days). In postnatal life, leptin receptor immunoreactivity was only evident after sexual maturation (after 35 days) and was absent in testes from sexually immature rats (less than 21 days). RT-PCR analysis would reveal leptin receptor expression in embryonic, prepubertal and adult rat testes and demonstrates the difference of sensitivity between these two methodologies. Leptin addition to adult rat Leydig cell cultures would inhibit hCG-stimulated testosterone production, but had no effect on the steroidogenic function of prepubertal Leydig cells and suggests that no functional Lepr are present in the prepubertal testes. Further studies also demonstrated that leptin acts as a direct inhibitory signal for testicular steroidogenesis and that this effect is due to suppression of several upstream factors (SF-1, StAR, and P450scc) in the steroidogenic pathway[240]. The administration of leptin for 5 days to adult male mice was investigated using a variety of techniques. Immunohistochemical testosterone staining revealed more intense staining in leptin treated than in control mice. Testicular weights and seminiferous tubule diameters were also increased by leptin administration. These results in the mouse indicate that leptin administration stimulates testicular function and testosterone synthesis. It is not clear, in these studies, whether the leptin effect is directly on the testes or through a hypothalamic-pituitary effect of leptin[241].

In men, there was no significant difference in histochemical staining of the testes between infertile and normal control males. There was leptin staining in seminiferous tubules and Leydig cells. These results suggest a leptin action as a central neuroendocrine effect rather than a direct effect on testicular tissue[242]. Glander et al[243] had also examined leptin and testes physiology in infertile male patients and individuals following vasectomy. The concentration of leptin in seminal plasma was significantly lower in normal semen samples than in that from infertility patients and showed a negative correlation with the percent of motile sperm. Leptin concentrations in serum showed no relationship to any sperm parameters, and in seminal plasma was unchanged following vasectomy. Leptin concentrations in seminiferous tubules may influence sperm motility. Using RT-PCR, Western blot and immunofluorescence techniques, Aquila and colleagues[244] have demonstrated that human sperm expresses leptin. There was a large difference in leptin secretion between uncapacitated and capacitated sperm. Greater leptin release from capacitated sperm suggests a functional role for sperm produced leptin in capacitation. Undoubtedly, future studies on direct actions of leptin in the testes will be important to understand leptin's role in testicular physiology.

The role of leptin in the male may extend beyond reproductive involvements. Mice lacking the androgen receptor (ARKO) were used to study the relationship between the androgen receptor (AR) and insulin resistance. In ARKO mice, a progressive reduced insulin sensitivity and impaired glucose tolerance was observed with advancing age. These mice also had an accelerated weight gain, hyperinsulinemia and hyperglycemia, as well as higher leptin levels. These studies demonstrate that the action of androgen at the AR has a role in the development of insulin resistance, which may contribute to the development of type 2 diabetes[245]. Moderately obese men have a decreased androgen profile with serum levels of total and free testosterone being suppressed. In massively obese men, there is a consistently low level of free testosterone. These investigators speculate that these results represent an action of leptin on LH pulse amplitude and serum LH levels, as well as possible negative actions of excess circulating leptin on testicular steroidogenesis[245]. Semen leptin concentrations are inversely correlated with serum testosterone levels and directly with serum leptin levels[246]. Additional studies are needed for a better understanding of the leptin-testes relationship and further studies in man may yield meaningful clinical information on this relationship.

10. CONCLUSIONS

After more than a decade of intense investigation by the scientific community, leptin has been shown to be a hormone with physiological implications that far surpass the influences on satiety and adiposity originally proposed. Therefore, as a modulator of energy homeostasis, leptin may significantly affect the advent of puberty, the regulation of menarche, and the enhancement of fertility. However, the polypeptide's direct regulatory effects on testicular, ovarian, uterine, and conceptus tissues, as well as its interactions with a fetal basis for adult health and disease, may constitute its most dramatic impacts on mammalian reproductive biology. In this capacity, the pleiotropic nature of leptin has proven to be the biggest surprise in our rapidly growing understanding of this "new" hormone and its expanding roles are proving to be somewhat removed from those regulating adipose metabolism and obesity. Indeed, as a new wave of investigators join the field, we might assume that the end of the story remains to be told and much more can be expected to be learned about the role(s) of leptin.

REFERENCES

1. Y. Zhang, R. Proenca, M. Maffei, M. Barone, L. Leopold and J.M. Friedman, Positional cloning of the mouse *obese* gene and its human homologue. Nature 372, 425-432 (1994).
2. F.F. Chehab, M.E. Lim, and R.Lu, Correction of the sterility defect in homozygous obese female mice by treatment with the human recombinant leptin. Nat. Gen. 12, 318-320 (1996).
3. F.F. Chehab, K.A. Mounzih, R. Lu, and N.E. Lim, Early onset of reproductive function in normal mice treated with leptin. Science 275, 88-90 (1997).
4. R.S. Ahima, J. Dushay, S.N. Flier, D. Prabakaran, and J.S. Flier, Leptin accelerates the onset of puberty in normal female mice. J. Clin. Invest. 99, 391-395 (1997).
5. S.G. Hassink, E. deLancey, D.V. Sheslow, S.M. Smith-Kirwin, D.M. O'Conner, R.V. Considine, I. Opentanova, K. Dostal, M.L. Spear, K. Leef, M. Ash, A.R. Spitzer, and V.L. Funanage, Placental leptin: an important new growth factor in intrauterine and neonatal development. Pediatrics 100, 1-6 (1997).
6. C. Bjorbaek, and B.B. Kahn, Leptin signaling in the central nervous system and the periphery. Rec. Prog. Horm. Res. 59, 305-331 (2004).
7. M. Maamra, M. Bidlingmaier, M-C. Postel-Vinay, Z. Wu, C.J. Strasburger, and R.J.M. Ross, Generation of human soluble leptin receptor by proteolytic cleavage of membrane-anchored receptors. Endocrinology 142, 4389-4393 (2001).

8. O. Gavrilova, V. Barr, B. Marcus-Samuels, and M. Reitman, Hyperleptinemia of pregnancy associated with the appearance of a circulating form of the receptor. J. Biol. Chem. 272, 30546-30551 (1997).
9. R.M. Seeber, J.T. Smith, and B.J. Waddell, Plasma leptin binding activity and hypothalamic leptin receptor expression during pregnancy and lactation. Biol. Reprod. 66, 1762-1767 (2002).
10. R.V. Considine, and J.F. Caro, Leptin and the regulation of body weight, Int.J. Biochem. Cell. Biol., 29, 1255-1272 (1997).
11. W.F. Blum, P. Englaro, A.M. Attanasio, W. Kiess, and W. Rascher, Human and clinical perspectives on leptin. Proc. Nutr. Soc., 57, 477-485 (1998).
12. J.F. Caro, J. Kolaczynski, M. Nyce, J. Ohannesian, I. Opentanova. W.H. Goldman, R.B. Lynn, P.L. Zhang, M.K. Sinha, and R.V. Considine, Decreased cerebrospinal-fluid/serum leptin ratio in obesity: a possible mechanism for leptin resistance. Lancet 348, 159-161 (1996).
13. M. Schwartz, E. Peskind, M. Raskind, E. Boyko, and D. Porte, Cerebrospinal fluid leptin levels: relationship to plasma levels and to adiposity in humans. Nat. Med., 2, 589-593 (1996).
14. M. Maffei, J. Halaas, E. Ravussin, R.E. Pratley, G.H. Lee, Y. Zhang, H. Fei, S. Kim, R. Lallone, and S. Ragnathan, Leptin levels in human and rodent: Measurement of plasma leptin and *ob* RNA in obese and weight-reduced subjects. Nat. Med. 1, 1155-1161 (1995).
15. R.V. Considine, M.K. Sinha, M.L. Heiman, A. Kriauciunas, T.W. Stephens, M.R. Nyce, J.P. Ohanensian, CC. Marco, McKee LJ, and T.L. Bauer, Serum immunoreactive-leptin concentrations in normal-weight and obese humans. N. Engl J. Med. 334, 292-295 (1996).
16. V.D. Castracane, R.R. Kraemer, M.A. Franken, G.R. Kraemer, and T. Gimpel, Serum leptin concentration in women: effect of age, obesity and estrogen administration. Fertil. Steril. 70, 472-477 (1998).
17. M. Rosenbaum, and R.L. Leibel, Clinical Review 107. Role of gonadal steroids in the sexual dimorphisms in body composition and circulating levels of leptin. J. Clin. Endocrinol. Metab. 84, 1784-1789 (1999).
18. C.T. Montague, J.B. Prins, L. Sanders, J.E. Digby, and S. O'Rahilly, Depot and sex-specific differences in human leptin mRNA expression. Diabetes 46, 342-347 (1997).
19. A.M. Lefebvre, M. Laville, N. Veg, J.P. Riou, L. van Gaal, J. Auwerx, and H. Vidal, Depot-specific differences in adipose tissue gene expression in lean and obese subjects. Diabetes 47, 98-103 (1998).
20. V. Van Harmelen, S. Reynisdotir, P. Eriksson, A. Thorne, J. Hoffstedt, J. Longvist and P. Arner, Leptin secretion from subcutaneous and visceral adipose tissue of women. Diabetes 47, 913-917 (1998).
21. H. Shimizu, Y. Shimomura, Y. Nakanishi, T. Futawatari, K. Ohtani, N. Sato, and M. Mori, Estrogen increases in vivo leptin in rats and human subjects. J. Endocrinol. 154, 285-292 (1997).
22. C.S. Mantzoros, J.S. Flier, and A.D. Rogol, A longitudinal assessment of hormonal and physical alterations during normal puberty in boys, V. Rising leptin levels may signal the onset of puberty. J. Clin. Endocrinol. Metab. 82, 1066-1070 (1997).
23. M.B. Horlick, M. Rosenbaum, M. Nicolson, L.S. Levine, B. Fedun, J. Wang, R.N. Pierson Jr., and R.L. Leibel, Effect of puberty on the relationship between circulating leptin and body composition. J. Clin. Endocrinol. Metab. 85, 2509-2518 (2000).
24. J..M. Elbers, H. Asscheman, J.C. Seidell, M. Frolich, A.E. Meinders, and L.J. Gooren, Reversal of the sex difference in serum leptin levels upon cross-sex hormone administration in transsexuals. J. Clin. Endocrinol. Metab. 82, 3267-3270 (1997).
25. M. Wabitsch, W.F. Blum, R. Muche, M. Braun, F. Hube, W. Rascher, E. Heinze,

W. Teller, and H. Hauner, Contribution of androgens to the gender difference in leptin production in obese children and adolescents. J. Clin Invest. 100, 808-813 (1997).

26. X. Casabiell, V. Pineiro, R. Peino, M. Lage, J.P. Camina, R. Gallego, L.G. Vallejo, C. Dieguez, and F.F. Casanueva, Gender differences in both spontaneous and stimulated leptin secretion by human omental adipose tissue in vitro: dexamethasone and estradiol stimulate leptin release in women, but not in men. J. Clin Endocrinol. Metab. 83, 2149-2155 (1998).

27. V. Pineiro, X. Casabiell, R. Peino, M. Lage, J.P. Camina, C. Menendez, J. Baltar, C. Diguez, and F.F. Casanueva, Dihydrotestosterone, stanazol, androstenedione and dehydroepiandrosterone sulphate inhibit leptin secretion in female but not male samples of omental adipose tissue in vitro: lack of effect of testosterone. J. Endocrinol. 160, 425-432 (1999).

28. W.H. Yu, M. Kimura, A. Walczewska, S. Karanth, and S.M. McCann, Role of leptin in hypothalamic-pituitary function. Proc. Natl. Acad. Sci. 94, 1023-1028 (1997).

29. R.K. Dearth, JK Hiney, and WL Dees, Leptin acts centrally to induce the prepubertal secretion of luteinizing hormone in the female rat. Peptides 21, 387-392 (2000).

30. W.H. Yu, A. Walczewska, S. Karanth, and S.M. McCann, Nitric oxide mediates leptin-induced luteinizing hormone-releasing hormone (LHRH) and LHRH and leptin-induced LH release from the pituitary gland. Endocrinology 138, 5055-5058 (1997).

31. A. Sahu, Leptin decreases food intake induced by melanin-concentrating hormone (MCH), galanin (GAL) and neuropeptide Y (NPY) in the rat. Endocrinology 139, 4739-4742 (1998).

32. M.L. Gottsch, D.K. Clifton, and R.A. Steiner, Galanin-like peptide as a link in the integration of metabolism and reproduction. Trends Endocrinol. Metab. 15, 215-221 (2004).

33. T. Ohtaki, S. Kumano, Y. Ishibashi, K. Ogi, H. Matsui, M. Harada, C. Kitada, T. Kurokawa, H. Onda, M. Fujino, Isolation and cDNA cloning of a novel galanin-like peptide (GALP) from porcine hypothalami. J. Biol. Chem. 274, 37041-37045 (1999).

34. A. Jureus, M.J. Cunningham, M.E. McClain, D.K. Clifton, and R.A. Steiner, Galanin-like peptide (GALP) is a target for regulation by leptin in the hypothalamus of the rat, Endocrinology 141, 2703-2706 (2000).

35. J.A. Larm, and A.L. Gundlach, Galanin-like peptide (GALP) mRNA is restricted to arcuate nucleus of hypothalamus in adult male rat brain. Neuroendocrinology 72, 67-71 (2000).

36. A. Jureus, M.J. Cunningham, D. Li, L.L. Johnson, S.M. Krasnow, D.N. Telemichael, D.K. Clifton, and R.A. Steiner, Distribution and regulation of galanin-like peptide (GALP) in the hypothalamus of the mouse. Endocrinology 142, 5140-5144 (2001).

37. A. Seth, S. Stanley, P. Jethwa, J. Gardiner, M. Ghatei, and S. Bloom, Galanin-like peptide stimulates the release of gonadotropin-releasing hormone in vitro and may mediate the effects of leptin on the hypothalamic-pituitary-gonadal axis. Endocrinology 145, 743-750 (2004).

38. M.J. Cunningham, J.M. Scarlett, and R.A. Steiner, Cloning and distribution of galanin-like peptide mRNA in the hypothalamus and pituitary of the macaque. Endocrinology 143, 755-763 (2002).

39. S. Kumano, H. Matsumoto, Y. Takatsu, J. Noguchi, C. Kitada, and T. Ohtaki, Changes in hypothalamic expression levels of galanin-like peptide in rat and mouse models support that it is a leptin-target peptide. Endocrinology 144, 2634-2643 (2003).

40. A.L. Gundlach, Galanin/GALP and galanin receptors: role in central control of feeding, body weight/obesity and reproduction? Eur. J. Pharmacol. 440, 255-268 (2002).

41. J.L. Cameron and C. Nosbisch, Suppression of pulsatile luteinizing hormone and testosterone secretion during short term food restriction in the adult male rhesus monkey (Macacca mulatta). Endocrinology 128, 1532-1540 (1991).
42. M.E. Lujan, A.A. Krzemien, R.L. Reid, and D.A. Van Vugt, Caloric restriction inhibits steroid-induced gonadotropin surges in ovariectomized rhesus monkeys. Endocrine 27, 25-32 (2005).
43. J. Steiner, N. LaPaglia, L. Kirsteins, M. Emanuele, and N. Emanuele, The response of the hypothalamic-pituitary-gonadal axis to fasting is modulated by leptin. Endocr. Res. 29, 107-117 (2003).
44. M.N. Maciel, D.A. Zieba, M. Amstalden, D.H. Keisler, J.P. Neves, and G.L. Williams, Leptin prevents fasting-mediated reductions in pulsatile secretion of luteinizing hormone and enhances its gonadotropin-releasing hormone-mediated release in heifers. Biol. Reprod. 70, 229-235 (2004).
45. L.J. Hardie, D.V. Rayner, S. Holmes, and P. Trayhurn, Circulating leptin levels are modulated by fasting, cold exposure and insulin administration in lean but not Zucker (fa/fa) rats as measured by ELISA. Biochem. Biophys. Res. Commun. 223, 660-665 (1996).
46. G. Boden, X. Chen, M. Mozzoli, and I. Ryan, Effect of fasting on serum leptin in normal human subjects. J. Clin. Endocrinol. Metab. 81, 3419-3423 (1996).
47. P.D. Finn, M.J. Cunningham, K-Y F Pau, H.G. Spies, D.K. Clifton, and R.A. Steiner, The stimulatory effect of leptin on the neuroendocrine reproductive axis of the monkey. Endocrinology 139, 4652-4662 (1998).
48. J. Lado-Abeal, Y.O. Lukyanenko, S. Swamy, R.C. Hermida, J.C. Hutson, and R.L. Norman, Short-term leptin infusion does not affect circulating levels of LH, testosterone or cortisol in food restricted pubertal male rhesus monkeys. Clin. Endocrinol. 51, 41-51 (1999).
49. J. Lado-Abeal, and R.L. Norman, Leptin and reproduction in the male. In: Leptin and Reproduction. Ed. by M.C. Henson and V.D. Castracane, Kluwer Academic/Plenum Publishers, New York, PP 117-117-129 (2003).
50. F. Machinal, M-N. Dieudonne, M-C. Leneveu, R. Pecquery, and Y. Giudicelli, In vivo and in vitro *ob* gene expression and leptin secretion in rat adipocytes: evidence for a regional specific regulation by sex steroid hormones, Endocrinology 140, 1567-1574 (1999).
51. N. Yoneda, S. Saito, M. Kimura, M. Yamada, M. Iida, T. Murakami, M. Irahara, K. Shima, and T. Aono, The influence of ovariectomy on *ob* gene expression in rats. Horm. Metab. Res. 30, 263-265 (1998).
52. S-C. Chu, Y-C. Chou, J-Y. Liu, C-H. Chen, J-C. Shyu, and F-P. Chou, Fluctuation of serum leptin level in rats after ovariectomy and the influence of estrogen supplement. Life Sci. 64, 2299-2306 (1999).
53. I.E. Messinis, S.D. Milingos, E. Alexandris, I. Kariotis, G. Kollios, and K. Seferiadis, Leptinconcentrations in normal women following bilateral ovariectomy. Hum. Reprod. 14, 913- 918 (1999).
54. F. Cella, G. Giordano, and R. Cordera, Serum leptin concentrations during the menstrual cycle in normal-weight women: effects of an oral triphasic estrogen-progestin medication. Eur. J. Endocrinol. 142, 174-178 (2000).
55. M. Yamada, M. Irahara, M. Tezuka, T. Murakami, K. Shima, and T. Aono, Serum leptin profiles in the normal menstrual cycles and gonadotropin treatment cycles. Gynecol. Obstet. Invest. 49, 119-123 (2000).
56. S.R. Lindheim, M.V. Sauer, F. Carmina, P.L. Chang, R. Zimmerman, and R.A. Lobo, Circulating leptin levels during ovulation induction: relation to adiposity and ovarian Morphology. Fertil. Steril. 73, 493-498 (2000).
57. L. Unkila-Kallio, S. Andersson, H.A. Koistinen, S.L. Karonen, O. Ylikorkala, and A. Tiitinen, Leptin during assisted reproductive cycles: the effect of ovarian stimulation

and of very early pregnancy. Human Reprod. 16, 657-662 (2001).

58. J.S. O'Neil, M.E. Burow, A.E. Green, J.A. McLachlan, and M.C. Henson, Effects of estrogen on leptin gene promoter activation in MCF-7 breast cancer and JEG-3 choriocarcinoma cells: selective regulation via estrogen receptors α and β, Mol. Cell. Endocrinol. 176, 67-75 (2001).

59. D. Islami, and P. Bischof, Leptin in the placenta, in: Leptin and Reproduction, edited by M.C. Henson and V.D. Castracane, Kluwer Academic/Plenum Publishers, New York, 2003, pp. 201-220.

60. E.D. Albrecht, G.W. Aberdeen, and G.J. Pepe, The role of estrogen in the maintenance of primate pregnancy. Am. J. Obstet. Gynecol. 182, 432-438 (2000).

61. P. Mystkowski, and M.W. Schwartz, Gonadal steroids and energy homeostasis in the leptin era. Nutrition 16, 937-946 (2000).

62. F. Geisthovel, N. Jochmann, A. Widjaja, R. Horn, and G. Brabant, Serum pattern of circulating free leptin, bound leptin, and soluble leptin receptor in the physiological menstrual cycle. Fertil. Steril. 81, 398-402 (2004).

63. R. Coya, P. Martul, J. Algorta, M.A. Aniel-Quiroga, M.A. Busturia, and R. Senaris, Progesterone and human placental lactogen inhibit leptin secretion on cultured trophoblast cells from human placenta's at term. Gynecol. Endocrinol. 21, 27-32 (2005).

64. M. Rocha, C. Bing, G. Williams, and M. Puerta, Physiologic estradiol levels enhance hypothalamic expression of the long form of the leptin receptor in intact rats. J. Nutr. Biochem. 15, 328-334 (2004).

65. K. Lindell, P.A. Bennett, Y. Itoh, I.C.A.F. Robinson, L.M.S. Carlsson, and B. Carlsson, Leptin receptor 5' untranslated regions in the rat: relative abundance, genomic organization and relation to putative response elements. Mol. Cell. Endocrinol. 172, 37-45 (2001).

66. I. S. Farooqi. Leptin and the onset of puberty: insights from rodent and human genetics. Semin. Reprod. Med. 20, 139-144 (2002).

67. C.C. Cheung, J.E. Thornton, J.L. Kuijper, D.S. Weigle, D.S. Clifton, and R.A Steiner, Leptin is a metabolic gate for the onset of puberty in the female rat. Endocrinology 138, 855-858 (1997).

68. N.M. Gruaz, M. Lalaoui, D.D. Pierroz, P. Englaro, P.C. Sizonenko, W.F. Blum, and M.L. Aubert, Chronic administration of leptin into the lateral ventricle induces sexual maturation in severely food-restricted female rats. J. Neuroendocrinol. 10, 627-633 (1998).

69. R.S. Ahima, D. Prabakaran, and J.S. Flier, Postnatal leptin surge and regulation of circadian rhythm of leptin by feeding. Implications for energy homeostasis and neuroendocrine function, J. Clin. Invest. 101, 1020-1027 (1998).

70. C. R. Barb, G.J. Hausman, and K. Czaja, Leptin: a metabolic signal affecting central regulation of reproduction in the pig. Domest. Anim. Endocrinol. 29, 186-192 (2005).

71. D.L. Foster, and S. Nagatani, Physiological perspectives on leptin as a regulator of reproduction: Role in timing puberty. Biol. Reprod. 60, 205-215 (1999).

72. H.E. Paczoska-Eliasiewicz, M. Proszkowiec-Weglarz, J. Proudman, T. Jacek, M. Mika, A. Sechman, J. Rzasa, and A. Gertler, Exogenous leptin advances puberty in domestic hen. Domest. Anim. Endocrinol. Epub ahead of print (2005).

73. R.V. Garcia-Mayor, M.A. Andrade, M. Rios, M. Lage, C. Dieguez, and F.F. Casanueva, Serum leptin levels in normal children: Relationship to age, gender, body mass index, pituitary-gonadal hormones and pubertal stage. J. Clin. Endocrinol. Metab. 82, 2849-2855 (1997).

74. S. Jaruratanasirikul, L. Mo-suwan, and L. Lebel, Growth pattern and age at menarche of obese girls in a transitional society. J. Pediatr. Endocrinol. Metab. 10, 487-490 (1997).

75. R.J. Teixeira, D. Ginsbarg, J. R. Freitas, G. Fucks, C.M. Silva, and M.A. Bordallo, Serum leptin levels in premature pubarche and prepubertal girls with and without obesity. J. Pediatr. Endocrinol. Metab. 10, 1393-1398 (2004).
76. M.T. Munoz, C. de la Piedra, V. Barrios, G. Garrido, and J. Argente, Changes in bone density and bone markers in rhythmic gymnasts and ballet dancers: implications for puberty and leptin levels. Eur. J. Endocrinol. 15, 491-496 (2004).
77. N.D. Quinton, R.E. Smith, P.E. Clayton, M.S. Gill, S. Shalet, Leptin binding activity changes with age: the link between leptin and puberty. J. Clin. Endocrinol. Metab. 84, 2336-2341 (1999).
78. J. Kratzsch, A. Lammert, A. Bottner, B. Seidel, G. Mueller, J. Thiery, J. Hebebrand, and W. Kiess, Circulating soluble leptin receptor and free leptin index during childhood puberty, and adolescence. Br. J. Clin. Endocrinol. Metab. 87, 4587-4594 (2002).
79. D.R. Mann, A.O. Johnson, T. Gimpel, and V.D. Castracane, Changes in circulating leptin, leptin receptor and gonadal hormones from infancy until advanced age in humans. J. Clin. Endocrinol. Metab. 88, 3339-3345 (2003).
80. H.F. Urbanski, and K.Y. Pau, A biphasic developmental pattern of circulating leptin in the male rhesus macaque (Macaca mulatta). Endocrinology 139, 2284-2286 (1998).
81. T.M. Plant and A.R. Durrant, Circulating leptin does not appear to provide a signal for triggering the initiation of puberty in the male rhesus monkey (Macaca mulatta). Endocrinology 138, 4505-4508 (1997).
82. D.R. Mann, M.A. Akinbami, K.G. Gould, and V.D. Castracane, A longitudinal study of leptin during development in the male rhesus monkey: the effect of body composition and season on circulating leptin levels. Biol. Reprod. 62, 285-291 (2000).
83. K.J. Suter, C.R. Pohl, and M.E. Wilson, Circulating concentrations of nocturnal leptin, growth hormone and insulin-like growth factor-1 increase before the onset of puberty in agonadal male monkeys: potential signals for the initiation of puberty. J. Clin. Endocrinol. Metab. 85, 808-814 (2000).
84. T.M. Plant, Leptin, growth hormone and the onset of primate puberty. J. Clin. Endocrinol. Metab. 86, 458-460 (2001).
85. K.J. Suter, C.R. Pohl, and M.E. Wilson, Growth signals and puberty. J. Clin. Endocrinol. Metab. 86, 460 (2001).
86. N. Okudan, H. Gokbel, K. Ucok, and A. Baltaci, Serum leptin concentrations and anaerobic performance do not change during the menstrual cycle of young females. Neuro. Endocrinol. Lett. 26, 297-300 (2005).
87. T. Tiermaa, V. Luukkaa, J. Rouru, M. Koulu, and R. Huupponen, Correlation between circulating leptin and luteinizing hormone during the menstrual cycle in normal-weight women. Europ. J. Endocrinol. 130, 190-194 (1998).
88. S.M. Stock, E.M. Sande, and K.A. Bremme, Leptin levels vary significantly during the menstrual cycle, pregnancy, and in vitro fertilization treatment: possible relation to estradiol. Fertil. Steril. 72, 657-662 (1999).
89. F. Geisthovel, N. Jochmann, A. Widjaja, R. Horn, and G. Brabant, Serum patterns of circulating free leptin, bound leptin, and soluble leptin receptor in the physiological menstrual cycle. Fertil. Steril. 81, 398-402 (2004).
90. N.D. Quinton, S.M. Laird, M.A. Okon, T.C. Li, R.F. Smith, R.J. Ross, and A.I. Blakemore, Serum leptin levels during the menstrual cycle of healthy fertile women. Br. J. Biomed. Sci. 56, 16-19 (1999).
91. M.G. Riad-Gabriel, .S.D. Jinagouda, A. Sharma, R. Boyadjian, and M.F. Saaf, Changes in plasma leptin during the menstrual cycle. Eur. J. Endocrinol. 139, 528-531 (1998).
92. P.A. Tataranni, M.B. Monroe, C.A. Dueck, S. A. Traub, M. Nicolson, M.M. Manore,,

K.S. Matt, and E. Ravussin, Adiposity, plasma leptin concentration and reproductive function in active and sedentary females, Int. J. Obes. Relat. Metab. Disord. 21, 818-821 (1997).

93. M.A. Franken, T. Gimpel, P. Dimarino, B. Tawwater, and V.D. Castracane. Serum leptin changes during the menstrual cycle of normal weight and obese women. 80th Ann. Meeting, Society Program and Abstracts, p. 398, Abst. # P3-50, (1998).

94. I.E. Messinis, I. Kariotis, S. Milingos, G. Kollios, and K. Seferiadis, Treatment of normal women with oestradiol plus progesterone prevents the decrease of leptin concentrations induced by ovariectomy. Human Reprod. 15, 2383-2387 (2000).

95. I.E. Messinis, I. Papageorgiou, S. Milingos, E. Asprodini, G. Kollios, and K. Seferiadis, Oestradiol plus progesterone treatment increases serum leptin concentrations in normal women. Human Reprod. 16, 1827-1832 (2001).

96. B. Imani, M.J. Eijkemans, F.H. de Jong, N.N. Payne, P. Bouchard, L.C. Juidice, and B.C. Fraser, Free androgen index and leptin are the most prominent endocrine predictors of ovarian response during clomiphene citrate induction of ovulation in normogonadotropic oligoamenorrheic infertility. J Clin. Endocrinol. Metab. 85, 676-682 (2000).

97. C.S. Mantzoros, D.W. Cramer, R.F. Liberman, and R.L. Barbieri, Predictive value of serum and follicular fluid leptin concentrations during assisted reproductive cycles in normal women and in women with polycystic ovarian syndrome. Human Reprod. 15, 539-544 (2000).

98. P. Fedorcsak, R. Storeng, P.O. Dale, T. Tanbo, P. Torjesen, J. Urbancsek, and T. Abyholm, Leptin and leptin binding activity in the preovulatory follicle of polycystic ovary syndrome patients. Scan. J. Clin. Lab. Invest. 60, 649-655, (2000).

99. T.L. Butzow, J.M. Moilanen, M. Lehtovirta, T. Tuomi, O Hovatta, R. Siegberg, G.G. Nilsson, and D. Apter, Serum and follicular fluid leptin during in vitro fertilization: relationship among leptin increase, body fat mass, and reduced ovarian response. J. Clin. Endocrinol. Metab. 84, 3135-3139 (1999).

100. Y. Zhao, D.O. Kreger, and J.D. Brannian, Serum leptin concentrations in women during gonadotropin stimulation cycles. J. Reprod Med. 45, 121-125 (2000).

101. J.D. Brannian, S.M. Schmidt, D.O. Kreger, and K.A. Hansen, Baseline non-fasting serum leptin concentration to BMI ratio is predictive of IVF outcomes. Human Reprod. 16, 1819-1826 (2001).

102. C. Dorn, J. Reinsberg, M. Kupka, H. van der Ven, and R.L. Schild, Leptin, VEGF, IGF-1, and IGFbp-3 concentrations in serum and follicular fluid of women undergoing in vitro fertilization. Arch. Gynecol. Obstet. 268, 187-193 (2003).

103. R. Chen, B. Fisch, A. Ben-Karoush, B. Kaplan, M.Hod, and R. Orvieto, Serum and follicular fluid leptin levels in patients undergoing controlled ovarian hyperstimulation for in vitro fertilization cycle. Clin Exp Obstet Gynecol. 31, 103-106 (2004).

104. C.K. Welt, J.L. Chan, J. Bullen, R. Murphy, P. Smith, A.M. DePaoli, A. Karalis, and C.S. Mantzoros. Recombinant human leptin in women with hypothalamic amenorrhea. New Eng. J. Med. 351, 987-997 (2004).

105. M.C. Henson, and V.D. Castracane, Leptin: roles and regulation in primate pregnancy. Semin. Reprod. Med. 20,113-122 (2002).

106. M.C. Henson, and V.D. Castracane, Leptin in pregnancy: an update. Biol.Reprod. 74, 218-229 (2006).

107. M.C. Henson, and V.D. Castracane, Leptin in primate pregnancy, in: Leptin and Reproduction, edited by M.C. Henson and V.D. Castracane (Kluwer Academic/Plenum Publishers, New York, 2003), pp. 239-263.

108. N. Sagawa, S. Yura, H. Itoh, H. Mise, K. Kakui, D. Korita, M. Takemura, M.A. Nuamah, Y. Ogawa, H. Masuzaki, K. Nakao, and S. Fujii, Role of leptin in pregnancy - a review. Placenta 23 (Suppl A, Trophoblast Res 16), S80-S86 (2002)

109. E. Domali, and I.E. Messinis, Leptin in pregnancy. J. Matern. Fetal. Neonatal. Med. 12, 222-230 (2002).
110. R. Bajoria, S.R. Sooranna, B.S. Ward, and R. Chatterjee, Prospective function of placental leptin at maternal-fetal interface. Placenta 23, 103-115 (2002).
111. J. Lepercq, J-C. Challier, M. Guerre-Millo, M. Cauzac, H. Vidal, and S. Hauguel-de Mouzon, Prenatal leptin production: evidence that fetal adipose tissue produces leptin. J. Clin. Endocrinol. Metab. 86, 2409-2413 (2001).
112. S. Yura, N. Sagawa, H. Mise, T. Mori, H. Masuzaki, Y. Ogawa, and K. Nakao, A positive umbilical venous-arterial difference of leptin level and its rapid decline after birth. Am. J. Obstet. Gynecol. 178, 926-930 (1998).
113. H. Masuzaki, Y. Ogawa, N. Sagawa, K. Hosoda, T. Matsumoto, H. Mise, H. Nishimura, Y. Yoshimasa, I. Tanaka, T. Mori, and K. Nakao, Non-adipose tissue production of leptin: leptin as a novel placenta-derived hormone in humans. Nat. Med. 3, 1029-1033 (1997).
114. N. Hoggard, J. Crabtree, S. Allstaff, D.R. Abramovich, and P. Haggarty, Leptin secretion to both the maternal and fetal circulations in the ex vivo perfused human term placenta. Placenta 22, 347-352 (2001).
115. G.M. Butterstein, and V.D. Castracane, The influence of the number of fetal/placental units on maternal serum leptin in the pregnant rat. Biol. Reprod. 66 (Suppl 1), 229 (2002).
116. V.D. Castracane, C. Hermann, and T.L. Gimpel, Serum leptin levels in multiple gestations indicating minimal placental leptin in maternal circulation. J. Soc. Gynecol. Invest. 9 (Program Suppl), 220A (2002).
117. M. Kawai, M. Yamaguchi, T. Murakami, K. Shima, Y. Murata, and K. Kishi, The placenta is not the main source of leptin production in pregnant rat: gestational profile of leptin in plasma and adipose tissues. Biochem. Biophys. Res. Commun. 240, 798-802 (1997).
118. E.K. Chien, M. Hara, M. Rouard, H. Yano, M. Phillippe, K.S. Polonsky, and G.I. Bell, Increase in serum leptin and uterine leptin receptor messenger RNA levels during pregnancy in rats. Biochem. Biophys. Res. Commun. 237, 476-480 (1997).
119. T. Tomimatsu, M. Yamaguchi, T. Murakami, K. Ogura, M. Sakata, N. Mitsuda, T. Kanzaki, H. Kurachi, M. Irahara, A. Miyake, K. Shima, T. Aono, and Y. Murata, Increase of mouse leptin production by adipose tissue after midpregnancy: gestational profile of serum leptin concentration. Biochem. Biophys. Res. Commun. 240, 213-215 (1997).
120. M.C. Henson, K.F. Swan, and J.S. O'Neil, Expression of placental leptin and leptin receptor transcripts in early pregnancy and at term. Obstet. Gynecol. 92, 1020-1028 (1998).
121. M.C. Henson, V.D. Castracane, J.S. O'Neil, T. Gimpel, K.F. Swan, A.E. Green, and W. Shi, Serum leptin concentrations and expression of leptin transcripts in placental trophoblast with advancing baboon pregnancy. J. Clin. Endocrinol. Metab. 84, 2543-2549 (1999).
122. V.D. Castracane, A.G. Hendrickx, and M.C. Henson, Serum leptin in nonpregnant and pregnant women and in old and new world nonhuman primates: a brief communication. Exp. Biol. Med. (Maywood) 230, 251-254 (2005).
123. J.A. Amico, A. Thomas, R.S. Crowley, and L.A. Burmeister, Concentrations of leptin in the serum of pregnant, lactating, and cycling rats and of leptin messenger ribonucleic acid in rat placental tissue. Life Sci. 63, 1387-1395 (1998).
124. M.D. Garcia, F.F. Casanueva, C. Dieguez, and R.M. Senaris, Gestational profile of leptin messenger ribonucleic acid (mRNA) content in the placenta and adipose tissue in the rat, and regulation of the mRNA levels of the leptin receptor subtypes in the hypothalamus during pregnancy and lactation. Biol. Reprod. 62, 698-703 (2000).
125. N. Hoggard, L. Hunter, R.G. Lea, P. Trayhurn, and J.G. Mercer, Ontogeny of the

expression of leptin and its receptor in the murine fetus and placenta. Br. J. Nutr. 83, 317-326 (2000).
126. N.M. Malik, N.D. Carter, C.A. Wilson, R.J. Scaramuzzi, M.J. Stock, and J.F. Murray, Leptin expression in the fetus and placenta during mouse pregnancy. Placenta 26, 47-52 (2005).
127. M.C. Henson, Pregnancy maintenance and the regulation of placental progesterone biosynthesis in the baboon. Hum. Reprod. Update 4, 389-405 (1998).
128. A.G. Comuzzie, S.A. Cole, L. Martin, K.D. Carey, M.C. Mahaney, J. Blangero, and J.L. VandeBerg, The baboon as a nonhuman primate model for the study of the genetics of obesity. Obes. Res. 11, 75-80 (2003).
129. S.A. Cole, L.J. Martin, K.W. Peebles, M.M. Leland, K. Rice, J.L. VandeBerg, J. Blangero, and A.G. Comuzzie, Genetics of leptin expression in baboons. Int. J. Obes. Rel. Metab. Disord. 27, 778-783 (2003).
130. C. Wang, M.S. Medan, K. Shimizu, C. Kojima, M. Itoh, G. Watanabe, and K. Taya, Section of leptin throughout pregnancy and early postpartum period in Japanese monkeys: placenta as another potential source of leptin. Endocrine 27, 75-82 (2005).
131. F. Akerman, Z.M. Lei, and C.V. Rao, Human umbilical cord and fetal membranes co-express leptin and its receptor genes. Gynecol. Endocrinol. 16, 299-306 (2002).
132. A.E. Green, J.S. O'Neil, K.F. Swan, R.P. Bohm Jr, M.S. Ratterree, and M.C. Henson, Leptin receptor transcripts are constitutively expressed in placenta and adipose tissue with advancing baboon pregnancy. Proc. Soc. Exp. Biol. Med. 223, 362-366 (2000).
133. S.R. Ladyman, and D.R. Grattan, Suppression of leptin receptor mRNA and leptin responsiveness in the ventromedial nucleus of the hypothalamus during pregnancy in the rat. Endocrinology 146, 3868-3874 (2005).
134. O. Zastrow, B. Seidel, W. Kiess, J. Thiery, E. Keller, A. Bottner, and J. Kratzsh, The soluble leptin receptor is crucial for leptin action: evidence from clinical and experimental data. Int. J. Obes. Relat. Metab. Disord. 27, 1472-1478 (2003).
135. G. Yang, H. Ge, A. Boucher, X. Yu, and C. Li, Modulation of direct leptin signaling by soluble leptin receptor. Mol. Endocrinol. 18, 1354-1362 (2004).
136. N. Kado, J. Kitawaki, H. Koshiba, H. Ishihara, Y. Kitaoka, M. Teramoto, and H. Honjo, Relationships between the serum levels of soluble leptin receptor and free and bound leptin in non-pregnant women of reproductive age and women undergoing controlled ovarian hyperstimulation. Hum. Reprod. 18, 715-720 (2003).
137. J. Krizova, V. Eretova, D. Haluzikova, K. Anderlova, S. Housova, E. Kotrilikova, and M. Haluzik, Soluble leptin receptor and leptin levels in pregnant women before and after delivery. Endocr. Res. 30, 379-385 (2004).
138. A. Lammert, W. Kiess, A. Bottner, A. Glasow, and J. Kratzsch, Soluble leptin receptor represents the main leptin binding activity in human blood. Biochem. Biophys. Res. Commun. 283, 982-988 (2001).
139. L. Huang, Z. Wang, and C. Li, Modulation of circulating leptin levels by its soluble receptor. J. Biol. Chem. 276, 6343-6349 (2001).
140. A. Lammert, G. Brockmann, U. Renne, W. Kiess, A. Bottner, J. Thiery, and J. Kratzsch, Different isoforms of the soluble leptin receptor in non-pregnant and pregnant mice. Biochem. Biophys. Res. Commun. 298, 798-804 (2002).
141. S. Schulz, C. Hackel, and W. Weise, Hormonal regulation of neonatal weight: placental leptin and leptin receptors. BJOG 107, 1486-1491 (2000).
142. D.E. Edwards, R.P. Bohm, Jr., J. Purcell, M.S. Ratterree, K.F. Swan, V.D. Castracane, and M.C. Henson, Two isoforms of the leptin receptor are enhanced in pregnancy-specific tissues and soluble leptin receptor is enhanced in maternal serum with advancing gestation in the baboon. Biol. Reprod. 71, 1746-1752 (2004).
143. P. Cameo, and A.T. Fazleabas, Expression of a new small soluble leptin receptor isoform in the primate decidua but not in the placenta. J. Soc. Gynecol. Invest. (Suppl) 12, abstract 671 (2005).

144. C.J. Ashworth, N. Hoggard, L. Thomas, J.G. Mercer, J.M. Wallace, and R.G. Lea, Placental leptin. Rev. Reprod. 5, 18-24 (2000).
145. P. Cameo, P. Bischof, and J.C. Calvo, Effect of leptin on progesterone, human chorionic gonadotropin and interleukin-6 secretion by human term trophoblast cells in culture. Biol Reprod 68, 472-477 (2003).
146. D. Islami, P. Bischof, and D. Chardonnens, Possible interactions between leptin, gonadotrophin-releasing hormone (GnRH-I and II) and human chorionic gonadotrophin (hCG). Eur. J. Obstet. Gynecol. Reprod. Biol. 110, 169-175 (2003).
147. M. Lappas, M. Permezel, and G.E. Rice, Leptin and adiponectin stimulate the release of proinflammatory cytokines and prostaglandins from human placenta and maternal adipose tissue via Nuclear Factor-κB, Peroxisomal Proliferator-Activated Receptor-γ and Extracellularly Regulated Kinase 1/2. Endocrinology 146, 3334-3342 (2005).
148. R.Coya, O. Gualillo, J. Pineda, M.C. Garcia, M.A. Busturia, A. Aniel-Quiroga, P. Martul, and R.M. Senaris, Effect of cyclic 3',5'-adenosine monophosphate, glucocorticoids, and insulin on leptin messenger RNA levels and leptin secretion in cultured human trophoblast. Biol. Reprod. 65, 814-819 (2001).
149. R.R. Gonzalez, P. Caballero-Campo, M. Jasper, A. Mercader, L. Devoto, A. Pellicer, and C. Simon, Leptin and leptin receptor are expressed in the human endometrium and endometrial leptin secretion is regulated by the human blastocyst. J. Clin. Endocrinol. Metab. 85, 4883-4888 (2000).
150. K. Kawamura, N. Sato, J. Fukuda, H. Kodama, J. Kumagai, H. Tanikawa, M. Murata, and T. Tanaka, The role of leptin during the development of mouse preimplantation embryos. Mol. Cell. Endocrinol. 202, 185-189 (2003).
151. J.A. Craig, H. Zhu, P.W. Dyce, L. Wen, and J. Li, Leptin enhances porcine preimplantation embryo development in vitro. Mol. Cell. Endocrinol. 229, 141-147 (2005).
152. R.R. Gonzalez, L. Devoto, A. Campana, and P. Bischof, Effects of leptin, interleukin-1α, interleukin-6, and transforming growth factor-β on markers of trophoblast invasive phenotype: integrins and metalloproteinases. Endocrine 15, 157-164 (2001).
153. M. Castellucci, R. De Matteis, A. Meisser, R. Cancello, Monsurro V, Islami D, Sarzani R, Marzioni D, Cinti S, and P. Bischof, Leptin modulates extracellular matrix molecules and metalloproteinases: possible implications for trophoblast invasion. Mol. Hum. Reprod. 6, 951-958 (2000).
154. F. Dominguez, A. Pellicer, and C. Simon, Paracrine dialogue in implantation. Mol. Cell. Endocrinol. 186, 175-181 (2002).
155. M. Boelhauve, F. Sinowatz, E. Wolf, and F.F. Paula-Lopes, Maturation of bovine oocytes in the presence of leptin improves development and reduces apotosis of in vitro produced
blastocysts. Biol. Reprod. Epub ahead of print as 10.1095/biolreprod.105.041103 (2005).
156. A. Cervero, J.A. Horcajadas, J. Martin, A. Pellicer, and C. Simon, The leptin system during human endometrial receptivity and preimplantation development. J. Clin. Endocrinol. Metab. 89, 2442-2451 (2004).
157. A. Cervero, J.A. Horcajadas, F. Dominguez, A. Pellicer, and C. Simon, Leptin system in embryo development and implantation: a protein in search of a function. Reprod. Biomed. Online 10, 217-223 (2005).
158. S.J. Yoon, K.Y. Cha, and K.A. Lee, Leptin receptors are down-regulated in uterine implantation sites compared to interimplantation sites. Mol. Cell. Endocrinol. 232, 27-35 (2005).
159. P. Cameo, and A. Fazleabas, Chorionic gonadotropin regulates leptin secretion in the baboon decidua. Society for the Study of Reproduction. Vancouver, BC, Abstract #502. (2004).

160. M.P. Ramos, B.R. Rueda, P.C. Leavis, and R.R. Gonzalez, Leptin serves as an upstream activator of an obligatory signaling cascade in the embryo-implantation process. Endocrinology 146, 694-701 (2005).
161. L.C. Schulz, and E.P. Widmaier, The effect of leptin on mouse trophoblast cell invasion. Biol. Reprod. 71, 1963-1967 (2004).
162. C.M. Steppan, and A.G. Swick, A role for leptin in brain development. Biochem. Biophys. Res. Commun. 256, 600-602 (1999).
163. N. Hoggard, P. Haggarty, L. Thomas, and R.G. Lea, Leptin expression in placental and fetal tissues: does leptin have a functional role? Biochem. Soc. Trans. 29, 57-63 (2001).
164. H. Christou, J.M. Connors, M. Ziotopoulou, V. Hatzidakis, E. Papathanassoglou, S.A. Ringer, and C.S. Mantzoros, Cord blood leptin and insulin-like growth factor levels are independent predictors of fetal growth. J. Clin. Endocrinol. Metab. 86, 935-938 (2001).
165. E. Petridou, C.S. Mantzoros, M. Belechri, A. Skalkidou, N. Dessypris, E. Papathoma, H. Salvanos, J.H. Lee, S. Kedikoglu, G. Chrousos, and D. Trichopoulos, Neonatal leptin levels are strongly associated with female gender, birth length, IGF-I levels and formula feeding. Clin. Endocrinol. (Oxf.) 2, 366-371 (2005).
166. H-C. Lo, L-Y. Tsao, W-Y. Hsu, H-N. Chen, W-K. Yu, and C-Y. Chi, Relation of cord serum levels of growth hormone, insulin-like growth factors, insulin-like growth factor binding proteins, leptin, and interleukin-6 with birth weight, birth length, and head circumference in term and preterm neonates. Nutrition 18, 604-608 (2002).
167. R.G. Lea, D. Howe, L.T. Hannah, O. Bonneau, L. Hunter, and N. Hoggard, Placental leptin in normal, diabetic and fetal growth-retarded pregnancies. Mol. Hum. Reprod. 6, 763-769 (2000).
168. S.R. Sooranna, S. Ward, and R. Bajoria, Discordant fetal leptin levels in monochorionic twins with chronic midtrimester twin-twin transfusion syndrome. Placenta 22, 392-398 (2001).
169. S.R. Sooranna, S. Ward, and R. Bajoria, Fetal leptin influences birth weight in twins with discordant growth. Pediatr. Res. 49, 667-672 (2001).
170. L. Yildiz, B. Avci, and M. Ingec, Umbilical cord and maternal blood leptin concentrations in intrauterine growth retardation. Clin. Chem. Lab. Med. 40, 1114-1117 (2002).
171. T-F. Chan, Y-F. Chung, H-S. Chen, J-H. Su, and S-SF. Yuan, Elevated amniotic fluid leptin levels in early second trimester are associated with earlier delivery and lower birthweight in twin pregnancy. Acta. Obstet. Gynecol. Scand. 83, 707-710 (2004).
172. D. Jaquet, A. Gaboriau, P. Czernichow, and C. Levy-Marchal, Relatively low serum leptin levels in adults born with intra-uterine growth retardation. Int. J. Obes. Relat. Metab. Disord. 25, 491-495 (2001).
173. O. Ogueh, S. Sooranna, K.H. Nicolaides, and M.R. Johnson, The relationship between leptin concentration and bone metabolism in the human fetus. J. Clin. Endocrinol. Metab. 5, 1997-1999 (2000).
174. J.O. Gordeladze, J.E. Reseland, and C.A. Drevon, Pharmacological interference with transcriptional control of osteoblasts: a possible role for leptin and fatty acids in maintaining bone strength and body lean mass. Curr. Pharm. Des. 7, 275-290 (2001).
175. F. Elefteriou, S. Takeda, K. Ebihara, J. Magre, N. Patano, C.A. Kim, Y. Ogawa, X. Liu, S.M. Ware, W.J. Craigen, J.J. Robert, C. Vinson, K. Nakao, J. Capeau, and G. Karsenty, Serum leptin level is a regulator of bone mass. Proc. Natl. Acad. Sci. USA 101, 3258-3263 (2004).
176. T. Whipple, N. Sharkey, L. Demers, and N. Williams, Leptin and the skeleton. Clin. Endocrinol. (Oxf.) 57, 701-711 (2002).
177. K. Kume, K. Satomura, S. Nishisho, E. Kitaoka, K. Yamanouchi, S. Tobiume, and M. Nagayama, Potential role of leptin in endochondral ossification. J. Histochem.

Cytochem. 50, 159-169 (2002).
178. M.R. Sierra-Honigmann, A.K. Nath, C. Murakami, G. Garcia-Cardena, A. Papapetropoulos, W.C. Sessa, L.A. Madge, J.S. Schechner, M.B. Schwabb, P.J. Polverini, and J.R. Flores-Riveros, Biological action of leptin as an angiogenic factor. Science 281, 1683-1686 (1998).
179. A. Bouloumie, K. Lolmede, C. Sengenes, J. Galitzky, and M. Lafontan, Angiogenesis in adipose tissue. Ann. Endocrinol. (Paris) 63, 91-95 (2002).
180. D. Islami, P. Bischof, and D. Chardonnens, Modulation of placental vascular endothelial growth factor by leptin and hCG. Mol. Hum. Reprod. 9, 395-398 (2003).
181. J.S. Torday, H. Sun, L. Wang, E. Torres, M.E. Sunday, and L.P. Rubin, Leptin mediates the parathyroid hormone-related protein paracrine stimulation of fetal lung maturation. Am. J. Physiol. Lung Cell. Mol. Physiol. 282, L405-L410 (2002).
182. J.S. Torday, and V.K. Rehan, Stretch-stimulated surfactant synthesis is coordinated by the paracrine actions of PTHrP and leptin. Am. J. Physiol. Lung Cell. Mol. Physiol. 283, L130-L135 (2002).
183. M.C. Henson, K.F. Swan, D.E. Edwards, G.W. Hoyle, J. Purcell, and V.D. Castracane, Leptin receptor expression in fetal lung increases in late gestation in the baboon: a model for human pregnancy. Reproduction 127, 87-94 (2004).
184. N. Kronfeld-Schor, J. Zhao, B.A. Silvia, E. Bicer, P.T. Matthews, R. Urban, S. Zimmerman, T.H. Kunz, and E.P. Widmaier, Steroid-dependent up-regulation of adipose leptin secretion in vitro during pregnancy in mice. Biol. Reprod. 63, 274-280 (2000).
185. M. Yamada, T. Matsuzaki, T. Iwasa, F. Shimizu, N. Tanaka, R. Ogata, M. Kiyokama, T. Yasui, M. Irahara, and T. Aono, Serum leptin levels in women throughout life; relationship to body mass index and serum estradiol levels. Jpn. J. Reprod. Endocrinol. 8, 55-60 (2003).
186. M. Monjo, E. Pujol, and P. Roca, Alpha-2 to beta-3 adrenoceptor switch in 3T3-L1 preadipocytes and adipocytes: modulation by testosterone, 17-beta estradiol, and progesterone. Am. J. Physiol. Endocrinol. Metab. 289, E145-E150 (2005).
187. M. Tanaka, S. Nakaya, T. Kumai, M. Watanabe, T. Tateishi, H. Shimizu, and S. Kobayashi, Effects of estrogen on serum leptin levels and leptin mRNA expression in adipose tissue in rats. Horm. Res. 56, 98-104 (2001).
188. J.S. O'Neil, A.E. Green, D.E. Edwards, K.F. Swan, T. Gimpel, V.D. Castracane, and M.C. Henson, Regulation of leptin and leptin receptor in baboon pregnancy: effects of advancing gestation and fetectomy. J. Clin. Endocrinol. Metab. 86, 2518-2524 (2001).
189. S. Bi, O. Gavrilova, D.W. Gong, M.M. Mason, and M. Reitman, Identification of a placental enhancer for the human leptin gene. J. Biol. Chem. 272, 30583-30588 (1997).
190. K. Ebihara, Y. Ogawa, N. Isse, K. Mori, N. Tamura, H. Masuzaki, K. Kohno, S. Yura, K. Hosoda, N. Sagawa, and K. Nakao, Identification of the human leptin 5' flanking sequences involved in the trophoblast-specific transcription. Biochem. Biophys. Res. Commun. 241, 658-663 (1997).
191. J.T. Smith, and B.J. Waddell, Leptin distribution and metabolism in the pregnant rat: transplacental leptin passage increases in late gestation but is reduced by excess glucocorticoids. Endocrinology 144, 3024-3030 (2003).
192. C.S. Wyrwoll, P.J. Mark, and B.J. Waddell, Directional secretion and transport of leptin and expression of leptin receptor isoforms in human placental BeWo cells. Mol. Cell. Endocrinol., Epub ahead of print as pmid 15955620 (2005).
193. A. Leal-Cerro, A. Soto, M.A. Martinez, C. Dieguez, and F.F. Casanueva, Influence of cortisol status on leptin secretion. Pituitary 4, 111-116 (2001).
194. A.J. Forhead, J. Thomas, J. Crabtree, N. Hoggard, D.S. Gardner, D.A. Giussani, and A.L. Fowden, Plasma leptin concentration in fetal sheep during late gestation:

ontogeny and effect of glucocorticoids. Endocrinology 143, 1166-1173 (2002).
195. Y. Faulconnier, C. Delavaud, and Y. Chilliard, Insulin and (or) dexamethasone effects on leptin production and metabolic activities of ovine adipose tissue explants. Reprod. Nutr. Dev. 43, 237-250 (2003).
196. B.S.J. Yuen, P.C. Owens, M.E. Symonds, D.H. Keisler, J.R. McFarlane, K.G. Kauter, and I.C. McMillen, Effects of leptin on fetal plasma adrenocorticotropic hormone and cortisol concentrations and the timing of parturition in the sheep. Biol. Reprod. 70, 1650-1657 (2004).
197. D.C. Howe, A. Gertler, and J.R.G. Challis, The late gestation increase in circulating ACTH and cortisol in the fetal sheep is suppressed by intracerebroventricular infusion of recombinant ovine leptin. J. Endocrinol. 174, 259-262 (2002).
198. S.M. Laird, N.D. Quinton, B. Anstie, T.C. Li, and A.I. Blakemore, Leptin and leptin binding activity in women with recurrent miscarriage: correlation with pregnancy outcome. Hum. Reprod. 16, 2008-2013 (2001).
199. T.G. Ramsay, and M.P. Richards, Hormonal regulation of leptin and leptin receptor expression in porcine subcutaneous adipose tissue. J. Anim. Sci. 82, 3486-3492 (2004).
200. J.T. Smith, and B.J. Waddell, Leptin receptor expression in the rat placenta: changes in Ob-Ra, Ob-Rb, and Ob-Re with gestational age and suppression by glucocorticoids. Biol. Reprod. 67, 1204-1210 (2002).
201. B.J. Waddell, and J.T. Smith, in: Leptin and Reproduction, edited by M.C. Henson and V.D. Castracane (Kluwer Academic/Plenum Publishers, New York, 2003) pp. 221-238.
202. R. Ishida-Takahashi, S. Uotani, T. Abe, M. Degawa-Yamauchi, T. Fukushima, N. Fujita, H. Sakamaki, H. Yamasaki, Y. Yamaguchi, and K. Eguchi, Rapid inhibition of leptin signaling by glucocorticoids in vitro and in vivo. J. Biol. Chem. 279, 19658-19664 (2004).
203. N. Anim-Nyame, S.R. Sooranna, P.J. Steer, and M.R. Johnson, Longitudinal analysis of maternal plasma leptin concentrations during normal pregnancy and pre-eclampsia. Hum. Reprod. 15, 2033-2036 (2000).
204. R.J. Teppa, R.B. Ness, W.R. Crombleholme, and J.M. Roberts, Free leptin is increased in normal pregnancy and further increased in preeclampsia. Metabolism 49, 1043-1048 (2000).
205. K. Linnemann, A. Malek, H. Schneider, and C. Fusch, Physiological and pathological regulation of feto/placento/maternal leptin expression. Biochem. Soc. Trans. 29, 86-90 (2001).
206. L.C. Chappell, P.T. Seed, A. Briley, F.J. Kelly, B.J. Hunt, D.S. Charnock-Jones, A.I. Mallet, and L. Poston, A longitudinal study of biochemical variables in women at risk of preeclampsia. Am. J. Obstet. Gynecol. 187, 127-136 (2002).
207. R.A. Odegard, L.J. Vatten, S.T. Nilsen, K.A. Salvesen, and R. Austgulen, Umbilical cord plasma leptin is increased in preeclampsia. Am. J. Obstet. Gynecol. 186, 427-432 (2002).
208. T. Reimer, D. Koczan, B. Gerber, D. Richter, H.J. Thiesen, and K. Friese, Microarray analysis of differentially expressed genes in placental tissue of pre-eclampsia: up-regulation of obesity-related genes. Mol. Hum. Reprod. 8, 674-680 (2002).
209. Y. Kocyigit, Y. Atamer, A. Atamer, A. Tuzcu, and Z. Akkus, Changes in serum levels of leptin, cytokines and lipoprotein in pre-eclamptic and normotensive pregnant women. Gynecol. Endocrinol. 19, 267-273 (2004).
210. A. Baksu, A. Ozkan, N. Goker, B. Baksu, and A. Uluocak, Serum leptin changes in preeclamptic pregnant women: relationship to thyroid-stimulating hormone, body mass index, and proteinuria. Am. J. Perinatol. 22, 161-164 (2005).
211. T.F. Chan, J.H. Su, Y.F. Chung, Y.H. Hsu, Y.T. Yeh, S.B. Jong, and S.S. Yuan, Amniotic fluid and maternal serum leptin levels in pregnant women who

subsequently develop preeclampsia. Eur. J. Obstet. Gynecol. Reprod. Biol. 108, 50-53 (2003).
212. G.A. Tommaselli, M. Pighetti, A. Nasti, A. D'Elia, M. Guida, C. Di Carlo, G. Bifulco, and C. Nappi, Serum leptin levels and uterine Doppler flow velocimetry at 20 weeks gestation as markers for the development of preeclampsia. Gynecol. Endocrinol. 19, 160-165 (2004).
213. M. Acromite, M. Ziotopoulou, C. Orlova, and C. Mantzoros, Increased leptin levels in preeclampsia: associations with BMI, estrogen and SHBG levels. Hormones 3, 46-52 (2004).
214. J. Challier, M. Galtier, T. Bintein, A. Cortez, J. Lepercq, and S. Hauguel-de Mouzon, Placental receptor isoforms in normal and pathological pregnancies. Placenta 24, 92-99 (2003).
215. R.H. Li, S.C. Poon, M.Y. Yu, and Y.F. Wong, Expression of placental leptin and leptin receptors in preeclampsia. Int. J. Gynecol. Pathol. 23, 378-385 (2004).
216. S. Iwagaki, Y. Yokoyama, L. Tang, Y. Takahashi, Y. Nakagawa, and T. Tamaya, Augmentation of leptin and hypoxia-inducible factor 1 alpha mRNAs in the preeclamptic placenta. Gynecol. Endocrinol. 18, 263-268 (2004).
217. N. Vitoratos, G. Chrystodoulacos, E. Salamalekis, D. Kassanos, E. Kouskouni, and G. Creatsas, Fetoplacental leptin levels and their relation to birth weight and insulin in gestational diabetic pregnant women. J. Obstet. Gynaecol. 22, 29-33 (2002).
218. T. Radaelli, A. Varastehpour, P. Catalano, and S. Hauguel-de Mouzon, Gestational diabetes induces placental genes for chronic stress and inflammatory pathways. Diabetes 52, 2951-2958 (2003).
219. J.G. Manderson, C.C. Patterson, D.R. Hadden, A.I. Traub, H. Leslie, and D.R. McCance, Leptin concentrations in maternal serum and cord blood in diabetic and nondiabetic pregnancy. Am. J. Obstet. Gynecol. 188, 1326-1332 (2003).
220. R.S. Lindsay, B.A. Hamilton, A.A. Calder, F.D. Johnstone, and J.D. Walker, The relation of insulin, leptin and IGF-1 to birthweight in offspring of women with type 1 diabetes. Clin. Endocrinol. (Oxf.) 61, 353-359 (2004).
221. M.P. Malee, A. Verma, G. Messerlian, R. Tucker, and B.R. Vohr, Association between maternal and child leptin levels 9 years after pregnancy complicated by gestational diabetes. Horm. Metab. Res. 34, 212-216 (2002).
222. M. Lappas, K. Yee, M. Permezel, and G.E. Rice, Release and regulation of leptin, resistin, and adiponectin from human placenta, fetal membranes, and maternal, adipose tissue and skeletal muscle from normal and gestational diabetes mellitus complicated pregnancies. J. Endocrinol. 186, 457-465 (2005).
223. T. Hytinantti, H.A. Koistinen, V.A. Koivisto, S.L. Karonen, E.M. Rutanen, and S. Andersson, Increased leptin concentration in preterm infants of pre-eclamptic mothers. Arch. Dis. Child. Fetal. Neonatal. Ed. 83, F13-F16 (2000).
224. T. Hytinantti, H.A. Koistinen, K. Teramo, S.L. Karonen, V.A. Koivisto, and S. Andersson, Increased fetal leptin in type I diabetes mellitus pregnancies complicated by chronic hypoxia. Diabetologia 43, 709-713 (2000).
225. A. Grosfeld, J. Andre, S. Hauguel-de Mouzon, E. Berra, J. Pouyssegur, and M. Guerre-Millo, Hypoxia-inducible factor I transactivates the human leptin gene promoter. J. Biol. Chem. 277, 42953-42957 (2002).
226. L. Poston, Does leptin play a role in preeclampsia?, in: Leptin and Reproduction, edited by M.C. Henson and V.D. Castracane (Kluwer Academic/Plenum Publishers, New York, 2003) pp. 299-310.
227. D.J.P. Barker, In utero programming of chronic disease. Clin. Sci. 95, 115-128 (1998).
228. D.J.P. Barker, J.G. Eriksson, T. Forsen, and C. Osmond, Fetal origins of adult disease: strength of effects and biological basis. Int. J. Epidemiol. 31, 1235-1239 (2002).

229. S.G. Bouret, S.J. Draper, and R.B. Simerly, Formation of projection pathways from the arcuate nucleus of the hypothalamus to hypothalamic regions implicated in the neural control of feeding behavior in mice. J. Neurosci. 24, 2797-2805 (2004).
230. S.G. Bouret, S.J. Draper, and R.B. Simerly, Trophic action of leptin on hypothalamic neurons that regulate feeding. Science 304, 108-110 (2004).
231. M.G. Ross, and M. Desai, Gestational programming: population survival effects of drought and famine during pregnancy. Am. J. Physiol. Regul. Integr. Comp. Physiol. 288, R97-R103 (2005).
232. A. Lecklin, M.G. Dube, R.N. Torto, P.S. Kalra, and S.P. Kalra, Perigestational suppression of weight gain with central leptin gene therapy results in lower weight F1 generation. Peptides 26, 1176-1187 (2005).
233. J. Matsuda, I. Yokota, M. Iida, T. Murakami, E. Naito, and Y. Kuroda, Serum leptin concentration in cord blood: relationship to birth weight and gender. J. Clin. Endocrinol. Metab. 82, 1642-1644 (1997).
234. T. Ertl, S. Funke, I. Sarkany, I. Szabo, W. Rascher, W.F. Blum, and E. Sulyok, Postnatal changes of leptin levels in full-term and preterm neonates: their relation to intrauterine growth gender and testosterone. Biol. Neonate 75, 167-176 (1999).
235. C. Maffeis, P. Moghetti, R. Vettor, A.M. Lombardi, S. Vecchini, and L. Tato. Leptin concentration in newborns' cord blood: relationship to gender and growth-regulating hormones. Int. J. Obes. Relat. Metab. Disord. 23, 943-947 (1999).
236. T. Laml, B.W. Hartmann, O. Preyer, E. Ruecklinger, G. Soeregi, and P. Wagenbichler, Serum leptin concentration in cord blood: relationship to birth weight and gender in pregnancies complicated by pre-eclampsia. Gynecol. Endocrinol. 14, 442-447 (2000).
237. S. Akcurin, S. Velipasaoglu, G. Akcurin, and M. Guntekin, Leptin profile in neonatal gonadtropin surge and relationship between leptin and body mass index in early infancy. J. Pediatr. Endocrinol. Metab. 18, 189-195 (2005).
238. M. Tena-Sempere, L. Pinilla, F.P. Zhang, L.C. Gonzalez, I. Huhtaniemi, F.F. Casanueva, C. Dieguez, and E. Aguilar, Developmental and hormonal regulation of leptin receptor (*Ob-R*) messenger ribonucleic acid expression in rat testis. Biol. Reprod. 64, 634-643 (2001).
239. M. Caprio, E. Fabbrini, G. Ricci S. Basciani, L. Gnessi, M. Arizzi, A.R. Carta, M.U. DeMartino, A.M. Isidori, G.V. Frajese, and A. Fabbri, Ontogenesis of leptin receptor in rat Leydig cells. Biol. Reprod. 68, 1199-1207 (2003).
240. M. Tena-Sempere, and M.L. Barreiro, Leptin in male reproduction: the testis paradigm. Mol. Cell. Endocrinol. 188, 9-13 (2002).
241. I. Kus, M. Sarsilimaz, S. Canpolat, B. Yilmaz, H. Kelestimur, N. Akpolat, and C. Ozogul, Immunohistochemical, histological and ultrastructural evaluation of the effects of leptin on testes in mice. Arch. Androl. 51, 395-405 (2005).
242. S. Soyupek, A. Armagan, T.A. Serel, M.B. Hoscan, H. Perk, E. Karaoz, and O. Candir, Leptin expression in the testicular tissue of fertile and infertile men. Arch. Androl. 51, 239-246 (2005).
243. H.J. Glander, A. Lammert, U. Paasch, A. Glasow, and J. Kratzsch, Leptin exists in tubuli seminiferi and in seminal plasma. Andrologia 34, 227-233 (2002).
244. S. Aquila, M. Gentile, E. Middea, S. Catalano, C. Morelli, V. Pezzi, and S. Ando, Leptin secretion in human ejaculated spermatozoa. J. Clin. Endocrinol. Metab. 90, 4753-4761 (2005).
245. N. Lima, H. Cavaliere, M. Knobel, A. Halpern, and G. Medeiros-Neto, Decreased androgen levels in massively obese men may be associated with impaired function of the gonadostat. Int. J. Obes. Relat. Metab. Disord. 24. 1433-1437 (2000).
246. H.U. von Sobbe, C. Koebnick, L. Jenne, and F. Kiesewetter, Leptin concentrations in semen are correlated with serum leptin levels and elevated in hypergonadotrophic hypogonadism. Andrologia 35, 233-237 (2003).

Chapter 10

LEPTIN AND CARDIOVASCULAR DISEASE

Kamal Rahmouni[1,2], Marcelo L. Correia[1,2,3], William G. Haynes[1,2,3]
[1]*Specialized Center of Research in Hypertension Genetics;* [2]*Department of Internal Medicine; and* [3]*General Clinical Research Center; University of Iowa, Iowa City, Iowa*

Abstract: Obesity is associated with increased cardiovascular morbidity and mortality, in part through development of hypertension. Recent observations suggest that the cardiovascular actions of leptin may help explain the link between excess fat mass and cardiovascular diseases. Leptin causes a significant increase in overall sympathetic nervous activity, which appears to be due to direct hypothalamic effects and is mediated by neuropeptides such as the melanocortin system and corticotrophin-releasing hormone. Renal sympathoactivation to leptin is preserved in presence of obesity, despite resistance to the metabolic effects of leptin. Such selective leptin resistance in the context of circulating hyperleptinemia could predispose to obesity-related hypertension. Some *in vitro* studies have suggested that leptin may have peripheral actions such as endothelium-mediated vasodilation that might oppose sympathetically induced vasoconstriction. However, we and others have shown that leptin does not have physiologically relevant direct vasodilator effects *in vivo*. The fact that chronic leptin administration or overexpression of leptin produces hypertension supports the concept that the chronic hemodynamic actions of leptin are predominantly related to sympathetic activation. Exploration of the sites and mechanisms of leptin resistance will provide novel therapeutic strategies for obesity, insulin resistance and hypertension.

Key words: hypertension; leptin resistance; sympathetic nervous system; renal function; vasculature, cardiac function.

1. INTRODUCTION

Obesity has become one of the most serious health problems in most industrialized societies. Weight gain is associated with a high risk of developing cardiovascular and metabolic diseases such as coronary heart disease, hypertension, diabetes and dyslipidemia. Epidemiological studies have documented a close relationship between body mass index and cardiovascular events[1-3]. The association between body weight and blood pressure has been found even in normotensive subjects with normal body mass index[4,5]. Subsequently, clinical studies have demonstrated that weight loss induced by low calorie diet or gastric bypass reduces arterial pressure and corrects diabetes and other co-morbidities associated with obesity[6,7]. Several experimental models of obesity-induced hypertension have been developed. Different species, including the dog, rabbit, rat and mouse develop obesity associated with an increase in blood pressure when fed a high fat diet[8-10]. Some genetic models of obesity, such as the Zucker fatty rat and agouti obese mouse, are also used as models of obesity hypertension[11,12].

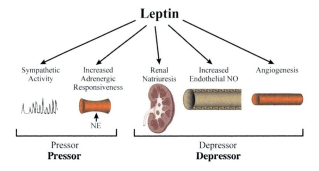

Figure 1. Cardiovascular actions of leptin. Leptin has central nervous system and peripheral actions that may alter blood pressure. Despite the potential depressor effects of leptin, experimental data suggests that the pressor, sympathetically mediated effect of leptin predominates.

Thus, a strong association between obesity and cardiovascular complications is well established. Although the precise mechanisms linking obesity and cardiovascular disease remain unclear, several mechanisms have been implicated including sympathoactivation and renal sodium retention. Leptin could potentially participate in these mechanisms. Indeed, although predominantly involved in the hypothalamic control of energy homeostasis, it is now recognized that leptin has broader effects. Several actions of leptin on cardiovascular homeostasis have been described (Figure 1), notably its effects on the autonomic nervous system. Also, several tissues besides the central nervous system express the leptin receptor, which appears involved in the modulation of physiological functions such as angiogenesis and arterial pressure and may have potential implications in cardiovascular disease.

2. LEPTIN AND SYMPATHETIC NERVOUS SYSTEM

2.1 Sympathetic effects of leptin

Consistent with its role in the regulation of energy expenditure, leptin was found to increase norepinephrine turnover in brown adipose tissue[13], suggesting activation of sympathetic outflow to this tissue. Using multi-fiber recording of regional sympathetic nerve activity (SNA) we evaluated the effects of leptin on the sympathetic outflow to different beds[14]. As expected, we found that intravenous administration of leptin in anesthetized Sprague-Dawley rats caused a significant and dose-dependent increase in SNA to brown adipose tissue (Figure 2). Unexpectedly, leptin caused also sympathoactivation to other beds not usually considered thermogenic, such as the kidney, hindlimb and adrenal. Satoh et al.[15] investigated the effect of leptin on circulating catecholamines and found that leptin administration caused a significant and dose-dependent increase in plasma concentration of norepinephrine and epinephrine.

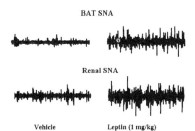

Figure 2. Effects of intravenous administration of leptin (1 mg/kg), as compared to vehicle, on SNA to brown adipose tissue (BAT) and kidney in Sprague Dawley rat. Leptin caused significant increase in both renal and BAT SNA.

We have shown that the leptin-induced regional increases in sympathetic nerve activity respond non-uniformly to baroreflex activation and hypothermia[16,17]. Leptin-induced increases in renal SNA can be suppressed by baroreflex activation, suggesting that the increase in renal SNA sub-serves circulatory functions. In contrast, leptin-induced brown adipose tissue sympathoactivation is not prevented by baroreflex activation, suggesting the recruitment of sympathetic fibers that serve thermogenic or metabolic, and not circulatory functions[16]. The effect of leptin on regional SNA response to hypothermia also differs between sympathetic fibers that serve circulatory or thermogenic functions. Leptin, at low doses that do not alter baseline SNA, acutely enhances sympathetic outflow to brown adipose tissue in response to hypothermia in lean rats. This effect is specific for thermogenic SNA because leptin does not affect the response of renal SNA to hypothermia[17].

Although some reports have shown that leptin could increase SNA through stimulation of peripheral afferent nerves[18,19], our data support the concept that sympathoactivation to leptin is due to its action in the central nervous system. First, leptin-induced sympathoexcitation is still apparent after transection of the sympathetic nerves distal to the recording site, and disappear after ganglion blockade with intravenous chlorisondamide[14]. These findings indicate that the increase in SNA is due to increased traffic in efferent post-ganglionic sympathetic nerves rather than afferent nerves. Second, direct administration of leptin to the 3rd cerebral ventricle, at sub-systemic doses, increases SNA[20] and dose-dependently increases plasma catecholamines[15]. Third, sympathoactivation to intravenous leptin can be completely abolished by selective lesioning of the hypothalamic arcuate nucleus[20]. The arcuate nucleus of the hypothalamus is also considered as a major site of leptin action to control body weight and food intake[21].

In humans, there is no direct evidence for a role of leptin in the regulation of sympathetic nervous system, because data from leptin administration in humans are absent. In non-human primates, however, leptin has been shown to activate the sympathetic nervous system, as assessed by an increase in circulating norepinephrine levels after single cerebroventricular administration of leptin[22]. Indirect evidence suggests that leptin may be important for the control of SNA in humans. A positive and significant correlation between muscle SNA and plasma leptin concentration has been reported in healthy, non-diabetic men[23]. Also, serum leptin levels are a strong positive determinant of resting metabolic rate, which is under sympathetic control, suggesting that action of leptin on SNA is a determinant of energy expenditure in human. In addition, Jeon et al.[24] have shown that the correlation between leptin and resting metabolic rate is lost in patients with a disrupted sympathetic nervous system caused by spinal cord injury. These patients had also a lower resting metabolic rate. Together, these findings strongly support the concept that leptin influences energy expenditure through the sympathetic nervous system in humans.

2.2 Sympathetic effects of leptin in obesity

Several lines of evidence suggest that obesity is associated with activation of the sympathetic nervous system. Plasma and urinary catecholamines are increased in obese humans as well as in obese animal models[25-27]. Using direct measurement with microneurography, several groups have shown increased SNA to skeletal muscle in obese subjects as compared to lean individuals[28,29]. Norepinephrine spillover techniques have demonstrated that human obesity is associated with increased SNA to a key organ of the cardiovascular homeostasis, the kidney[30]. Elevated renal SNA is also reported in animal models of obesity, including rat on high fat diet[31].

These findings demonstrate that enhanced SNA is a common feature of obesity, which would play a major role in obesity-induced hypertension and cardiovascular diseases[32]. However, the mechanisms responsible of the increased SNA in obesity remain unknown.

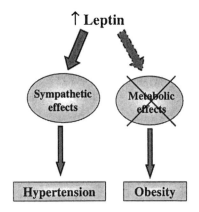

Figure 3. Concept of selective leptin resistance: there is resistance to the appetite and weight reducing actions of leptin, but preservation of the sympathetic actions. This phenomenon might explain in part how hyperleptinemia could be accompanied by obesity (partial loss of appetite and metabolic actions of leptin), but still contribute to sympathetic overactivity and hypertension because of preservation of the sympathetic actions of leptin to some organs involved in the blood pressure regulation such as the kidney.

Obesity is known to be associated with circulating hyperleptinemia, reflecting resistance to leptin because despite the high circulating levels of leptin such subjects remain obese[33]. Under these circumstances, in order for leptin to have a role in obesity-related hypertension, one must postulate that any leptin resistance is selective, with preservation of sympathetic responsiveness. Indeed, we have demonstrated that in some animal models, including agouti mice and diet-induced obesity, leptin resistance is selective with sparing of the effects of leptin on renal SNA. For example, in agouti mice, the anorexic and weight-reducing effects of leptin were less in the obese mice compared to lean littermates, but the increase in renal SNA in response to leptin was similar in both lean and obese mice[34,35]. Eikelis et al.[36] have recently shown the existence of a strong correlation between leptin plasma concentration and renal SNA across a broad range of leptin values in men of widely differing adiposity. This indicates that leptin may be the main cause of sympathoactivation associated with obesity in animal models, but also in humans (Figure 3).

2.3 Mechanisms of leptin-induced sympathetic activation

The receptor-mediated sympathoexcitatory effect of leptin is supported by the absence of SNA response to leptin in the obese Zucker rats[14], but it was not clear which form of the leptin receptor was involved since Zucker rats lack all forms of the leptin receptor. We recently demonstrated an absence of renal SNA response to leptin in db/db mice, which indicate that the effects of leptin on sympathetic outflow are mediated by the long-form

Ob-Rb of the leptin receptor[37].

As mentioned above the leptin receptor has divergent signaling capacities and modulates the activity of different intracellular enzymes. Although STAT signaling was thought to be the main pathway that mediates the leptin action in the hypothalamus, PI_3 kinase has been found to play a pivotal role in the effect of leptin on food intake[38]. Our group has demonstrated that PI_3 kinase also plays a major role in the transduction of leptin-induced changes in renal sympathetic outflow. We compared renal sympathoactivation to leptin before and after intracerebral administration of PI_3 kinase inhibitors. Both LY294002 and wortmannin markedly attenuated the increase in renal SNA induced by leptin, without affecting sympathoactivation to stimulation of melanocortin system[39]. The role of PI_3 kinase and other pathways in leptin-induced sympathoactivation to different other beds including brown adipose tissue, hindlimb, and adrenal gland remain unknown. Leptin likely controls sympathetic nerve activity in a tissue-specific manner, for several reasons. First, as mentioned above, activation of arterial baroreceptors and hypothermia modulates differentially leptin-induced sympathoactivation to the kidney and brown adipose tissue[16,17]. Second, in diet-induced obese mice, brown adipose tissue and lumbar SNA responses to leptin are attenuated as compared to lean mice, whereas leptin-induced increases in renal SNA occur with the same time-course and magnitude in both diet-induced obese and lean mice[40].

Several hypothalamic neuropeptides, monoamines, and other transmitter substances have been identified as candidate mediators of leptin action in the hypothalamus. These include melanocortins, neuropeptide Y (NPY), corticotrophin releasing hormone (CRH), Melanin-concentrating hormone and cocaine-and amphetamine-regulated transcript[21]. Therefore, leptin could cause regional sympathoactivation through stimulation of different neuropeptides. In the neural melanocortin system, α-melanocyte stimulating hormone (α-MSH) is derived from propiomelanocortin and acts mainly on melanocortin-4 receptors (MC-4R). Both renal and lumbar sympathoactivation to leptin seems mediated by the melanocortin system because blockade of melanocortin receptors with SHU9119[41] or agouti protein[42] inhibits the renal and lumbar SNA response to leptin. However, SHU9119 does not block leptin-induced sympathoactivation to brown adipose tissue[41]. Using a MC-4R knockout mouse, we recently confirmed that the renal SNA response to leptin is mediated by MC-4R. Indeed, we have shown a gene dose effect, with MC4-R heterozygotes having 50% of the normal response to leptin, and homozygote knockouts having no renal SNA response to leptin[37]. The interrelationship between leptin and the melanocortin system appears to be more complex than first thought, because absence of the leptin receptor in db/db mice attenuates the renal SNA response to stimulation of the MC-3/4R with MTII[37]. This was not expected because the melanocortin system was considered downstream to leptin. Although the mechanisms of this attenuated SNA response to MTII in db/db remain unknown, a potential mechanism relates to the increased expression of the agouti related protein in these mice[43], which is known to at least partially block melanocortin receptors in the brain.

The increase in brown adipose tissue SNA seems to depend on other neuropeptides than the melanocortin system. Given that intracerebral CRH increases SNA to brown adipose tissue, we investigated the role of this system in leptin-induced sympathoactivation to this tissue. Our results show that a CRH receptor antagonist blocked leptin-induced sympathoactivation to brown adipose tissue, but not to the kidney[44]. In summary, leptin appears to causes regional sympathoactivation via different neuropeptide pathways, with some evidence suggesting that melanocortins mediate renal sympathoactivation and CRH mediates brown adipose tissue SNA response to leptin.

3. LEPTIN AND BLOOD PRESSURE

3.1 Pressor effects of leptin

Leptin induced activation of SNA to organs such as the kidney was the first indication of the potential role of this hormone in regulation of blood pressure. The sympathetic nervous system is an important component in the control of renal function[45] and long-term renal sympathetic stimulation by leptin would be expected to raise arterial pressure by causing vasoconstriction and by increasing renal tubular sodium reabsorption. Dunbar et al.[46] have shown that the sympathoactivation to leptin is followed by a slow but progressive increase in mean arterial pressure. Shek et al.[47] demonstrated that intravenous infusion of leptin at a dose that increases plasma leptin from 1 to 94 ng/ml for 12 days increases arterial pressure and heart rate, despite a decrease in food intake that would be expected to decrease arterial pressure. Leptin-induced increases in arterial pressure are probably due to a central neural action of this hormone because intracerebroventricular administration of leptin mimics the effects of its systemic administration[48]. The substantial dose-dependent increase in heart rate as well as the greater response to air-jet stress observed in leptin-treated rats supports central activation of the sympathetic nervous system[48]. Finally, blockade of the adrenergic system inhibits the pressor response to leptin[49].

Further evidence for the pressor effects of leptin derives from the studies of transgenic mice over-expressing leptin in the liver[50]. These mice had ten fold increases in plasma leptin and decreased body weight. Despite the decreased body weight, the transgenic mice over-expressing leptin had significantly higher arterial pressure than non-transgenic littermates. The transgenic mice also had increased urinary excretion of norepinephrine, a marker of sympathetic nervous system. The increase in arterial pressure was normalized after alpha-adrenergic or ganglionic blockade, again demonstrating the importance of the sympathetic nervous system in the pressor effects of leptin.

We evaluated arterial pressure in obese, leptin deficient ob/ob mice and their wild type, lean controls[12]. Despite body weights nearly twice as high as their lean controls, the leptin deficient ob/ob mice had lower arterial pressure. Aizawa-Abe et al.[50] subsequently reported that administration of leptin to ob/ob mice (so-called leptin reconstitution) increased systolic blood pressure by as much as 25 mmHg despite decreases in food intake and body weight. These findings demonstrate that leptin contributes physiologically to the regulation of arterial pressure.

In contrast to leptin deficient ob/ob mice, agouti yellow obese mice have elevated arterial pressure despite the fact that the agouti mice have milder obesity than the ob/ob mice[12]. Obesity induced by high fat diet is also associated with an increase in arterial pressure[9,31,40]. The presence of high circulating levels of leptin associated with the selectivity in leptin resistance; i.e., preserved ability of leptin to increase renal SNA (Figure 3), could explain the hypertension in these different models of obesity. Interestingly, we recently demonstrated that preservation of renal SNA response to leptin translates into a preservation of the arterial pressure response in a murine model of diet-induced obesity (high fat diet). Indeed, arterial pressure in diet-induced obese mice was responsive to leptin, because 12 days of leptin treatment caused a significant increase in arterial pressure. The leptin-induced arterial pressure increase was of the same magnitude in obese (about 10 mmHg) as lean control mice (about 11 mm Hg)[40]. These findings enhance the potential pathophysiologic significance of the phenomenon of selective leptin resistance.

Other mechanisms may also contribute to the development of obesity-related hypertension. For example, in vitro studies have shown that leptin causes oxidative stress in cultured endothelial cells by increasing the generation of reactive oxygen species[51,52]. Leptin has also been shown to stimulate the secretion of proinflammatory cytokines, such as tumor necrosis factor-alpha and interleukin-6 that are known to promote hypertension[53].

As it has been described for renal SNA, the melanocortin system appears to mediate the effect of leptin on blood pressure. First, pharmacological activation of melanocortin receptors for 14 days caused significant increases in arterial pressure despite the decreases in food intake and body weight[54]. Second, inhibition of the melanocortin receptors blocks the increase in blood pressure induced by leptin[42,55].

In order to investigate whether the increase in arterial pressure induced by leptin is due to enhanced salt-sensitivity we studied the effects of a high-salt diet on the pressor responses of intracerebroventricular administration of leptin. The increase in arterial pressure was similar in leptin-treated rats fed a low- or high-salt diet, indicating that leptin-dependent mechanisms in the central nervous system do not alter arterial pressure sensitivity to salt[48].

In humans, several studies have shown that plasma leptin is related to blood pressure in both normotensive and hypertensive subjects[56,57] and a positive correlation has been observed between longitudinal changes in the leptin and arterial pressure[58]. Farooqi et al.[59] have reported that replacement leptin therapy in a child with congenital leptin deficiency for one year caused a drastic decrease in body weight (16 kg). This weight loss would be expected to substantially lower arterial pressure, but the arterial pressure did not change. These observations are consistent with a pressor action of leptin offsetting the depressor action of weight loss.

3.2   Depressor effects of leptin

Recently, several studies have suggested that leptin may have direct vascular effects that tend to decrease arterial pressure. The vascular endothelium is an important component in the control of arterial pressure homeostasis[60]. Endothelial cells release several vasoactive factors, of which nitric oxide (NO) is perhaps the most important with potent vasodilator action. Functionally competent leptin receptors are present on endothelial cells[61] and leptin administration in rat causes a dose-dependent increase in NO metabolite concentrations. In one study in anesthetized rats, infusion of leptin during inhibition of NO synthesis increased arterial pressure[62]. Leptin also decreased arterial pressure after suppression of sympathetic influence using ganglionic blockade[62] or chemical symapathectomy[63]. Furthermore, in vitro studies have shown that leptin evoke an endothelium-dependent relaxation of arterial rings[63,64]. Therefore, it has been argued that these vasodilator effects of leptin might oppose its neurogenic pressor action.

In contrast to these reports, Gardiner et al.[65] found no evidence for a vasodilator action of leptin in conscious rats. These authors showed that leptin do not change blood flow in different beds including renal, mesenteric and abdominal arteries, and presence of NO synthase inhibitor, L-NAME, failed to unmask any pressor effect of leptin[65]. Similarly, we found that leptin does not have substantial direct or indirect vasodilator effects in vivo. Indeed, leptin, at concentration sufficient to increase sympathetic nerve outflow, did not change arterial pressure or blood flow measured from the mesenteric, lower aortic and renal arteries[66]. Blockade of the adrenergic system or NO synthase did not reveal any pressor effect of leptin[66]. Furthermore, leptin did not alter the sympathetically mediated vasomotor response in hindlimb or kidney to stimulation of the splanchnic sympathetic nerve trunk[67]. Kuo et al.[68] found that blockade of NO synthesis augmented the heart rate and renal vascular and glomerular responses to leptin, but did not substantially augment the pressor response to leptin. Thus, the role of

NO in the blood pressure responses to leptin remains controversial, but the consistent negative results of studies in conscious animals argue against a meaningful stimulation of NO generation.

4. RENAL EFFECTS OF LEPTIN

Besides the indirect action of leptin on the renal function via sympathoactivation, leptin could exert a direct effect on the kidney. In the rat, leptin receptor expression was found in the inner zone of the medulla and pyramid, associated with the vascular structures, tubules and ducts[69]. Several investigators have shown that acute administration of leptin in anesthetized or conscious normotensive lean rats produces significant increases in sodium excretion and urine volume without significant effects on renal blood flow, glomerular filtration rate or potassium excretion[70-72]. As expected, these saluretic effects of leptin where blunted in the Zucker rat[73], but also in high fat diet obese rat[72]. Surprisingly, spontaneously hypertensive rats were also refractory to the diuretic and natriuretic effects of leptin due perhaps to enhanced renal SNA, because renal denervation restored the saluretic response of these rats to leptin[73]. A study by Shek et al.[47] suggested that the natriuretic action of leptin is not operative at physiological levels because a chronic increase in leptin concentrations within the physiological range in rats did not produce natriuresis despite an increase in arterial pressure. This study[47] provided no support for a significant natriuretic action of leptin, and instead suggested that leptin may actually produce a modest anti-natriuretic effect (probably due to the activation of the renal SNA) that opposes pressure natriuresis.

However, leptin appears to have an important role in obesity-induced renal damage such as glomerular hyperfiltration and increased urinary albumin loss. In glomerular endothelial cells, leptin directly stimulates cellular proliferation, transforming growth factor-beta$_1$ (TGF-beta$_1$) synthesis, and type IV collagen production. Conversely, in mesangial cells, leptin upregulates synthesis of the TGF-beta type II receptor, but not TGF-beta$_1$, and stimulates glucose transport and type I collagen production[74]. Chronic leptin treatment induces glumerosclerosis and proteinuria in normal rats[74]. Therefore, leptin may be of relevance to the development of glomerular pathology associated with obesity.

5. CARDIOMYOPATHY AND LEPTIN

Obese individuals are at increased risk for development of chronic heart failure. The pathologic hallmarks of obesity-related cardiomyopathy are ventricular dilation, attributed to hypervolemia, combined with myocyte hypertrophy. The mechanisms inducing myocardial hypertrophy are poorly understood and may result from increased hemodynamic stress and humoral factors. Hyperleptinemia could potentially contribute to myocardial hypertrophy. In hypertensive men, myocardial wall thickness is associated with plasma leptin, independent of body composition and blood pressure[75].

Leptin has been proposed to alter the proliferative properties of cardiomyocytes. However, the available evidence for this action of leptin is controversial. Leptin receptors have been isolated in neonatal rat ventricular myocytes. In vitro exposure of these cells to leptin induces substantial increases in the expression of α-skeletal actin (250%) and myosin light chain-2 (300%)[76]. Moderate increases in cell surface area and protein synthesis were also observed.

Contrasting with these results, leptin-deficient ob/ob mice and leptin receptor-deficient db/db mice develop echocardiographic and histological cardiomyocyte hypertrophy that is reversed by leptin replacement in the ob/ob mice[77]. Blood pressures were similar in obese mice and control lean littermates. So differences in ventricular mass could not be attributed to blood pressure. Leptin replacement causes weight loss in the ob/ob mice. To control for the effects of weight loss on myocyte hypertrophy, a group of untreated ob/ob mice was food restricted to match the calorie intake of the leptin-treated group (pair-feeding). Although weight loss was similar in both groups, complete reversion of echocardiographic ventricular hypertrophy was only observed in the leptin-treated animals. Myocyte size decreased in both groups but to a greater extent in mice treated with leptin. These results indicate that disruption of leptin signaling might cause myocardial hypertrophy. Therefore, it is possible that local leptin resistance rather than hyperleptinemia may contribute to obesity-related myocardial hypertrophy.

Modulation of proliferative properties of cardiomyocytes is not the only effect of leptin on the myocardium. Leptin attenuates cardiomyocyte contractility, in vitro, through NO-dependent mechanisms[78]. Nevertheless, it has also been shown that the negative inotropic action of leptin is abrogated in cardiomyocytes collected from hyperleptinemic spontaneously hypertensive rats as compared with normotensive Wistar rats[79]. Leptin-dependent increases in NO are also blunted in spontaneously hypertensive rat cardiomyocytes, despite normal density of leptin receptors. Thus, spontaneously hypertensive rat cardiomyocytes appear to develop resistance to the negative inotropic effect of leptin. Leptin resistance in this case could be viewed as a protective adaptation in order to preserve cardiomyocyte function despite increased hemodynamic load of severe hypertension in hyperleptinemic spontaneously hypertensive rats.

6. THROMBOSIS AND LEPTIN

Experimental evidence mostly from animals suggests that leptin could be an important pro-coagulant factor. Thrombi originating from arterial lesions in ob/ob mice are unstable as compared with littermate controls. Leptin replacement normalizes thrombi formation in ob/ob mice. Furthermore, aggregation of platelets is attenuated in ob/ob and db/db mice but leptin normalizes platelet aggregation only in ob/ob mice[80]. The time for thrombus formation is prolonged in ob/ob and db/db mice after carotid lesioning[81]. Moreover, bone marrow transplant from db/db mice to normal mice delays thrombi formation in the transplant recipients, suggesting that platelet leptin receptors are important for normal thrombogenesis. Leptin also increases human platelet aggregation in vitro by a receptor-dependent mechanism[82]. In addition, leptin modestly decreases the expression of thrombomodulin, an anti-coagulant protein, in cultured human umbilical vein endothelial cells[82].

Fibrinolysis may also be modulated in part by leptin. One human study, adjusted for differences in adiposity and age, found a significant association between leptin and decreased tissue plasminogen activator activity, and high plasminogen activator inhibitor-1 activity, in men and post-menopausal women[83]. These pro-thrombotic actions of leptin could potentially contribute to the increased risk of obese subjects in developing acute coronary events and also venous thrombosis and pulmonary thromboembolism.

7. CONCLUSION

The epidemic of obesity has led to an unwelcome upsurge of cardiovascular diseases including diabetes and hypertension. The mechanisms of obesity-related cardiovascular diseases are not fully understood, but the discovery of leptin and its effects on cardiovascular system may provide a partial explanation. Leptin has diverse cardiovascular actions, though sympathoactivation is probably the most important. The concept of selective leptin resistance may explain how leptin could contribute to obesity-related hypertension despite loss of its metabolic effects. Thus, it is possible that excess leptin may contribute to cardiovascular complications despite metabolic leptin resistance.

REFERENCES

1. H.B. Hubert, M. Feinleib, P.M. McNamara, and W.P. Castelli, Obesity as an independent risk factor for cardiovascular disease: a 26-year follow-up of participants in the Framingham Heart Study, *Circulation* **67**, 968–977 (1983).
2. R.F. Kushner, Body weight and mortality, *Nutrit. Rev.* **51**, 127–136 (1993).
3. P.G. Kopelman, Obesity as a medical problem, *Nature* **404**, 635–643 (2000).
4. R. Stamler, J. Stamler, W.F. Riedlinger, G. Algera, and R.H. Roberts, Weight and blood pressure. Findings in hypertension screening of 1 million Americans, *JAMA* **240**, 1607–1610 (1978).
5. N. Mikhai, and M.L. Tuck, Epidemiological and clinical aspects of obesity related hypertension, *J. Clin. Hypertens.* (Greenwich) **2**, 41–45 (2000).
6. J.L. Carson, M.E. Ruddy, A.E. Duff, N.J. Holmes, R.P. Cody, and R.E. Brolin, The effect of gastric bypass surgery on hypertension in morbidly obese patients, *Arch. Intern. Med.* **154**, 193–200 (1994).
7. R.J. Richards, V. Thakur, and E. Reisin, Obesity-related hypertension: its physiological basis and pharmacological approaches to its treatment, *J. Hum. Hypertens.* **10**, S59–S64 (1996).
8. L.N. Kaufman, M.M. Peterson, and S.M. Smith, Hypertension and sympathetic hyperactivity induced in rats by high-fat or glucose diets, *Am. J. Physiol.* **260**, E95–E100 (1991).
9. E. Mills, C.M. Kuhn, M.N. Feinglos, and R. Surwit, Hypertension in CB57BL/6J mouse model of non-insulin-dependent diabetes mellitus, *Am. J. Physiol.* **264**, P73–R78 (1993).
10. J.P. Montani, V. Antic Z. Yang, and A. Dulloo, Pathways from obesity to hypertension: from the perspective of a vicious triangle, *Intl. J. Obes. Relat. Metab. Disord.* **26**, S28–S38 (2002).
11. T.W. Kurtz, R.C. Morris, and H.A. Pershadsingh, The Zucker fatty rat as a genetic model of obesity and hypertension, *Hypertension* **13**, 896–901 (1989).
12. A.L. Mark, R.A. Shaffer, M.L. Correia, D.A. Morgan, C.D. Sigmund, and W.G. Haynes, Contrasting blood pressure effects of obesity in leptin-deficient ob/ob mice and agouti yellow obese mice, *J. Hypertens.* **17**, 1949–1953 (1999).
13. S. Collins, C.M. Kuhn, A.E. Petro, A.G. Swick, B.A. Chrunyk, and R.S. Surwit, Role of leptin in fat regulation, *Nature* **380**, 677 (1996).
14. W.G. Haynes, D.A. Morgan, S.A. Walsh, W.I. Sivitz, and A.L. Mark, Receptor-mediated regional sympathetic nerve activation by leptin, *J. Clin. Invest.* **100**, 270–278 (1997).
15. N. Satoh, Y. Ogawa, G. Katsuura, Y. Numata, T. Tsuji, M. Hayase, K. Ebihara, H. Masuzaki, K. Hosoda, Y. Yoshimasa, and K. Nakao, Sympathetic activation of leptin via the ventromedial hypothalamus: leptin-induced increase in catecholamine secretion, *Diabetes* **48**, 1787–1793 (1999).
16. M. Hausberg, D.A. Morgan, M.A. Chapleau, W. I. Sivitz, A.L. Mark, and W.G. Haynes, Differential modulation of leptin-induced sympathoexcitation by baroreflex activation, *J. Hypertens.* **20**, 1633–1641 (2002).
17. M. Hausberg, D.A. Morgan, J.L. Mitchell, W. I. Sivitz, A.L. Mark, and W.G. Haynes, Leptin potentiates thermogenic sympathetic responses to hypothermia: a receptor-mediated effects, *Diabetes* **51**, 2434–2440 (2002).
18. A. Niijima, Afferent signals from leptin sensors in the white adipose tissue of the epididymis, and their reflex effect in the rat, *J. Auton. Nerv. Syst.* **27**(73), 19–25 (1998).

19. M. Tanida, S. Iwashita, Y. Ootsuka, N. Terui, and M. Suzuki, Leptin injection into white adipose tissue elevates renal sympathetic nerve activity dose-dependently through the afferent nerves pathway in rats, *Neurosci. Lett.* **293**, 107–110 (2000).
20. W.G. Haynes, Interaction between leptin and sympathetic nervous system in hypertension, *Curr. Hypertens. Rep.* **2**, 311–318 (2000).
21. M.W. Schwartz, S.C. Woods, D. Porte Jr, R.J. Seeley, and D.G. Baskin, Central nervous system control of food intake, *Nature* **404**, 661–671 (2000).
22. M. Tang-Christensen, P.J. Havel, R.R. Jacobs, P.J. Larsen, and J.L. Cameron, Central administration of leptin inhibits food intake and activates the sympathetic nervous system in rhesus macaques, *J. Clin. Endocrinol. Metab.* **84**, 711–717 (1999).
23. S. Snitker, R.E. Pratley, M. Nicolson, P.A. Tataranni, and E. Ravussin, Relationship between muscle sympathetic nerve activity and plasma leptin concentration, *Obes. Res.* **5**, 338–340 (1997).
24. J.Y. Jeon, R.D. Steadward, G.D. Wheeler, G. Bell, L. McCargar, and V. Harber, Intact sympathetic nervous system is required for leptin effects on resting metabolic rate in people with spinal cord injury, *J. Clin. Endocrinol. Metab.* **88**, 402–407 (2003).
25. J.R. Sowers, L.A. Whitfield, R.A. Catania, N. Stern, M.L. Tuck, L. Dornfeld, and M. Maxwell, Role of the sympathetic nervous system in blood pressure maintenance in obesity, *J. Clin. Endocrinol. Metab.* **54**, 1181–1186 (1982).
26. J.B. Young, and L. Landsberg, Diet-induced changes in sympathetic nervous system activity: possible implications for obesity and hypertension, *J. Chronic Dis.* **35**, 879–886 (1982).
27. A.P. Rocchini, C.P. Moorhead, S. Deremer, and D. Bondi, Pathogenesis of weight-related pressure changes in blood pressure in dogs, *Hypertension* **13**, 922–928 (1989).
28. P. Vollenweider, D. Randin, L. Tappy, E. Jequier, P. Nicod, and U. Scherrer, Impaired insulin-induced sympathetic neural activation and vasodilation in skeletal muscle in obese humans, *J. Clin. Invest.* **93,** 2365–2371 (1994).
29. G. Grassi, G. Seravalle, B.M. Cattaneo, G.B. Bolla, A. Lanfranchi, M. Colombo, C. Giannattasio, A. Brunani, F. Cavagnini, and G. Mancia, Sympathetic activation in obese normotensive subjects, *Hypertension* **25**, 560–563 (1995).
30. M. Vaz, G. Jennings, A. Turner, H. Cox, G. Lambert, and M. Esler, Regional sympathetic nervous activity and oxygen consumption in obese normotensive human subjects, *Circulation* **96**, 3423–3429 (1997).
31. S. Iwashita, M. Tanida, N. Terui, Y. Ootsuka, M. Shu, D. Kang, and M. Suzuki, Direct measurement of renal sympathetic nervous activity in high-fat diet-related hypertensive rats, *Life Sci.* **71**(5), 537–546 (2002).
32. J.E. Hall, D.A. Hildebrandt, J. Kuo, and S. Fitzgerald, Role of sympathetic nervous system and neuropeptides in obesity hypertension, *Braz. J. Med. Biol. Res.* **33**, 605–618 (2000).
33. R.V. Considine, M.K. Sinha, M.L. Heiman, A. Kriauciunas, T.W. Stephens, M.R. Nyce, J.P. Ohannesian, C.C. Marco, L.J. McKee, T.L. Bauer, and J.F. Caro, Serum immunoreactive-leptin concentrations in normal-weight and obese humans, *N. Engl. J. Med.* **334**, 292–295 (1996).
34. M.L. Correia, W.G. Haynes, K. Rahmouni, D.A. Morgan, and A.L. Mark, The concept of selective leptin resistance: evidence from agouti yellow obese mice, *Diabetes* **51**, 439–442 (2002).
35. K. Rahmouni, W.G. Haynes, D.A. Morgan, and A.L. Mark, Selective resistance to central neural administration of leptin in agouti obese mice, *Hypertension* **39**, 486–490 (2002).

36. N. Eikelis, M. Schlaich, A. Aggarwal, D. Kaye, and M. Esler, Interactions between leptin and the human sympathetic nervous system, *Hypertension* **41**, 1072–1079 (2003).
37. K. Rahmouni, W.G. Haynes, D.A. Morgan, and A.L. Mark, Role of melanocortin-4 receptors in mediating renal sympathoactivation to leptin and insulin, *J. Neurosci.* **23** (14), 5998–6004 (2003).
38. K.D. Niswender, and M.W. Schwartz, Insulin and leptin revisited: adiposity signals with overlapping physiological and intracellular signaling capabilities, *Front. Neuroendocrinol.* **24**, 1–10 (2003).
39. K. Rahmouni, W.G. Haynes, D.A. Morgan, and A.L. Mark, Intracellular mechanisms involved in leptin regulation of sympathetic outflow, *Hypertension* **41**, 763–767 (2003).
40. K. Rahmouni, D.A. Morgan, G.A. Morgan, A.L. Mark, and W.G. Haynes, Role of selective leptin in hypertension in diet-induced obesity hypertension, *Diabetes* **54**, 2012-2018 (2005).
41. W.G. Haynes, D.A. Morgan, A. Djalali, W.I. Sivitz, and A.L. Mark, Interactions between the melanocortin system and leptin in control of sympathetic nerve traffic, *Hypertension* **33**, 542–547 (1999).
42. J.C. Dunbar, and H. Lu, Leptin-induced increase in sympathetic nervous and cardiovascular tone is mediated by proopiomelanocortin (POMC) products, *Brain Res. Bull.* **50**, 215–221 (1999).
43. J. Korner, E. Savontaus, S.C. Chua Jr, R.L. Leibel, and S.L.J. Wardlaw, Leptin regulation of Agrp and NPY mRNA in the rat hypothalamus. *Neuroendocrinology* **13**, 959–966 (2001).
44. M.L. Correia, D.A. Morgan, J.L. Mitchell, W.I. Sivitz, A.L. Mark, and W.G. Haynes, Role of corticotrophin-releasing factor in effects of leptin on sympathetic nerve activity and arterial pressure, *Hypertension* **38**, 384–388 (2001).
45. G.F. DiBona, and U.C. Kopp, Neural control of renal function, *Physiol. Rev.* **77**, 75–197 (1997).
46. J.C. Dunbar, Y. Hu, and H. Lu, Intracerebroventricular leptin increases lumbar and renal sympathetic nerve activity and blood pressure in normal rats, *Diabetes* **46**, 2040–2043 (1997).
47. E.W. Shek, M.W. Brands, and J.E. Hall, Chronic leptin infusion increases arterial pressure, *Hypertension* **32**, 376–377 (1998).
48. M.L. Correia, D.A. Morgan, W.I. Sivitz, A.L. Mark, and W.G. Haynes, Leptin acts in the central nervous system to produce dose-dependent changes in arterial pressure, *Hypertension* **37**, 936–942 (2001).
49. M. Carlyle, O.B. Jones, J.J. Kuo, and J.E. Hall, Chronic cardiovascular and renal actions of leptin: role of adrenergic activity, *Hypertension* **39**, 496–501 (2002).
50. M. Aizawa-Abe, Y. Ogawa, H. Masuzaki, K. Ebihara, N. Satoh, H. Iwai, N. Matsuoka, T. Hayashi, K. Hosoda, G. Inoue, Y. Yoshimasa, and K. Nakao, Pathophysiological role of leptin in obesity-related hypertension, *J. Clin. Invest.* **105**, 1243–1252 (2000).
51. A. Bouloumie, T. Marumo, M. Lafontan, and R. Busse, Leptin induces oxidative stress in human endothelial cells, *FASEB J.* **13**, 1231–1238 (1999).
52. S.I. Yamagishi, D. Edelstein, X.L. Du, Y. Kaneda, M. Guzman, and M. Brownlee, Leptin induces mitochondrial superoxide production and monocyte chemoattractant protein-1 expression in aortic endothelial cells by increasing fatty acid oxidation via protein kinase A. *J. Biol. Chem.* **276**, 25096–25100 (2001).
53. S. Loffreda, S.Q. Yang, H.Z. Lin, C.L. Karp, M.L. Brengman, D.J. Wang, A.S. Klein, S. Margetic, C. Gazzola, G.G. Pegg, and R.A. Hill, Leptin regulates proinflammatory immune responses. *FASEB J.* **12**, 57–65 (1998).

54. J.J. Kuo, A.A. Silva, and J.E. Hall, Hypothalamic melanocortin receptors and chronic regulation of arterial pressure and renal function, *Hypertension* **41**, 768–774 (2003).
55. A.A. Da Silva, J.J. Kuo, and J.E. Hall, Role of hypothalamic melanocortin 3/4-receptors in mediating chronic cardiovascular, renal, and metabolic actions of leptin, *Hypertension* **43**, 1312-1317 (2004).
56. H. Hirose, I. Saito, M. Tsujioka, M. Mori, H. Kawabe, and T. Saruta, The obese gene product, leptin: possible role in obesity-related hypertension in adolescents, *J. Hypertens.* **16**, 2007-2012 (1998).
57. U. Schorr, K. Blaschke, S. Turan, A. Distler, and A.M. Sharma, Relationship between angiotensinogen, leptin and blood pressure levels in young normotensive men, *J. Hypertens.* **16**, 1475-1480.
58. K. Itoh, K. Imai, T. Masuda, S. Abe, M. Tanaka, R. Koga, H. Itoh, T. Matsuyama, S. Iwashita, M. Tanida, N. Terui, Y. Ootsuka, M. Shu, D. Kang, and M. Suzuki, Relationship between changes in serum leptin levels and blood pressure after weight loss, *Hyperten. Res.* **25**, 881–886 (2002).
59. I.S. Farooqi, S.A. Jebb, G. Langmack, E. Lawrence, C.H. Cheetham, A.M. Prentice, I.A. Hughes, M.A. McCamish, and S. O'Rahilly, Effects of recombinant leptin therapy in a child with congenital leptin deficiency, *N. Engl. J. Med.* **341**, 879–884 (1999).
60. F. Contreras, M. Rivera, J. Vasquez, M.A. De la Parte, and M. Velasco, Endothelial dysfunction in arterial hypertension, *J. Hum. Hypertens.* **14**, S20–S25 (2000).
61. M.R. Sierra-Honigmann, A.K. Nath, C. Murakami, G. Garcia-Cardena, A. Papapetropoulos, W.C. Sessa, L.A. Madge, J.S. Schechner, M.B. Schwabb, P.J. Polverini, and J.R. Flores-Riveros Jr., Biological action of leptin as an angiogenic factor, *Science* **28**, 1683–1686 (1998).
62. G. Fruhbeck, Pivotal role of nitric oxide in the control of blood pressure after leptin administration, *Diabetes* **48**, 903–908 (1999).
63. G. Lembo, C. Vecchione, L. Fratta, G. Marino, V. Trimarco, G. d'Amati, and B. Trimarco, Leptin induces direct vasodilation through distinct endothelial mechanisms, *Diabetes* **49** (2), 293–297 (2000).
64. K. Kimura, K. Tsuda, A. Baba, T. Kawabe, S. Boh-oka, M. Ibata, C. Moriwaki, T. Hano, and I. Nishio, Involvement of nitric oxide in endothelium-dependent arterial relaxation by leptin, *Biochem. Biophys. Res. Commun.* **273**, 745–749 (2000).
65. S.M. Gardiner, P.A. Kemp, J.E. March, and T. Bennett, Regional haemodynamic effects of recombinant murine or human leptin in conscious rats, *Br. J. Pharmacol.* **130**, 805–810 (1999).
66. J.L. Mitchell, D.A. Morgan, M.L. Correia, A.L. Mark, W.I. Sivitz, and W.G. Haynes, Does leptin stimulate nitric oxide to oppose the effects of sympathetic activation? *Hypertension* **38**, 1081–1086 (2001).
67. A. Jalali, D.A. Morgan, W.I. Sivitz, M.L. Correia, A.L. Mark, and W.G. Haynes, Does leptin cause functional peripheral sympatholysis? *Am. J. Hypertens.* **14**, 615–618 (2001).
68. J.J. Kuo, O.B. Jones, and J.E. Hall, Inhibition of NO synthesis enhances chronic cardiovascular and renal actions of leptin, *Hypertension* **37**, 670–676 (2001).
69. C. Serradeil-Le Gal, D. Raufaste, G. Brossard, B. Pouzet, E. Marty, J.P. Maffrand, and G. Le Fur, Characterization and localization of leptin receptors in the rat kidney. *FEBS Lett.* **404**, 185–191 (1997).
70. E.K. Jackson, P. and Li P, Human leptin has natriuretic activity in the rat, *Am. J. Physiol.* **272**, F333–F338 (1997).
71. D. Villarreal, G. Reams, R.H. Freeman, and A. Taraben, Renal effects of leptin in normotensive, hypertensive, and obese rats, *Am. J. Physiol.* **275**, R2056–R2060 (1998).

72. J. Beltowski, G. Wjcicka, D. Gorny, and A. Marciniak, Human leptin administered intraperitoneally stimulates natriuresis and decreases renal medullary Na+, K+-ATPase activity in the rat — impaired effect in dietary-induced obesity, *Med. Sci. Monit.* **8**, BR221–BR229 (2002).
73. D. Villarreal, G. Reams, and R.H. Freeman, Effects of renal denervation on the sodium excretory actions of leptin in hypertensive rats, *Kidney Intl.* **58**, 989–994 (2000).
74. G. Wolf, A. Hamann, D.C. Han, U. Helmchen, F. Thaiss, F.N. Ziyadeh, and R.A. Stahl, Leptin stimulates proliferation and TGF-ß expression in renal glomerular endothelial cells: Potential role in glomerulosclerosis, *Kidney Intl.* **56**, 860–872 (1999).
75. G. Paolisso, M.R. Tagliamonte, M. Galderisi, G.A. Zito, A. Petrocelli, C. Carella, O. de Divitiis, and M. Varricchio, Plasma leptin level is associated with myocardial wall thickness in hypertensive insulin-resistant men, *Hypertension* **34**, 1047–1052 (1999).
76. V. Rajapurohitam, X.T. Gan, L.A. Kirshenbaum, and M. Karmazyn, The obesity-associated peptide leptin induces hypertrophy in neonatal rat ventricular myocytes, *Circ. Res.* **93**, 277-279 (2003).
77. L.A. Barouch, D.E. Berkowitz, R.W. Harrison, *et al.*, Disruption of leptin signaling contributes to cardiac hypertrophy independently of body weight in mice, *Circulation* **108**, 754-759 (2003).
78. M.W. Nickola, L.E. Wold, P.B. Colligan, G.J. Wang, W.K. Samson, and J. Ren, Leptin attenuates cardiac contraction in rat ventricular myocytes. Role of NO. *Hypertension* **36**, 501-505 (2000).
79. L.E. Wold, D.P. Relling, J. Duan, F.L. Norby, and J. Ren, Abrogated leptin-induced cardiac contractile response in ventricular myocytes under spontaneous hypertension: role of Jak/STAT pathway, *Hypertension* **39**, 69–74 (2002).
80. S. Konstantinides, K. Schafer, S. Koschnick, and D.J. Loskutoff, Leptin-dependent platelet aggregation and arterial thrombosis suggests a mechanism for atherothrombotic disease in obesity, *J. Clin. Invest.* **108**, 1533-1540 (2001).
81. P.F. Bodary, R.J. Westrick, K.J. Wickenheiser, Y. Shen, and D.T. Eitzman, Effect of leptin on arterial thrombosis following vascular injury in mice, *JAMA* **287**, 1706-1709 (2002).
82. I. Maruyama, M. Nakata, and K. Yamaji, Effect of leptin in platelet and endothelial cells. Obesity and arterial thrombosis, *Ann. N. Y. Acad. Sci.* **902**, 315-319 (2000).
83. S. Soderberg, T. Olsson, M. Eliasson, O. Johnson, and B. Ahren, Plasma leptin levels are associated with abnormal fibrinolysis in men and postmenopausal women, *J. Intern. Med.* 1999, **245**, 533-543 (1999).

Chapter 11

LEPTIN AND CANCER

Delia-Marina Alexe[1] and Eleni Petridou[1,2]
[1]*Department of Hygiene and Epidemiology, Athens University Medical School, Athens, Greece* [2]*Department of Epidemiology, Harvard School of Public Health, Boston, MA*

Abstract: Because obesity is an established risk factor in various cancers and leptin plays a significant role in the physiopathology of obesity, the exploration of leptin's link to cancer risk is of considerable importance. We have reviewed the reported findings on the role of leptin in the pathogenesis of a series of different forms of cancer, which have been more intensively studied, namely those related to human reproduction (breast, endometrial, ovarian and prostate cancer), cancers of the gastrointestinal tract (esophagus, gastric and colon cancer) and leukemias.

Key words: leptin; obesity; cancer; carcinogenesis

1. INTRODUCTION

Leptin (from the Greek word "leptos," meaning thin), a peptide hormone of 16kDa and 167 amino acids, is the product of the "obesity" (*ob*) gene, discovered in 1994[1]. A mutation in this gene was associated with severe obesity and type II diabetes in mice; thus, leptin was initially viewed as a way to cure obesity and received a lot of attention from both the scientific community and the media[1,2]. Human obesity, however, is a much more complex condition and it is not mainly due to a deficit in leptin[2]. In fact, most people who suffer from obesity, not related to the very rare condition of a defect in the *ob* gene, actually have hyperleptinemia[3]; therefore, the new challenge is to explore the underlying mechanisms of leptin sensitivity, namely to determine what makes the hypothalamus of these individuals resistant to leptin.

In humans, the *ob* gene is located on chromosome 7q31.3, whereas in mice it is on chromosome 6^4. Leptin is synthesized mainly by adipose tissue but it is also produced by a variety of cells, including placental cells, and secretory cells of the mammary epithelium[5]. Digestive epithelia, including gastric mucosa and liver, have also been recently recognized as sources of leptin[6]. Once synthesized, leptin is not stored in large pools in the adipose cell, but it is secreted through a consecutive pathway[7]. It acts through a receptor from the class I cytokine receptor family, which has at least six isoforms (Ob-Ra to Ob-Rf)[2]. The specific actions of all isoforms of Ob receptors still remain unknown. Leptin signaling is mediated mainly through the long form of Ob-Rb, but involvement of the short form Ob-Rb has also been indicated.[8]

The knowledge about the biological actions of leptin has increased considerably during the last years and its role in the regulation of other important physiology in humans has been widely recognized. It has been demonstrated that the actions of leptin are not limited to the regulation of food intake by signaling satiety, but that this hormone is also involved in the overall regulation of the metabolism, including energy expenditure and body temperature, the reproductive function and other physiologic functions, such as immunity and hematopoesis[9]. Moreover, other factors that play an important role in the regulation of appetite, such as ghrelin, have been identified[10].

Leptin acts both at central (hypothalamic) and peripheral levels as an important regulator of body weight and metabolism by increasing energy consumption and loss of adipose tissue mass as well as of the reproductive function. At hypothalamic level, leptin acts on the centers that control feeding behavior and hunger, energy expenditure and body temperature, as well as on those generating information concerning the nutritional status of the organism[11]. It inhibits the synthesis of neuropeptide Y and counteracts the effect of anandamide, thus decreasing the sensation of hunger and food consumption[12].

Leptin is involved in the regulation of reproductive function via the gonadotropin-releasing hormone (GnRH), thus affecting the luteinizing and follicle stimulating hormones (LH, FSH)[13]. It has been shown that exercise-induced hypothalamic amenorrhea and anorexia nervosa are associated with low concentrations of leptin, while the administration of this hormone can restore ovulatory menstrual cycles and improve reproductive, thyroid, and IGF hormones and bone markers in hypothalamic amenorrhea[14].

T lymphocytes and vascular endothelial cells also express leptin receptors, marking the involvement of this hormone in angiogenesis and inflammatory function[15, 16]. Leptin also acts on human bone marrow stromal cells to enhance the differentiation to osteoblasts[17].

Studies with obese and non-obese humans found a strong positive correlation of serum leptin concentrations with the percentage of body fat, and a higher concentration of *ob mRNA* in fat from obese compared to lean mass subjects [3, 18]. Among healthy full-term newborn, leptin has been strongly associated with female gender, birth length, and insulin like growth factor I (IGF-I) levels[19]. An intriguing finding that needs to be further explored is that newborns fed with formula milk have higher levels of leptin compared to those exclusively breast-fed[19]. This could have implications in later life, considering the impact of leptin in the pathology of obesity and its possible associations with insulin resistance and cancer risk.

Obesity is a pathological status characterized by hyperinsulinemia and insulin resistance, low levels of IGF binding protein and high levels of free insulin like growth factor-I (IGF-I)[20]. Insulin may enhance leptin release and elevate circulating leptin levels[21]. Furthermore, it appears that obese individuals develop resistance to leptin, as high levels of leptin are observed in these cases[22]. The pathway of insulin-mediated neoplasia may include the stimulation of cell proliferation through the alteration of the IGF-I axis, inhibition of apoptosis, and altered sex hormone milieu [20]. Leptin has been found to act as a growth factor in different tissues via the signal transducer and activator of transcription (STAT), increasing the proliferation of a variety of cancer cells (esophageal, breast and prostate cancer cells) and exercising antiapoptotic effects [9, 23, 24]. Leptin has also been shown to induce cell migration and expression of growth factors in human prostate cancer cells [23, 25], to promote the invasiveness of kidney and colonic epithelial cells[26] and to be involved in angiogenesis[27].

Because obesity is an established risk factor in various cancers[28] and leptin plays a significant role in the physiopathology of obesity, the exploration of leptin's link to cancer risk is of considerable importance. We have reviewed the reported findings on the role of leptin in the pathogenesis of a series of different forms of cancer, which have been more intensively studied, namely those related to human reproduction (breast, endometrial, ovarian and prostate cancer), cancers of the gastrointestinal tract (esophagus, gastric and colon cancer) and leukemias.

2. LEPTIN AND HUMAN REPRODUCTION RELATED CANCERS

2.1 Breast Cancer

Obesity is an established risk factor for breast cancer in postmenopausal women. Compared to women with normal or low body mass index (BMI), obese women after the menopause have a higher incidence of breast cancer, more advanced disease at diagnosis, an increased rate of metastasis and a poor response to both chemotherapy and radiotherapy [29, 30]. Obesity is also correlated with a poor prognosis of estrogen-receptor positive breast cancers in postmenopausal women [29, 31].

The pathogenic link between obesity and postmenopausal breast cancer depends on the production of estrogens after the menopause by adipose tissue cells. Estrogens act on breast cells, stimulating their proliferation and thus creating an environment conducive to growth enhancement[29]. Hyperinsulinemia, hyperleptinemia and high IGF-I levels seem to contribute to breast carcinogenesis. Insulin appears to have a mitogenic effect on malignant cells by binding to and signaling through the insulin and IGF-I receptors [32]; moreover, insulin may enhance the production of leptin, another potential growth factor for breast and breast cancer cells [21, 22, 33].

Leptin is expressed in physiological breast cells, in breast cancer cell lines, and particularly in estrogen-receptor positive (ER-positive) breast cancer cells, as well as in solid tumors [34-39]. In the normal breast, it has an important role in the development of the mammary gland. Mice lacking leptin or leptin receptors have poorly developed mammary glands[40]. Leptin was recently detected in the nipple aspirate fluid, correlated with the serum levels of leptin in premenopausal, but not postmenopausal women. There was no association, however, of the presence of leptin in nipple aspirate fluid or serum leptin levels with breast cancer risk[41].

Both ductal breast tumors and benign lesions such as hyperplasia express leptin as well as the tissue in the vicinity of the malignant ductal breast lesion[33], whereas a recent study showed that receptors of leptin are overexpressed in malignant cells[42]. Distant metastases were present in one out of three of cases of Ob-R positive tumors with leptin overexpression but in none of the tumors that lacked Ob-R expression or leptin overexpression, suggesting an involvement of leptin in the promotion of carcinogenesis and metastasis[42].

Leptin promotes the growth of both normal and malignant cells by activating signal transducer and activator of transcription 3 (STAT3) and extracellular regulated kinase (ERK) 1/2 pathways[36,43-45]. In ER-positive cancer cells leptin stimulates their proliferation via the activation of the of mitogen-activated protein kinase (MAPK)[37]. In addition, leptin induces mRNA expression of aromatase activity via the AP-1 pathway, and directly activates estrogen receptors alpha (ERα), thus increasing the production of estrogens and promoting estrogen-dependent breast cancer progression without the direct involvement of estrogen natural ligand[44,45]. Thus, leptin seems to contribute to the development of estrogen-independent tumors, which is translated into resistance to estrogen therapy and a worse prognosis. In support of this hypothesis comes the experimental evidence of leptin interference with the effects of the antiestrogen ICI 182, 780 by acting on ERα in MCF-7 breast cancer cells[39].

The presence of leptin receptor gene polymorphism was investigated as a potential mechanism underlying the high risk factor for breast cancer in postmenopausal obese women; the results, however, were inconclusive[46]. Leptin levels were also measured in women carriers of BRCA1. Postmenopausal BRCA1 mutation carriers had significantly lower leptin levels, but the involvement of leptin as a link between this mutation and the high risk of malignancy of the breast is not considered likely[47].

There are only few epidemiological studies focusing on the role of leptin in breast cancer and their findings are inconsistent. Petridou et al reported no evidence for an association between leptin and postmenopausal breast cancer; among pre-menopausal Greek women, however, there was a statistically significant inverse association of leptin with breast cancer[48]. Mantzoros et al studied the effect of leptin on the risk of pre-menopausal breast cancer in situ and found that leptin did not increase this risk substantially[49]. Furthermore, no effect of serum leptin on the angiogenic activity and metastasis in breast cancer patients was found in another study[50]. The results of a prospective study evaluating the role of leptin in prediganosis plasma among postmenopausal women enrolled in the Northern Sweden Health and Disease Cohort found no significant association with breast cancer risk[51].

On the contrary, a recent case-control study of newly diagnosed women with breast cancer reported higher leptin levels among Chinese women with breast cancer and a significant increase in the leptin/ adiponectin ratio compared to healthy controls[52]. Importantly, the leptin/ adiponectin ratio was positively correlated with tumor size, indicating the presence of a more aggressive cancer in these cases[52]. Higher leptin levels in patients with breast cancer compared to controls, independently of the menopausal status of patients, along with abnormal levels of insulin, triglicerides, APOA 1 and reduced level of serum HDL-C, were also found in another study among Chinese women[53].

Leptin seems to reflect the hormonal status in patients with breast cancer, as hyperleptinemia has been associated with elevated blood plasma concentrations of progesterone and estradiol, and high tissue levels of receptors for both estrogen and progesterone[54]. While the laboratory findings suggest that leptin is involved in the growth of breast cancer cells, the epidemiological evidence is still inconclusive.

2.2 Other Gynecological Cancers

Leptin might be a potential regulator for ovarian cancer, as leptin receptors (both short and long isoforms) were identified in ovarian surface epithelium and ovarian cancer cell lines; in addition, administration of leptin resulted in growth stimulation of BG-1 cells, an activation of ERK1/2 and inhibition of constitutive phosphorylation of p38 MAPK[55]. In patients with ovarian cancer, increased leptin levels were reported, associated with higher circulating follicle-stimulating hormone (FSH)[56]. A blood test based on the simultaneous quantification of leptin and three other analytes (prolactin, osteopontin, and IGF-I) was evaluated for the early detection of epithelial ovarian cancer [57]. While no single protein could distinguish the cancer group from the healthy controls, the combination of four analytes reached a 95% sensitivity, 95% positive predictive value, 95% specificity and 94% negative predictive value[57]. In another gynecological cancer, namely endometrial cancer, the expression of aberrant leptin receptor has been reported along with elevated serum leptin [58, 59].

2.3 Prostate Cancer

Leptin is a regulator of the reproductive function of the organism, promoting the actions of GnRH; thus it affects the production and activity of sexual hormones [13, 14, 60]. Sex steroid hormones, and particularly androgens, have been investigated in relation to the etiology of prostate cancer and especially the growth and progression of prostate cancer, but whether an association does exist between these hormones and prostate cancer has been difficult to demonstrate in epidemiological studies[61-63]. Obesity, another factor that is characterized by alterations of the balance of sexual hormones, has also been examined as a potential risk factor for prostate cancer but the results are still inconclusive.

Prostate cancer cells DU 145 and PC-3 express mRNA for leptin receptors huOb-Ra and huOB-Rb [64,65]. As shown by *in vitro* studies, leptin acts as a growth factor for prostate cancer cells and it is also involved in the suppression of apoptosis, migration and angiogenesis [22, 23, 64-67]. Importantly, leptin seems to promote the growth of the androgen-independent prostate cancer cells (DU 145 and PC-3) but not of androgen-dependent cells (LNCaP-FGC); thus, this hormone could be involved in the development of hormone resistance in the natural history of prostate cancer[65]. Moreover, it has been reported that interleukin (IL) 6 and IGF-I act in an additive way on leptin stimulation of cell proliferation, a mechanism that could contribute to the occurrence of androgen independence by prostate cancer cells [65, 66].

While these laboratory studies point to the existence of a possible pathophysiological link between increased bioactivity of leptin and the risk of developing prostate cancer, epidemiological studies documenting the role of leptin in prostate cancer have reported conflicting results. Lagiou et al have found no significant association of leptin levels with a higher risk of prostate cancer or benign prostatic hyperplasia in elderly men. There was no correlation between serum leptin levels and estradiol, testosterone, sex-hormone-binding globulin and IGF-I[68]. Freedland et al reported no correlation between serum leptin and the pathological stage of prostate cancer among men treated with radical prostatectomy [69]. In contrast, Chang et al found higher levels of leptin in patients with tumors of large volume, while the levels of leptin were independent of testosterone[70]. Higher risk for prostate cancer was also found among Chinese men with a waist-to-hip ratio (WHR) higher than 0.87, suggesting that leptin may interact with markers related to abdominal obesity to increase the risk of prostate cancer[71]. An association between moderately increased leptin levels and the development of prostate cancer was reported in a prospective study where blood samples were taken at the time when the subjects were free of disease[72]. After investigating the consistency of these findings in a later study, however, the authors found no support for the hypothesis that elevated levels of circulating leptin are associated with overall increased risk of prostate cancer[73].

The association between obesity, a situation characterized by high levels of leptin, and prostate cancer has been investigated in a number of epidemiological studies; however, there is no clear evidence to support a strong pathogenic link between obesity and prostate cancer. While the results of some of these studies support a higher incidence of prostate malignancy in obese people, other studies indicate no association or an inverse association with obesity [74]. There are some findings that the association between BMI and cancer risk might be age dependent and that people younger than 60 years with a higher BMI might have a lower risk for prostate cancer possibly due to their lower androgen levels[75].

More consistent is the evidence concerning the relationship between a higher BMI and a more aggressive form of prostate cancer[69, 74, 76]. Taking into account *in vitro* observations that leptin may promote the androgen-independent growth of prostate cancer[65, 66] and the independence of leptin from testosterone levels [68, 70], it is possible that higher leptin in obese people could contribute to the evolution of tumor cells into more aggressive androgen-resistant forms. Further studies are needed, however, in order to clarify the influence of leptin on both prostate cancer risk and the prognosis of this malignancy.

3. LEPTIN AND GASTROINTESTINAL TRACT CANCERS

3.1 Gastric Cancer

Leptin is present throughout the gut, in the stomach and salivary glands and leptin receptors have been detected in gastric mucosal biopsies, cultured human gastric epithelial cells, and gastric cancer cells[77, 78]. Normal gastric cells in rodents and humans produce leptin [78-80] and four isoforms of Ob receptors have been identified at this level[77]. It should be noted that leptin remains stable even at pH 2, which supports the hypothesis that it has important paracrine and endocrine functions and the potential to reach the intestine in an active form [6, 77, 78].

Gastric leptin seems to play a key role in the neuroendocrine regulation of satiety through vagal pathways[81]. It may control meal size and the regulation of small intestine mobility through a positive feedback loop with cholecystokinin[82,83] and it may also help the cytoprotection of gastric mucosa[84]. Leptin regulates the secretion of pepsinogen and of gastric hormones, such as gastrin and somatostatin, and it may also be involved in gut inflammatory processes[77, 85].

It was recently reported that gastric cancer cells exhibit strong expression of both leptin and receptors for leptin[86]. In contrast to normal gastric cells where the *Ob* receptor is present in the progenitor zone cells, in gastric cancer tissues this receptor is present in the basement membrane of almost all cells. Leptin induces gastric cancer cell proliferation *in vitro* by activating janus kinase/signal transducer and activator of transcription (JAK-STAT) signaling pathways and increasing ERK2 phosphorylation in gastric cancer cells; thus, blocking these pathways can be seen as a potential therapeutical measure that would inhibit the proliferation of gastric carcinoma cells[86].

Helicobacter pylori (H. pylori) chronic infection is a component cause of gastric adenocarcinoma[87]. The expression of gastric leptin is increased in patients with chronic gastritis due to H. pylori, as shown by the analysis of surgically resected human stomach tissues and biopsy specimens[88, 89]. This probably reflects the involvement of gastric leptin in the immune and proinflammatory processes at this level. H. pylori infection seems also to decrease serum ghrelin, another adiposity signal [90]. These alterations could increase the risk of carcinogenesis in patients with H. pylori infection.

Clinical studies have reported a significant decrease in serum leptin concentrations in patients with advanced upper gastrointestinal cancer [91-93]. It has been suggested that the concentrations of serum leptin might be directly related to cancer cachexia, thus serum leptin would have the potential of being a reliable parameter for assessing nutritional status in patients with neoplasm[92]. There is increasing evidence, however, that the decrease in serum leptin is independent from the weight loss, as this finding was observed in gastric cancer patients with and without weight loss[92, 93]. Circulating leptin concentrations in patients with cancer do not seem to be influenced by the presence of an inflammatory response, as no correlation was found with the levels of interleukin 6 and C-reactive protein[94, 95]. In cachexia, chronic high growth hormone and low insulin levels may play an important role in the inhibition of leptin secretion and weight loss[93].

3.2 Colon Cancer

Leptin and its Ob-Rb receptors have been identified in human colon cells, colonic epithelial crypts, polyps, colonic tumor resections, and adjacent mucosa[96]. The contribution of leptin to the proliferation and migration of normal human colonic epithelial cells has been demonstrated *in vitro*[96, 97]. This hormone is also involved in the repair of inflamed or wounded digestive mucosa, as well as the healing of colon anastomosis in rats[98].

Epidemiological evidence supports the role of obesity and high fat diet in colon cancer but the mechanisms remain unknown[99]. High-fat diet increases serum leptin and there are findings in support of the theory that enhancement of colon cell proliferation and carcinogenesis by high fat diet may be mediated through elevated serum leptin[100-101].

An elevated risk of carcinogenesis due to increased levels of IGF-I and insulin in obesity has been proposed[20]. Serum leptin levels are increased in obese people, who seem to develop resistance to leptin[22]. Hyperleptinemia may contribute to stimulation of cellular proliferation and inhibition of apoptosis, and promotion of angiogenesis. However, the exact involvement of leptin in carcinogenesis remains largely unknown.

Colon cancer cells exhibit receptors for leptin[99, 102, 103]. As indicated, findings from a number of *in vitro* and *in vivo* studies support the hypothesis that leptin promotes the proliferation of colon cancer cells through its involvement in cellular growth, cell migration and angiogenesis[102, 103]. Leptin acts via the stimulation MAPK activity and nuclear factor-kappaB (NF-κB) pathway to promote the proliferation of these cells and their invasive capacity at early stages of neoplasia[97, 103, 104]. It inhibits the apoptosis of colon cancer cells and it has been reported that it counteracts the inhibitory effect of sodium butyrate on the proliferation of HT-29 colon cancer cells[103].

Hirose et al reported that hyperleptinemia and hyperinsulinemia enhance azoxymethane-AOM induced premalignant lesions of the colon in db/db mice[105]. A recent study exploring the *in vitro* effect of leptin on the proliferation of human colon cancer cells and *in vivo* on the growth of HT-29 xenografts in nude mice and the development of intestinal tumors in ApcMin/+ mice, found a leptin-dose dependent stimulation of cell DNA synthesis and growth in all cell lines. Hyperleptinemia, however, was not correlated with an increase of tumor volume or weight and tumor Ki-67 index was even inhibited[102]. Furthermore, the reduction of the development of the initial precancerous lesions induced by azoxymethane by leptin has also been reported in the rat colonic mucosa[106, 107].

In clinico-epidemiological studies, higher serum leptin levels have been associated with a three fold higher risk for colon cancer among men, while no association with rectal cancer was reported. Leptin concentrations were more strongly associated with cancers of the left colon than those of the right[108, 109]. It is worth noting that these studies examined prospectively the risk of colon cancer according to leptin levels in persons that were healthy at the time of blood sample collection.

In contrast, case control studies comparing the levels of leptin between patients with colon cancer and healthy controls reported significantly *lower* serum leptin levels in patients[95, 110]. It was suggested that leptin could act as a marker of cachexia/ weight loss in patients with cancer[92]. However, the low levels of leptin were observed even though the BMI of the colon cancer patients were not different from that of the control group, while serum leptin levels of early-stage patients did not differ from those of advanced-stage patients, nor was there any difference in the serum leptin levels of patients who did and who did not receive chemotherapy[110]. These findings indicate that, as with gastric cancer, there might be other mechanisms that could be involved in the body weight loss in patients with colon cancer.

3.3 Esophageal Cancer

There is very little evidence on the role of leptin in the causation of the adenocarcinoma of the esophagus, cancer that has a rapid increase in its incidence, probably linked to the increase in the obesity. It has been reported that leptin increases the proliferation of Barrett's associated esophageal adenocarcionoma cell lines SEG-1 and BIC-1 by nonapoptotic mechanisms, but further research is needed[111].

4. LEPTIN AND LEUKEMIAS

Leptin is involved in the hematopoetic process as a promoter of normal myeloid and erythroid development[112]. White blood cell count is correlated with body fat, thus with leptin, in humans[113]. As part of the cytokine family along with interkeukins, leptin plays an important role in the regulation of immune function. It promotes the induction of T lymphocytes and monocytes/ macrophages (activation and proliferation), and the production of proinflammatory cytokines[114-122]. It also has a trophic effect on monocytes, preventing apopstosis via the p42/44 MAPK pathway [116] and seems to play an important role in natural killer cell (NK) development and activation[123]. Leptin receptors (the isoform Ob-Ra) have also been identified on human polymorphonuclear neutrophils (PMN) where leptin seems to indirectly activate these cells via the induction of tumor necrosis factor alpha (TNF-alpha) and also to stimulate their chemotaxis[117, 124].

Leptin is required for normal lymphopoiesis[125]. Reduced leptin levels due to nutritional deprivation cause a high susceptibility to infection, as this condition is associated with thymic atrophy [117, 126, 127]. Administration of leptin to mice has been shown to reverse this immunosuppressive effect of acute starvation; thus, leptin seems to link the nutritional status to immune function of the organism[127].

There is increasing evidence about the association of obesity, expressed as high BMI, with a higher risk for acute myeloid leukemia (AML)[128], and particularly acute promyelocytic leukemia[129]. High BMI also appears to be a predictive factor for increased treatment-related toxicity and fatality in cases of leukemia[130]. There is also some evidence about a higher risk for chronic myeloid leukemia and chronic lymphoid leukemia in obese people[131-133]. Leptin might be the link between obesity and these forms of leukemia, promoting the proliferation of leukemic cells and stimulating their invasive capacity.

Receptors for leptin have been identified in several myeloid and lymphoid leukemic cell lines[134-135]. Specific binding for leptin was identified in the cell lines K562, HEL, MO7E and CML6. In cases of chronic myeloid leukemia, there was a higher expression of mRNA for leptin receptors in blast crisis than in chronic phase. Interestingly, leptin receptor gene expression decreased in differentiated cells[134].

Leptin has been shown to stimulate the proliferation of AML cells and to also have an anti-apoptotic effect[134-136]. It increases the number of progenitor cells and spontaneous AML blast proliferation [135, 137] as well as AML blast release of IL-1beta, IL6, TNF-alpha and granulocyte-macrophage colony stimulating factor (GM-CSF)[137]. Interestingly, while normal promyelocytes lack receptor expression, leukemic promyelocytes express both short and long form of Ob-R isoforms[135]. The frequency of expression of receptors for leptin was found higher in recurrent than in newly diagnosed cases of AML[135]. In the light of these findings, the inhibition of binding of leptin to its receptors seems a possible adjunct therapy in AML [138].

An elevation of serum leptin levels in patients with AML compared to healthy controls was reported in a recent study and the difference was partly accounted for by the higher BMI of cases[139]. These findings are in line with the results of the in vitro observation concerning the implication of leptin in the pathogenesis of AML. On the contrary, no correlation or an inverse correlation of leptin levels with the risk of acute lymphoblastic leukemia (ALL) was reported [139, 140].

Increased serum level of leptin was reported in former ALL patients following cranial irradiation along with growth hormone deficiency[141-143]. These patients have an increased risk for developing obesity and insulin resistance, and a high cardiovascular risk[142, 143]. Is seems possible that the development of leptin resistance could be an important pathogenic mechanism, since treatment with growth hormone does not change hyperleptinaemia, hyperinsulinaemia and the impaired insulin sensitivity[143, 144].

It has been suggested that leptin resistance could be provoked by hypothalamic radiation at young ages [145] but hyperleptinemia also occurs during treatment of ALL without cranial irradiation so there might be other pathogenic mechanisms besides the impaired response of hypothalamus to leptin[144]. A polymorphism in the leptin receptor has been found to possibly influence the susceptibility to obesity in female survivors of childhood ALL and especially those submitted for cranial radiation[145].

5. LEPTIN AND OTHER CANCERS

Studies concerning the role of leptin in the causation of other cancers are scarce nor has there been, so far, hard evidence on whether its role is associated mostly with obesity-related cancers. Thus, in renal cancer, higher levels or leptin were correlated with a better prognosis[146]. In patients with lung cancer, circulating leptin concentrations are not altered in weight-losing cancer patients and are inversely related to the intensity of the inflammatory response[147]. Notably, leptin receptors have also been identified in human pituitary adenomas[148].

6. CONCLUSIONS

Obesity significantly contributes to the total burden of mortality from most forms of cancer. Steroid hormones, as well as insulin and insulin-like growth hormones seem to be involved in the biological process of carcinogenesis, however, the evidence concerning the exact involvement of these hormones is still inconclusive. Leptin, a hormone that is intimately linked to adipose tissue, has been incriminated as a contributing factor in carcinogenesis, studied mainly as a possible underlying mechanism, linking obesity with cancer. There is some evidence, however, that leptin may also be involved in cancers that are not related with obesity, such as gastric cancer but the underlying mechanisms are still obscure.

Leptin has properties of a growth factor in different tissues, both physiological and malignant, and has been reported to have antiapoptotic effects and to promote cell invasiveness and angiogenesis. In vitro studies have shown that malignant cell lines, such as gastric, colon, prostate and breast cancer cells, as well as acute myeloid leukemic cells express receptors for leptin and respond in a dose-dependent way to the administration of leptin. In prostate cancer cells, leptin seems to contribute to the occurrence of androgen independence. Leptin may also play a role in the development of estrogen- independence in estrogen-receptor positive breast cancer, and it seems to interfere with antiestrogen therapy. If the two latter findings are confirmed, possible therapeutic solutions targeting leptin pathways, contributing to the improvement of prognosis of androgen-independent prostate or estrogen-independent breast tumors, could be sought.

The evidence from clinico-epidemiological studies in support of the laboratory findings about the role of leptin in carcinogenesis, however, is largely lacking. Elevated serum leptin levels seem to be associated with a higher risk for colon cancer among men. There is some evidence that the increased risk for AML in people with hyperleptinemia might reflect the action of leptin as a link between obesity and this forms of leukemia, promoting the proliferation of leukemic cells and stimulating their invasive capacity. In prostate cancer, epidemiological reports show that higher levels of leptin may be related to worse prognosis than to increased risk for developing the disease. Inconclusive are also the findings concerning the involvement of leptin in the carcinogenesis of the mammary gland.

Another concern is that most of the clinico-epidemiological studies that have found an association are of case-control design and they have not adequately controlled for fat mass or other potential confounders. Although leptin increases IGF and has growth potential as summarized in this chapter, its effect seems permissive that it may exert its role only in the range of very low to normal leptin levels, with no additional effect in the range of normal to high leptin levels. Therefore, further studies with more robust epidemiologic design, preferably prospective cohort investigations, are needed to evaluate in a more specific way, hypotheses generated by laboratory data.

REFERENCES

1. Y. Zhang, R. Proenca, M. Maffei, M. Barone, L. Leopold and J.M. Friedman. Positional cloning of the mouse obese gene and its human homologue. *Nature*, **372**, 425-432 (1994).
2. J. Auwerxand and B. Staels. Leptin. *Lancet*, **351**, 737-742 (1998).
3. R.V. Considine, M.K. Sinha, M.L. Heiman, A. Kriauciunas, T.W. Stephens, M.R. Nyce, J.P. Ohannesian, C.C. Marco, L.J. McKee, T.L. Bauer and J.F. Caro. Serum immunoreactive-leptin concentrations in normal-weight and obese humans. *N Engl J Med*, **334**, 292-295 (1996).
4. OMIM (Online Mendelian Inheritance in Man, John Hopkins University). Leptin; lep. Available online at:
http://www.ncbi.nlm.nih.gov/entrez/dispomim.cgi?id=164160
5. M. Baratta. Leptin--from a signal of adiposity to a hormonal mediator in peripheral tissues. *Med Sci Monit*, **8**, RA282-92 (2002).
6. S. Guilmeau, M. Buyse and A. Bado. Gastric leptin: a new manager of gastrointestinal function. *Curr Opin Pharmacol*, **4**, 561-566 (2004).
7. S.R. Bornstein, M. Abu-Asab, A. Glasow, G. Path, H. Hauner, M. Tsokos, G.P. Chrousos and W.A. Scherbaum. Immunohistochemical and ultrastructural localization of leptin and leptin receptor in human white adipose tissue and differentiating human adipose cells in primary culture. *Diabetes*, **49**, 532-538 (2000).

8. R. Pai, C. Lin, T. Tran and A Tarnawski. Leptin activates STAT and ERK2 pathways and induces gastric cancer cell proliferation. *Biochem Biophys Res Commun*, **331**, 984-992 (2005).
9. L. Huang and C. Li. Leptin: a multifunctional hormone. *Cell Res*, **10**, 81-92 (2000).
10. M. Kojima, H. Hosoda, Y. Date, M. Nakazato, H. Matsuo and K. Kangawa. Ghrelin is a growth-hormone-releasing acylated peptide from stomach. *Nature*, **402**, 656-660 (1999).
11. A. Hamann and S. Matthaei. Regulation of energy balance by leptin. *Exp Clin Endocrinol Diabetes*, **104**, 293-300 (1996).
12. V. Di Marzo, S.K. Goparaju, L. Wang, J. Liu, S. Batkai, Z. Jarai, F. Fezza, G.I. Miura, R.D. Palmiter, T. Sugiura and G. Kunos. Leptin-regulated endocannabinoids are involved in maintaining food intake. *Nature*, **410**, 822-825 (2001).
13. S. Greisen, T. Ledet, N. Moller, J.O. Jorgensen, J.S. Christiansen, K. Petersen and P. Ovesen. Effects of leptin on basal and FSH stimulated steroidogenesis in human granulosa luteal cells. *Acta Obstet Gynecol Scand*, **79**, 931-935 (2000).
14. J.L. Chan and C.S. Mantzoros. Role of leptin in energy-deprivation states: normal human physiology and clinical implications for hypothalamic amenorrhea and anorexia nervosa. *Lancet*, **366**, 74-85 (2005).
15. B. Siegmund, J.A. Sennello, J. Jones-Carson, F. Gamboni-Robertson, H.A. Lehr, A. Batra, I. Fedke, M. Zeitz and G. Fantuzzi. Leptin receptor expression on T lymphocytes modulates chronic intestinal inflammation in mice. *Gut*, **53**, 965-972 (2004).
16. M.R. Sierra-Honigmann, A.K. Nath, C. Murakami, G. Garcia-Cardena, A. Papapetropoulos, W.C. Sessa, L.A. Madge, J.S. Schechner, M.B. Schwabb, P.J. Polverini and J.R. Flores-Riveros. Biological action of leptin as an angiogenic factor. *Science*, **281**, 1683-1686 (1998).
17. T. Thomas, F. Gori, S. Khosla, M.D. Jensen, B. Burguera and, B.L. Riggs. Leptin acts on human marrow stromal cells to enhance differentiation to osteoblasts and to inhibit differentiation to adipocytes. *Endocrinology*, **140**, 1630-1638 (1999).
18. M. Maffei, J. Halaas, E. Ravussin, R.E. Pratley, G.H. Lee, Y. Zhang, H. Fei, S. Kim, R. Lallone, S. Ranganathan, P.A. Kern and J.M. Friedman. Leptin levels in human and rodent: measurement of plasma leptin and ob RNA in obese and weight-reduced subjects. *Nat Med*, **1**, 1155-1161 (1995).
19. E. Petridou, C.S. Mantzoros, M. Belechri, A. Skalkidou, N. Dessypris, E. Papathoma, H. Salvanos, J.H. Lee, S. Kedikoglou, G. Chrousos and D. Trichopoulos. Neonatal leptin levels are strongly associated with female gender, birth length, IGF-I levels and formula feeding. *Clin Endocrinol (Oxf)*, **62**, 366-371 (2005).
20. K. Gupta, G. Krishnaswamy, A. Karnad and A.N. Peiris. Insulin: a novel factor in carcinogenesis. *Am J Med Sci*, **323**,140-145 (2002).
21. H. Askari, J. Liu and S. Dagogo-Jack. Hormonal regulation of human leptin in vivo: Effects of hydrocortisone and insulin. *Int J Obes Relat Metab Disord*, **24**, 1254-1259 (2000).
22. P. Somasundar, D.W. McFadden, S.M. Hileman and L. Vona-Davis. Leptin is a growth factor in cancer. *J Surg Res*, **116**, 337-349 (2004).
23. P. Somasundar, A.K. Yu, L. Vona-Davis and D.W. McFadden. Differential effects of leptin on cancer in vitro. *J Surg Res*, **113**, 50-55 (2003).
24. N.M. Morton, V. Emilsson, Y.L. Liu and M.A Cawthorne. Leptin action in intestinal cells. *J Biol Chem*, **273**, 26194-26201 (1998).

25. K.A. Frankenberry, P. Somasundar, D.W. McFadden and L.C. Vona-Davis. Leptin induces cell migration and the expression of growth factors in human prostate cancer cells. *Am J Surg*, **188**, 560-565 (2004).
26. S. Attoub, V. Noe, L. Pirola, E. Bruyneel, E. Chastre, M. Mareel, M.P. Wymann and C. Gespach. Leptin promotes invasiveness of kidney and colonic epithelial cells via phosphoinositide 3-kinase-, rho-, and rac-dependent signaling pathways. *FASEB J*, **14**, 2329-2338 (2000).
27. A, Markowska, K, Malendowicz and K. Drews. The role of leptin in breast cancer. *Eur J Gynaecol Oncol*, **25**, 192-194 (2004).
28. F. Bianchini, R. Kaaks and H. Vainio. Overweight, obesity, and cancer risk. *Lancet Oncol,* **3**, 565-574 (2002).
29. A.R. Carmichael and T. Bates. Obesity and breast cancer: a review of the literature. *Breast*, **13**, 85-92 (2004).
30. D.J. Hunter and W.C. Willett. Diet, body size, and breast cancer. *Epidemiol Rev,* **15**, 110-132 (1993).
31. K. Yoo, K. Tajima, S. Park, D. Kang, S. Kim, K. Hirose, T. Takeuchi and S. Miura. Postmenopausal obesity as a breast cancer risk factor according to estrogen and progesterone receptor status (Japan). *Cancer Lett,* **167**, 57-63 (2001).
32. C. Mantzoros, E. Petridou, N. Dessypris, C. Chavelas, M. Dalamaga, D.M. Alexe, Y. Papadiamantis, C. Markopoulos, E. Spanos, G. Chrousos and D. Trichopoulos. Adiponectin and breast cancer risk. *J Clin Endocrinol Metab,* **89**, 1102-1107 (2004).
33. F. Caldefie-Chezet, M. Damez, M. de Latour, G. Konska, F. Mishellani, C. Fusillier, M. Guerry, F. Penault-Llorca, J. Guillot and M.P. Vasson. Leptin: A proliferative factor for breast cancer? Study on human ductal carcinoma. *Biochem Biophys Res Commun*, **334**, 737-741 (2005).
34. Y. Chilliard, M. Bonnet, C. Delavaud, Y. Faulconnier, C. Leroux, J. Djiane and F. Bocquier. Leptin in ruminants. Gene expression in adipose tissue and mammary gland, and regulation of plasma concentration. *Domest Anim Endocrinol,* **21**, 271-295 (2001).
35. S.N. O'Brien, B.H. Welter and T.M. Price. Presence of leptin in breast cell lines and breast tumors. *Biochem Biophys Res Commun*, **259**, 695-698 (1999).
36. X. Hu, S.C. Juneja, N.J. Maihle and M.P. Cleary. Leptin--a growth factor in normal and malignant breast cells and for normal mammary gland development. *J Natl Cancer Inst*, **94**, 1704-1711 (2002).
37. K. Laud, I. Gourdou, L. Pessemesse, J.P. Peyrat and J. Djiane. Identification of leptin receptors in human breast cancer: functional activity in the T47-D breast cancer cell line. *Mol Cell Endocrinol*, **188**, 219-226 (2002).
38. M.N. Dieudonne, F. Machinal-Quelin, V. Serazin-Leroy, M.C. Leneveu, R. Pecquery and Y. Giudicelli. Leptin mediates a proliferative response in human MCF7 breast cancer cells. *Biochem Biophys Res Commun*, **293**, 622-628 (2002).
39. C. Garofalo, D. Sisci and E. Surmacz. Leptin interferes with the effects of the antiestrogen ICI 182,780 in MCF-7 breast cancer cells. *Clin Cancer Res,* **10**, 6466-6475 (2004).
40. M.P. Cleary, J.P. Grande, S.C. Juneja and N.J. Maihle. Diet-induced obesity and mammary tumor development in MMTV-neu female mice. *Nutr Cancer*, **50**, 174-180 (2004).
41. E.R. Sauter, C. Garofalo, J. Hewett, J.E. Hewett, C. Morelli and E. Surmacz. Leptin expression in breast nipple aspirate fluid (NAF) and serum is influenced by body

mass index (BMI) but not by the presence of breast cancer. *Horm Metab Res*, **36**, 336-340 (2004).
42. M. Ishikawa, J. Kitayama and H. Nagawa. Enhanced expression of leptin and leptin receptor (OB-R) in human breast cancer. *Clin Cancer Res,* **10**, 4325-4331 (2004).
43. N. Yin, D. Wang, H. Zhang, X. Yi, X. Sun, B. Shi, H. Wu, G. Wu, X. Wang and Y. Shang. Molecular mechanisms involved in the growth stimulation of breast cancer cells by leptin. *Cancer Res,* **64**, 5870-5875 (2004).
44. S. Catalano, S. Marsico, C. Giordano, L. Mauro, P. Rizza, M.L. Panno and S. Ando. Leptin enhances, via AP-1, expression of aromatase in the MCF-7 cell line. *J Biol Chem*, **278**, 28668-28676 (2003).
45. S. Catalano, L. Mauro, S. Marsico, C. Giordano, P. Rizza, V. Rago, D. Montanaro, M. Maggiolini, M.L. Panno and S. Ando. Leptin induces, via ERK1/ERK2 signal, functional activation of estrogen receptor alpha in MCF-7 cells. *J Biol Chem*, **279**, 19908-19915 (2004).
46. H.Y. Woo, H. Park, C.S. Ki, Y.L. Park and W.G. Bae. Relationships among serum leptin, leptin receptor gene polymorphisms, and breast cancer in Korea. *Cancer Lett*. (article in press) (2005).
47. I. Rzepka-Gorska, B. Tarnowski, A. Chudecka-Glaz and B. Gorski. BRCA1 mutation, leptin and estrogen levels in breast cancer patients. *Eur J Gynaecol Oncol,* **26**, 205-206 (2005).
48. E. Petridou, Y. Papadiamantis, P. Markopoulos, E. Spanos, N. Dessypris and D. Trichopoulos. Leptin and insulin growth factor I in relation to breast cancer (Greece). *Cancer Causes Control,* **11**, 383-388 (2000).
49. C.S. Mantzoros, K. Bolhke, S. Moschos and D.W. Cramer. Leptin in relation to carcinoma in situ of the breast: a study of pre-menopausal cases and controls. *Int J Cancer,* **80**, 523 (1999).
50. U. Coskun, N. Gunel, F.B. Toruner, B. Sancak, E. Onuk, O. Bayram, O. Cengiz, E. Yilmaz, S. Elbeg and S. Ozkan. Serum leptin, prolactin and vascular endothelial growth factor (VEGF) levels in patients with breast cancer. *Neoplasma,* **50**, 41-46 (2003).
51. P. Stattin, S. Soderberg, C. Biessy, P. Lenner, G. Hallmans, R. Kaaks and T. Olsson. Plasma leptin and breast cancer risk: a prospective study in northern Sweden. *Breast Cancer Res Treat,* **86**, 191-196 (2004).
52. D.C. Chen, Y.F. Chung, Y.T. Yeh, H.C. Chaung, F.C. Kuo, O.Y. Fu, H.Y. Chen, M.F. Hou and S.S. Yuan. Serum adiponectin and leptin levels in Taiwanese breast cancer patients. *Cancer Lett* (article in press) (2005).
53. C. Han, H.T. Zhang, L. Du, X. Liu, J. Jing, X. Zhao, X. Yang and B. Tian. Serum levels of leptin, insulin, and lipids in relation to breast cancer in china. *Endocrine,* **26**, 19-24 (2005).
54. L. Tessitore, B. Vizio, D. Pesola, F. Cecchini, A. Mussa, J.M. Argiles and C. Benedetto. Adipocyte expression and circulating levels of leptin increase in both gynaecological and breast cancer patients. *Int J Oncol,* **24**, 1529-1535 (2004).
55. J.H. Choi, S.H. Park, P.C. Leung and K.C. Choi. Expression of leptin receptors and potential effects of leptin on the cell growth and activation of mitogen-activated protein kinases in ovarian cancer cells. *J Clin Endocrinol Metab,* **90**, 207-210 (2005).
56. L. Tessitore, B. Vizio, D. Pesola, F. Cecchini, A. Mussa, J.M. Argiles and C. Benedetto. Adipocyte expression and circulating levels of leptin increase in both gynaecological and breast cancer patients. *Int J Oncol,* **24**, 1529-1535 (2004).

57. G. Mor, I. Visintin, Y. Lai, H. Zhao, P. Schwartz, T. Rutherford, L. Yue, P. Bray-Ward and D.C. Ward. Serum protein markers for early detection of ovarian cancer. *Proc Natl Acad Sci U S A*, **102**, 7677-7682 (2005).
58. S.S. Yuan, K.B. Tsai, Y.F. Chung, T.F. Chan, Y.T. Yeh, L.Y. Tsai and J.H. Su. Aberrant expression and possible involvement of the leptin receptor in endometrial cancer. *Gynecol Oncol*, **92**, 769-775 (2004).
59. E. Petridou, M. Belechri, N. Dessypris, P. Koukoulomatis, E. Diakomanolis, E. Spanos and D. Trichopoulos. Leptin and body mass index in relation to endometrial cancer risk. *Ann Nutr Metab*, **46**, 147-151 (2002).
60. C.K. Welt, J.L. Chan, J. Bullen, R. Murphy, P. Smith, A.M. DePaoli, A. Karalis and C.S. Mantzoros. Recombinant human leptin in women with hypothalamic amenorrhea. *N Engl J Med*, **351**, 987-997 (2004).
61. M.C. Bosland. The role of steroid hormones in prostate carcinogenesis. *J Natl Cancer Inst Monogr*, **27**, 39-66 (2000).
62. E.A. Platz and E. Giovannucci. The epidemiology of sex steroid hormones and their signaling and metabolic pathways in the etiology of prostate cancer. *J Steroid Biochem Mol Biol*, **92**, 237-253 (2004).
63. P. Soronen, M. Laiti, S. Torn, P. Harkonen, L. Patrikainen, Y. Li, A. Pulkka, R. Kurkela, A. Herrala, H. Kaija, V. Isomaa and P. Vihko. Sex steroid hormone metabolism and prostate cancer. *J Steroid Biochem Mol Biol*, **92**, 281-286 (2004).
64. P. Somasundar, K.A. Frankenberry, H. Skinner, G. Vedula, D.W. McFadden, D. Riggs, B. Jackson, R. Vangilder, S.M. Hileman and L.C. Vona-Davis. Prostate cancer cell proliferation is influenced by leptin. *J Surg Res*, **118**, 71-82 (2004)
65. M. Onuma, J.D. Bub, T.L. Rummel and Y. Iwamoto. Prostate cancer cell-adipocyte interaction: leptin mediates androgen-independent prostate cancer cell proliferation through c-Jun NH2-terminal kinase. *J Biol Chem*, **278**, 42660-42667 (2003).
66. K.A. Frankenberry, P. Somasundar, D.W. McFadden and L.C. Vona-Davis. Leptin induces cell migration and the expression of growth factors in human prostate cancer cells. *Am J Surg*, **188**, 560-565 (2004).
67. G.A. Bray. The underlying basis for obesity: relationship to cancer. *J Nutr*, **132**, 3451S-3455S (2002).
68. P. Lagiou, L.B. Signorello, D. Trichopoulos, A. Tzonou, A. Trichopoulou and C.S. Mantzoros. Leptin in relation to prostate cancer and benign prostatic hyperplasia. *Int J Cancer*, **76**, 25-28 (1998)
69. S.J. Freedland, L.J. Sokoll, L.A. Mangold, D.J. Bruzek, P. Mohr, S.K. Yiu, J.I. Epstein and A.W. Partin. Serum leptin and pathological findings at the time of radical prostatectomy. *J Urol*, **173**, 773-776 (2005).
70. S. Chang, S.D. Hursting, J.H. Contois, S.S. Strom, Y. Yamamura, R.J. Babaian, P. Troncoso, P.S. Scardino, T.M. Wheeler, C.I. Amos and M.R. Spitz. Leptin and prostate cancer. *Prostate*, **46**, 62-67 (2001).
71. A.W. Hsing, S. Chua Jr, Y.T. Gao, E. Gentzschein, L. Chang, J.Deng and F.Z. Stanczyk. Prostate cancer risk and serum levels of insulin and leptin: a population-based study. *J Natl Cancer Inst*, **93**, 783-789 (2001).
72. P. Stattin, S. Soderberg, G. Hallmans, A. Bylund, R. Kaaks, U.H. Stenman, A. Bergh and T. Olsson. Leptin is associated with increased prostate cancer risk: a nested case-referent study. *J Clin Endocrinol Metab*, **86**, 1341-1345 (2001).
73. P. Stattin, R. Kaaks, R. Johansson, R. Gislefoss, S. Soderberg, H. Alfthan, U.H. Stenman, E. Jellum and T. Olsson. Plasma leptin is not associated with prostate cancer risk. *Cancer Epidemiol Biomarkers Prev*, **12**, 474-475 (2003).

74. C.L. Amling. Relationship between obesity and prostate cancer. *Curr Opin Urol,* **15**, 167-171 (2005).
75. E. Giovannucci, E.B. Rimm, Y. Liu, M. Leitzmann, K. Wu, M.J. Stampfer and W.C. Willett. Body mass index and risk of prostate cancer in U.S. health professionals. *J Natl Cancer Inst,* **95**, 1240-1244 (2003).
76. S.O. Andersson, A. Wolk, R. Bergstrom, H.O. Adami, G .Engholm, A. Englund and O. Nyren. Body size and prostate cancer: a 20-year follow-up study among 135006 Swedish construction workers. *J Natl Cancer Inst,* **89**, 385-389 (1997).
77. H. Mix, A. Widjaja, O. Jandl, M. Cornberg, A. Kaul, M. Goke, W. Beil, M. Kuske, G. Brabant, M.P. Manns and S. Wagner. Expression of leptin and leptin receptor isoforms in the human stomach. *Gut,* **47**, 481-486 (2000).
78. S. Cinti, R.D. Matteis, C. Pico, E. Ceresi, A. Obrador, C. Maffeis, J. Oliver and A. Palou. Secretory granules of endocrine and chief cells of human stomach mucosa contain leptin. *Int J Obesity,* **24**, 789-793 (2000).
79. A. Bado, S. Levasseur, S. Attoub, S. Kermorgant, J.P. Laigneau, M.N. Bortoluzzi, L. Moizo, .T Lehy, M. Guerre-Millo, Y. Le Marchand-Brustel and M.J. Lewin. The stomach is a source of leptin. *Nature,* **394**, 790-793 (1998).
80. I. Sobhani, A. Bado, C. Vissuzaine, M. Buyse, S. Kermorgant, J.P. Laigneau, S. Attoub, T. Lehy, D. Henin, M. Mignon and M.J. Lewin. Leptin secretion and leptin receptor in the human stomach. *Gut,* **47**, 178-183 (2000).
81. S. Guilmeau, M. Buyse and A. Bado. Gastric leptin: a new manager of gastrointestinal function. *Curr Opin Pharmacol,* **4**, 561-566 (2004).
82. S. Guilmeau, M. Buyse, A. Tsocas, J.P. Laigneau and A. Bado. Duodenal leptin stimulates cholecystokinin secretion: evidence of a positive leptin-cholecystokinin feedback loop. *Diabetes,* **52**, 1664-1672 (2003).
83. J.M. Kiely, S.J. Graewin, H.A. Pitt and D.A. Swartz-Basile. Leptin increases small intestinal response to cholecystokinin in leptin-deficient obese mice. *J Surg Res,* **124**, 146-150 (2005).
84. R. Schneider, S.R. Bornstein, G.P. Chrousos, S. Boxberger, G. Ehninger and M. Breidert. Leptin mediates a proliferative response in human gastric mucosa cells with functional receptor. *Horm Metab Res,* **33**, 1-6 (2001).
85. M.J. Lewin and A. Bado. Gastric leptin. *Microsc Res Tech,* **53**, 372-376 (2001).
86. R. Pai, C. Lin, T. Tran and A. Tarnawski. Leptin activates STAT and ERK2 pathways and induces gastric cancer cell proliferation. *Biochem Biophys Res Commun,* **331**, 984-992 (2005).
87. P.B. Ernst and B.D. Gold. The disease spectrum of Helicobacter pylori: the immunopathogenesis of gastroduodenal ulcer and gastric cancer. *Annu Rev Microbiol,* **54**, 615-640 (2000).
88. T. Azuma, H. Suto, Y. Ito, M. Ohtani, M. Dojo, M. Kuriyama and T. Kato. Gastric leptin and Helicobacter pylori infection. *Gut,* **49**, 324-329 (2001).
89. Y. Nishi, H. Isomoto, S. Uotani, C.Y. Wen, S. Shikuwa, K. Ohnita, Y. Mizuta, A. Kawaguchi, K. Inoue and S. Kohno. Enhanced production of leptin in gastric fundic mucosa with Helicobacter pylori infection. *World J Gastroenterol,* **11**, 695-699 (2005).
90. H. Isomoto, H. Ueno, Y. Nishi, C.Y. Wen, M. Nakazato and S. Kohno. Impact of Helicobacter pylori infection on ghrelin and various neuroendocrine hormones in plasma. *World J Gastroenterol,* **11**, 1644-1648 (2005).
91. H. Dulger, S. Alici, M.R. Sekeroglu, R. Erkog, H. Ozbek, T. Noyan and M. Yavuz. Serum levels of leptin and proinflammatory cytokines in patients with gastrointestinal cancer. *Int J Clin Pract,* **58**, 545-549 (2004).

92. B. Zhu, S. Liu, J. Liu and F. Wan. Effect of serum leptin on nutritional status of patients with cancer. *Wei Sheng Yan Jiu,* **31**,100-102 (2002).
93. Q. Huang, X. Zhang, Z.W. Jiang, B.Z. Liu, N. Li and J.S. Li. Hypoleptinemia in gastric cancer patients: relation to body fat mass, insulin, and growth hormone. *JPEN J Parenter Enteral Nutr,* **29**, 229-235 (2005).
94. A.M. Wallace, A. Kelly, N. Sattar, C.S. McArdle and D.C. McMillan. Circulating concentrations of "free" leptin in relation to fat mass and appetite in gastrointestinal cancer patients. *Nutr Cancer,* **44**,157-160 (2002).
95. A.M. Wallace, N. Sattar and D.C. McMillan. Effect of weight loss and the inflammatory response on leptin concentrations in gastrointestinal cancer patients. *Clin Cancer Res,* **4**, 2977-2979 (1998).
96. S. Attoub, V. Noe, L. Pirola, E. Bruyneel, E. Chastre, M. Mareel, M.P. Wymann and C. Gespach. Leptin promotes invasiveness of kidney and colonic epithelial cells via phosphoinositide 3-kinase-, rho-, and rac-dependent signaling pathways. *FASEB J,* **14**, 2329-2338 (2000).
97. J.C. Hardwick, G.R. Van Den Brink, G.J. Offerhaus, S.J. Van Deventer and M.P. Peppelenbosch. Leptin is a growth factor for colonic epithelial cells. *Gastroenterology,* **121**, 79-90 (2001).
98. A. Tasdelen, C. Algin, E. Ates, H. Kiper, M. Inal and F. Sahin. Effect of leptin on healing of colonic anastomoses in rats. *Hepatogastroenterology,* **51**, 994-997 (2004).
99. M. Shike. Body weight and colon cancer. *Am J Clin Nutr,* **63**, 442S-444S (1996).
100. A.J. FitzGerald, N. Mandir and R.A. Goodlad. Leptin, cell proliferation and crypt fission in the gastrointestinal tract of intravenously fed rats. *Cell Prolif,* **38**, 25-33 (2005).
101. Z. Liu, T. Uesaka, H. Watanabe and N. Kato. High fat diet enhances colonic cell proliferation and carcinogenesis in rats by elevating serum leptin. *Int J Oncol,* **19**, 1009-1014 (2001).
102. T. Aparicio, L. Kotelevets, A. Tsocas, J.P. Laigneau, I. Sobhani, E. Chastre and T. Lehy. Leptin stimulates the proliferation of human colon cancer cells in vitro but does not promote the growth of colon cancer xenografts in nude mice or intestinal tumorigenesis in ApcMin/+ mice. *Gut,* **54**, 1136-1145 (2005)
103. P. Rouet-Benzineb, T. Aparicio, S. Guilmeau, C. Pouzet, V. Descatoire, M. Buyse and A. Bado. Leptin counteracts sodium butyrate-induced apoptosis in human colon cancer HT-29 cells via NF-kappaB signaling. *J Biol Chem,* **279**, 16495-16502 (2004).
104. M. Bahceci, A.Tuzcu, M. Akkus, M. Yaldiz and A. Ozbay. The effect of high-fat diet on the development of obesity and serum leptin level in rats. *Eat Weight Disord,* **4**, 128-32 (1999).
105. Y. Hirose, K. Hata, T. Kuno, K. Yoshida, K. Sakata, Y. Yamada, T. Tanaka, B.S. Reddy and H. Mori. Enhancement of development of azoxymethane-induced colonic premalignant lesions in C57BL/KsJ-db/db mice. *Carcinogenesis,* **25**, 821-825 (2004).
106. T. Aparicio, S. Guilmeau, H. Goiot, A. Tsocas, J.P. Laigneau, A .Bado, I. Sobhani and T. Lehy. Leptin reduces the development of the initial precancerous lesions induced by azoxymethane in the rat colonic mucosa. *Gastroenterology,* **126**, 499-510 (2004).
107. D.E. Stein and J.G. Kral. Leptin reduces the development of the initial precancerous lesions induced by azoxymethane in the rat colonic mucosa. *Gastroenterology,* **127**, 1867-1868 (2004).

108. P. Stattin, A. Lukanova, C. Biessy, S. Soderberg, R. Palmqvist, R. Kaaks, T. Olsson and E. Jellum. Obesity and colon cancer: does leptin provide a link? *Int J Cancer*, **109**, 149-152 (2004).
109. P. Stattin, R. Palmqvist, S. Soderberg, C. Biessy, B. Ardnor, G. Hallmans, R. Kaaks and T. Olsson. Plasma leptin and colorectal cancer risk: a prospective study in Northern Sweden. *Oncol Rep*, 10, 2015-2021 (2003).
110. F. Arpaci, M.I. Yilmaz, A. Ozet, H. Ayta, B. Ozturk, S. Komurcu and M. Ozata. Low serum leptin level in colon cancer patients without significant weight loss. *Tumori*, **88**, 147-149 (2002).
111. P. Somasundar, D. Riggs, B. Jackson, L. Vona-Davis and D.W. McFadden. Leptin stimulates esophageal adenocarcinoma growth by nonapoptotic mechanisms. *Am J Surg*, **186**, 575-578 (2003).
112. M. Hino, T. Nakao, T. Yamane, K. Ohta, T. Takubo and N. Tatsumi. Leptin receptor and leukemia. *Leuk Lymphoma*, 36,457-461 (2000).
113. C.A. Wilson, G. Bekele, M. Nicolson, E. Ravussin and R.E. Pratley. Relationship of the white blood cell count to body fat: role of leptin. *Br J Haematol*, **99**, 447-451 (1997).
114. V. Sanchez-Margalet, C. Martin-Romero, J. Santos-Alvarez, R. Goberna, S. Najib and C. Gonzalez-Yanes. Role of leptin as an immunomodulator of blood mononuclear cells: mechanisms of action. *Clin Exp Immunol*, **133,** 11-9 (2003).
115. S. Najib and V. Sanchez-Margalet. Human leptin promotes survival of human circulating blood monocytes prone to apoptosis by activation of p42/44 MAPK pathway. *Cell Immunol*, **220**, 143-149 (2002).
116. V. Sanchez-Margalet, C. Martin-Romero, J. Santos-Alvarez, R. Goberna, S. Najib and C. Gonzalez-Yanes. Role of leptin as an immunomodulator of blood mononuclear cells: mechanisms of action. *Clin Exp Immunol*, **133**, 11-9 (2003).
117. H. Zarkesh-Esfahani, A.G. Pockley, Z. Wu, P.G. Hellewell, A.P. Weetman and R.J. Ross. Leptin indirectly activates human neutrophils via induction of TNF-alpha. *J Immunol*, **172**, 1809-1814. 2004
118. C. Gabay, M. Dreyer, N. Pellegrinelli, R. Chicheportiche and C.A. Meier. Leptin directly induces the secretion of interleukin 1 receptor antagonist in human monocytes. *J Clin Endocrinol Metab*, **86**, 783-791 (2001).
119. C. Martin-Romero, J. Santos-Alvarez, R. Goberna and V. Sanchez-Margalet. Human leptin enhances activation and proliferation of human circulating T lymphocytes. *Cell Immunol*, **199**, 15-24 (2000).
120. V. Sanchez-Margalet, C. Martin-Romero. Human leptin signaling in human peripheral blood mononuclear cells: activation of the JAK-STAT pathway. Cell Immunol. 2001;211:30-6.
121. C. Martin-Romero, J. Santos-Alvarez, R. Goberna and V. Sanchez-Margalet. Human leptin enhances activation and proliferation of human circulating T lymphocytes. *Cell Immunol*, **199**, 15-24 (2000).
122. J. Santos-Alvarez, R. Goberna and V. Sanchez-Margalet. Human leptin stimulates proliferation and activation of human circulating monocytes. *Cell Immunol*, **194**, 6-11 (1999).
123. Z. Tian, R. Sun, H. Wei and B. Gao. Impaired natural killer (NK) cell activity in leptin receptor deficient mice: leptin as a critical regulator in NK cell development and activation. *Biochem Biophys Res Commun*, **298**, 297-302 (2002).
124. F. Caldefie-Chezet, A. Poulin and M.P. Vasson. Leptin regulates functional capacities of polymorphonuclear neutrophils. *Free Radic Res*, **37**, 809-814 (2003).

125. B.D. Bennett, G.P. Solar, J.Q. Yuan, J. Mathias, G.R. Thomas and W. Matthews. A role for leptin and its cognate receptor in hematopoiesis. *Curr Biol*, **6**, 1170-1180 (1996).
126. G. Matarese. Leptin and the immune system: how nutritional status influences the immune response. *Eur Cytokine Netw*, **11**, 7-14 (2000).
127. G.M. Lord, G. Matarese, J.K. Howard, R.J. Baker, S.R. Bloom and R.I. Lechler. Leptin modulates the T-cell immune response and reverses starvation-induced immunosuppression. *Nature*, **394**, 897-901 (1998).
128. J.A. Ross, E. Parker, C.K. Blair, J.R. Cerhan and A.R. Folsom. Body mass index and risk of leukemia in older women. *Cancer Epidemiol Biomarkers Prev*, **13**, 1810-1813 (2004).
129. E. Estey, P. Thall, H. Kantarjian, S. Pierce, S. Kornblau and M. Keating. Association between increased body mass index and a diagnosis of acute promyelocytic leukemia in patients with acute myeloid leukemia. *Leukemia*, **11**, 1661-1664 (1997).
130. G. Meloni, A. Proia, S. Capria, A. Romano, G. Trape, S.M. Trisolini, M. Vignetti and F. Mandelli. Obesity and autologous stem cell transplantation in acute myeloid leukemia. *Bone Marrow Transplant*, **28**, 365-367 (2001).
131. K. Kasim, P. Levallois, B. Abdous, P. Auger and K.C. Johnson. Lifestyle factors and the risk of adult leukemia in Canada. *Cancer Causes Control*, **16**, 489-500 (2005).
132. C. Samanic, G. Gridley, W.H. Chow, J. Lubin, R.N. Hoover and J.F. Fraumeni Jr. Obesity and cancer risk among white and black United States veterans. *Cancer Causes Control*, **15**, 35-43 (2004).
133. S.Y. Pan, K.C. Johnson, A.M. Ugnat, S.W. Wen, Y. Mao; Canadian Cancer Registries Epidemiology Research Group. Association of obesity and cancer risk in Canada. *Am J Epidemiol*, **159**, 259-268 (2004).
134. T. Nakao, M. Hino, T. Yamane, Y. Nishizawa, H. Morii and N. Tatsumi. Expression of the leptin receptor in human leukaemic blast cells. *Br J Haematol*, **102**, 740-745 (1998).
135. M. Konopleva, A. Mikhail, Z. Estrov, S. Zhao, D. Harris, G. Sanchez-Williams, S.M. Kornblau, J. Dong, K.O. Kliche, S. Jiang, H.R. Snodgrass, E.H. Estey and M. Andreeff. Expression and function of leptin receptor isoforms in myeloid leukemia and myelodysplastic syndromes: proliferative and anti-apoptotic activities. *Blood*, **93**, 1668-1676 (1999).
136. Y. Tabe, M. Konopleva, J. Igari and M. Andreeff. Spontaneous migration of acute promyelocytic leukemia cells beneath cultured bone marrow adipocytes with matched expression of the major histocompatibility complex. *Rinsho Byori*, **52**, 642-648 (2004).
137. O. Bruserud, T.S. Huang, N. Glenjen, B.T. Gjertsen and B. Foss. Leptin in human acute myelogenous leukemia: studies of in vivo levels and in vitro effects on native functional leukemia blasts. *Haematologica*, **87**, 584-595 (2002).
138. P.O. Iversen, C.A. Drevon and J.E. Reseland. Prevention of leptin binding to its receptor suppresses rat leukemic cell growth by inhibiting angiogenesis. *Blood*, **100**, 4123-4128 (2002).
139. N.A. Hamed, O.A. Sharaki and M.M. Zeidan. Leptin in acute leukaemias: relationship to interleukin-6 and vascular endothelial growth factor. *Egypt J Immunol*, **10**, 57-66 (2003).

140. H. Wex, E. Ponelis, T. Wex, R. Dressendorfer, U. Mittler and P. Vorwerk. Plasma leptin and leptin receptor expression in childhood acute lymphoblastic leukemia. *Int J Hematol,* **76**, 446-452 (2002).
141. B.M. Brennan, A. Rahim, W.F. Blum, J.A. Adams, O.B. Eden and S.M. Shalet. Hyperleptinaemia in young adults following cranial irradiation in childhood: growth hormone deficiency or leptin insensitivity? *Clin Endocrinol (Oxf),* **50**, 163-169 (1999).
142. K. Link, C. Moell, S. Garwicz, E. Cavallin-Stahl, J. Bjork, U. Thilen, B. Ahren and E.M. Erfurth. Growth hormone deficiency predicts cardiovascular risk in young adults treated for acute lymphoblastic leukemia in childhood. *J Clin Endocrinol Metab,* **89**, 5003-5012 (2004).
143. B. Bulow, K. Link, B. Ahren, A.S. Nilsson and E.M. Erfurth. Survivors of childhood acute lymphoblastic leukaemia, with radiation-induced GH deficiency, exhibit hyperleptinaemia and impaired insulin sensitivity, unaffected by 12 months of GH treatment. *Clin Endocrinol (Oxf),* **61**, 683-691 (2004).
144. J.H. Davies, B.A. Evans, E. Jones, W.D. Evans, M.E. Jenney and J.W. Gregory. Osteopenia, excess adiposity and hyperleptinaemia during 2 years of treatment for childhood acute lymphoblastic leukaemia without cranial irradiation. *Clin Endocrinol (Oxf),* **60**, 358-365 (2004).
145. J.A. Ross, K.C. Oeffinger, S.M. Davies, A.C. Mertens, E.K. Langer, W.R. Kiffmeyer, C.A. Sklar, M. Stovall, Y. Yasui and L.L. Robison. Genetic variation in the leptin receptor gene and obesity in survivors of childhood acute lymphoblastic leukemia: a report from the Childhood Cancer Survivor Study. *J Clin Oncol,* **22**, 3558-3562 (2004).
146. T. Rasmuson, K. Grankvist, J. Jacobsen, T. Olsson and B. Ljungberg. Serum insulin-like growth factor-1 is an independent predictor of prognosis in patients with renal cell carcinoma. *Acta Oncol,* **43**, 744-748 (2004).
147. M.R. Aleman, F. Santolaria, N. Batista, M. de La Vega, E. Gonzalez-Reimers, A. Milena, M. Llanos and J.L. Gomez-Sirvent. Leptin role in advanced lung cancer. A mediator of the acute phase response or a marker of the status of nutrition? *Cytokine,* **19**, 21-26 (2002).
148. M.T. Kristiansen, L.R. Clausen, S. Nielsen, O. Blaabjerg, T. Ledet, L.M. Rasmussen and J.O. Jorgensen. Expression of leptin isoforms and effects of leptin on the proliferation and hormonal secretion in human pituitary adenomas. *Horm Res,* **62**, 129-136 (2004).

Chapter 12

LIPODYSTROPHY: The experiment of nature to study leptin

Rexford S. Ahima[1] and Malaka B. Jackson[2]
University of Pennsylvania School of Medicine, [1]Department of Medicine, Division of Endocrinology, Diabetes and Metabolism, Philadelphia, Pennsylvania; [2]Division of Endocrinology, Children's Hospital of Philadelphia, Philadelphia, Pennsylvania

Abstract: Lipodystrophic syndromes consist of a heterogeneous group of disorders characterized by generalized or partial loss of adipose tissue, and are commonly associated with severe insulin resistance, diabetes mellitus, hyperlipidemia and hepatic steatosis. In women, other features may include acanthosis nigricans, hirsutism and oligomenorrhea. Inherited lipodystrophy first recognized more than one hundred years ago is rare, while acquired lipodystrophy associated with antiretroviral drug treatment now accounts for the majority of cases. Our understanding of the mechanisms underlying lipodystrophies has been enhanced by advances in molecular genetics, as well as studies in rodents and humans linking lipid and glucose abnormalities to deficiency of adipose secreted hormones, in particular leptin. This review focuses on the classification of human lipodystrophy, mouse models which resemble the human condition, metabolic and hormonal changes observed in this disorder, and the role of leptin in the pathophysiology and treatment of lipodystrophy.

Key words: Adipose tissue; adipokine; leptin; adiponectin; fatty acid oxidation

1. INTRODUCTION

Lipodystrophy in humans is characterized by distinctive patterns of adipose tissue loss that can be either inherited or acquired. Of the inherited lipodystrophies, currently there are four major classifications in which the molecular derangement has been identified. These are congenital generalized lipodystrophy (CGL), familial partial lipodystrophy - the Dunnigan variety and in association with PPARγ gene mutations, and lipodystrophy associated with mandibuloacral dysplasia. The acquired forms of lipodystrophy are by far more common than the inherited ones. Acquired lipodystrophy is seen in association with protease inhibitor and other antiretroviral drugs used to treat the human immunodeficiency virus (HIV) infection. Additionally, patients with acquired partial and generalized lipodystrophy have been described, and appear to have an autoimmune etiology (reviewed by Garg[1]). Both inherited and acquired lipodystrophies are associated with varying degrees of insulin resistance, diabetes, hyperlipidemia, steatosis and neuroendocrine deficits.

Mice have been generated that mimic fat loss, metabolic and hormonal abnormalities in lipodystrophy. As will be discussed later, the first indication that adipose derived hormones may be involved in the pathogenesis of metabolic derangement in lipodystrophy, came from the laboratory of Brown and Goldstein[2]. Infusion of recombinant leptin to attain physiological levels, partially reversed insulin resistance, diabetes and hyperlipidemia in a mouse model of congenital lipoatrophy[2]. This finding was subsequently confirmed in other lipodystrophic murine models and later in humans [3-9]. In the latter, leptin not only improved glucose and lipid levels, but also decreased hepatomegaly and restored deficits of the pituitary-gonadal axis. Here, we will discuss the classification of human and murine lipodystrophy, associated metabolic and hormonal abnormalities, and how lipodystrophy provides a paradigm for unraveling the role of leptin and various adipocyte hormones in the regulation of energy balance, neuroendocrine axis, glucose and lipids.

2. INHERITED LIPODYSTROPHIES

2.1 Congenital Generalized Lipodystrophy

This autosomal dominant disorder was first described in the 1950s by Berardinelli and Seip[10]. To date, about 250 patients have been identified with either type 1 or type 2 congenital generalized lipodystrophy (CGL). However, it is likely that many cases go undiagnosed and it has been suggested that the worldwide prevalence of this disorder is nearly 1 in 10 million, affecting people from various racial origins (reviewed by Garg[1]).

Clinically, CGL patients have almost complete adipose tissue loss that results in a muscular appearance that is evident at birth. Additionally, a prominent navel or an umbilical hernia may be present. During childhood, affected children have an increased growth velocity, advancement of bone age and an insatiable appetite[10,11]. Subsequently, acanthosis nigricans appears in the axilla, groin, neck and truncal regions. Some affected female patients will develop clitorimegaly and polycystic ovarian syndrome. Additionally, these women have difficulty with conception. Conversely, fertility appears to be preserved in affected males. Other clinical features common to both types of CGL are hepatosplenomegaly, an acromegalic appearance and post-pubertal lytic lesions in the appendicular bones. A few patients have mild mental retardation and hypertrophic cardiomyopathy[1,10,11]. The hepatomegaly observed in CGL is secondary to fatty infiltration and eventually leads to the development of a cirrhotic liver. As early as infancy, hypertriglyceridemia and hyperinsulinemia can be observed. Elevated triglyceride levels can result in recurrent episodes of pancreatitis. CGL often predisposes to a non-ketotic form of diabetes mellitus either during or after adolescence, and diabetic complications later on.

Genetic mutations have been identified in the majority of the known kindreds with CGL, and form the basis for classifying affected individuals into three subtypes – Type 1 CGL, Type 2 CGL, and CGL without an identified genetic mutation[12,13]. Type 1 CGL has been associated with an abnormal 1-acylglycerol-3-phosphate-*O*-acyltransferase 2 (AGPAT2) gene linked to chromosome 9q34[12,13]. Five AGPAT isoforms are involved in the generation of triglycerides and phospholipids. AGPAT1 is highly expressed in liver and skeletal muscle, while AGPAT2 is abundant in omental adipose tissue. It has been postulated that AGPAT2 deficiency results in a decrease in adipose triglyceride synthesis or secondarily causes a decline in the availability of phospholipids required for intracellular signaling and membrane functions. The depletion of triglyceride is manifest in adipocytes in bone marrow, subcutaneous, abdominal and intrathoracic regions, with sparing of adipose tissue depots that serve the purpose of cushioning or protection in the orbits, joints, palms, soles, perineum, vulva and perinephric regions[11].

Conversely, patients with Type 2 CGL have adipose depletion in the above cushion areas as well as in metabolically active adipose tissues[1,11]. Mutations in the *seipen* gene or Berardinelli-Seip congenital lipodystrophy 2 (BSCL2) gene on chromosome 11q13 have been identified in affected kindreds with Type 2 CGL[14-16]. Phenotype-genotype studies in 45 affected kindreds revealed an early onset of diabetes with a mean age of 10 years[14-17]. Moreover, Type 2 CGL patients were more likely to develop cardiomyopathy. Additionally, half of the Type 2 CGL patients were noted to have mild mental retardation, which was not observed in patients with AGPAT2 gene mutations[17]. This differential manifestation is consistent with increased expression of the *seipen* in the brain, suggesting a role of the gene in cognitive function. Leptin is significantly lower in Type 2 CGL females than Type 1 CGL, although there appears to be no difference in leptin levels among the men with either type of CGL. Moreover, lytic lesions in appendicular bones are primarily observed in patients with *AGPAT2* gene mutations[17].

2.2 Familial Partial Lipodystrophy – Dunnigan Variety

Familial partial lipodystrophy (FPL) is an autosomal dominant disorder[18]. Patients can be distinguished from those with CGL based on a normal fat distribution at birth and throughout childhood. Moreover, FPL patients rarely develop acanthosis nigricans or polycystic ovarian syndrome. With the onset of puberty, FPL patients begin to lose fat mass mostly from the arms and legs[18-21]. Women often develop a Cushingoid habitus as they gain excess central adiposity in the face, neck and abdomen[19]. As the disease progresses, there is variable loss of adipose tissue from the chest and frontal abdominal region[19,20]. Given the overall muscular appearance, FPL is more difficult to diagnose in men than women. Metabolic derangements are also more frequently observed in females[19,20]. Diabetes occurs after 20 years of age and has been associated with increased fat deposition in non-lipodystrophic regions. High density lipoprotein (HDL) cholesterol is decreased and triglyceride is often elevated in these patients. Extreme elevations in triglyceride levels can result in episodes of acute pancreatitis[19-21]. Although steatohepatitis has been reported, secondary hepatic cirrhosis is rare. Elevated triglyceride levels are associated with increased extra-hepatic fat deposition, as manifested by loss of subcutaneous adipose tissue and increased abdominal and intermuscular fat deposition in the extremities on magnetic resonance imaging[19-21].

FPL-Dunningan variety has been linked to a missense mutation of the *LMNA* gene on chromosome 1q21-22, which encodes lamins A and C[22-28]. Lamins belong to the intermediate filament family and function to stabilize the nuclear envelope and associate with chromatin. It has been suggested that *LMNA* mutations cause adipocyte loss and metabolic derangement by disturbing nuclear function, with subsequent cell death or alteration of interactions between lamin and transcription factors, e.g. sterol regulatory element-binding protein 1c (SREBP1c)[29,30]. Although this idea is supported by the fact that fibroblasts from affected patients show a chaotic nuclear lamina meshwork and aberrant nuclear blebbing, it is still not clear how these abnormalities lead to selective fat loss[29,30]. Moreover, studies have demonstrated no difference between lamin A and C expression in omental adipocytes when compared to adipocytes from subcutaneous, abdominal or neck areas[31].

2.3 Familial Partial Lipodystrophy – PPARγ gene mutation

Peroxisome proliferator-activated receptor (PPAR)-γ is a transcription factor critical to adipogenesis. A number of patients with missense mutations in *PPARγ* have been identified[32-35]. Phenotypically these patients have severe insulin resistance, hyperglycemia, hypertriglyceridemia and hypertension. An elderly patient heterozygous for Arg397Cys missense mutation was noted to be hirsute, with severe loss of subcutaneous adipose tissue in her arms, legs and face, and sparing of truncal adipose tissue[34]. In contrast to CGL, the age of onset and pattern of adipose loss in *PPARγ* mutation is less predictable. It has been proposed that the formation of a salt bridge between the arginine 397 position and glutamic acid 324 may be disrupted, but how this missense mutation of *PPARγ* results in the lipodystrophic phenotype is unclear[33].

2.4 Lipodystrophy associated with mandibuloacral dysplasia

Mandibuloacral dysplasia is a rare autosomal recessive disease[36-40]. In addition to lipodystrophy, these patients have hypoplasia of the mandible and clavicle, contractures, bird-like facies with dental abnormalities, mottled skin and alopecia[36-40]. Lipodystrophy may appear as the loss of subcutaneous fat in the arms and legs (type A), or a more global loss (type B). Some affected patients have been found to be homozygous for a *LMNA* mutation or compound heterozygous at the zinc metalloproteinase gene, which is involved in post-translational proteolytic processing of prelamin A[41]. However, other patients do not have mutations in either gene, suggesting that additional, unidentified loci are involved. As in other cases on lipodystrophy, lipid and glucose abnormalities are present in this disorder[36-40].

2.5 Other Inherited Human Lipodystrophies

A form of lipodystrophy that occurs in association with short stature, ocular depression, abnormal iris and corneal development, hyperextensible joints and delayed teething has been described[42]. These patients have normal fat distribution on the legs, but exhibit loss of fat from the face and arms, with sporadic truncal involvement. In neonatal progeroid syndrome, affected individuals inherit a form of lipodystrophy in an autosomal recessive pattern characterized by near complete loss of subcutaneous adipose tissue, with gluteal and sacral sparing[43].

3. ACQUIRED LIPODYSTROPHIES

3.1 HIV Lipodystrophy

Abnormalties in body composition, ranging from fat loss (lipoatrophy) in the periphery, and excess nuchal and abdominal adiposity, have been reported in a high as 40-50% of ambulatory HIV-infected patients receiving combination antiretroviral therapy[44,45]. The prevalence may be even higher, depending on the group of patients, sex, age and race, as well as the type and duration of antiretroviral treatment[45]. Subcutaneous lipoatrophy is most prominent in the face, limbs, and buttocks but can also occur in the trunk. Central fat deposition often occurs in visceral fat. Excess adiposity may also be localized in the breasts and over the dorsal aspect of the neck, resulting in a "buffalo hump"[44]. Fatty infiltration is often increased within the muscle and liver[45].

Prospective studies have demonstrated initial increases in limb fat during the first few months of antiretroviral therapy, followed by a progressive decline during the ensuing three years[46]. The type of antiretroviral drugs and duration of treatment are strongly associated with the severity of lipodystrophy[45,47,48]. Combination therapy with nucleoside analogue reverse-transcriptase inhibitors and a protease inhibitor is strongly associated with lipodystrophy[49]. Protease inhibitors are thought to induce fat loss by inhibiting sterol regulatory enhancer–binding protein 1 (SREBP1)–mediated dimerization and activation of adipocyte retinoid X receptor (RXR) and peroxisome PPAR, and possibly PPAR coactivator 1[45]. In vitro studies have shown that protease inhibitors prevent lipogenesis and adipocyte differentiation and enhance lipolysis[48].

Among the nucleoside analogues, stavudine is most commonly associated with lipodystrophy, especially when used in combination with didanosine (45). Nucleoside analogues may predispose to mitochondrial injury, and can also inhibit adipogenesis and differentiation, increase lipolysis and synergize with the toxic effects of protease inhibitors[45]. Older age, acquired immunodeficiency syndrome (AIDS) infection and reduced CD4+ cell count, all confer a higher risk of lipodystrophy. Increased circulating fatty acids and impaired fatty acid oxidation contribute to increased intramyocellular lipid content, hepatic steatosis and insulin resistance.

Hypercholesterolemia and hypertriglyceridemia is prevalent in patients receiving combination therapy of protease inhibitor, nonnucleoside reverse-transcriptase inhibitor, and nucleoside reverse-transcriptase inhibitors. Typically, insulin resistance develops but without acanthosis nigricans, and rarely progresses to hyperglycemia[45].

3.2 Acquired Partial Lipodystrophy

Acquired generalized lipodystrophy (APL), also known as Barraquer-Simons syndrome, is a rare disorder described in less than 300 patients of various ethnic backgrounds[1]. Affected individuals lose subcutaneous adipose tissue in a cephalo-caudal manner, i.e. from the face and upper extremities, during childhood and adolescence. In females, fat deposition is increased in the hips and legs. Interestingly, patients with APL seldom develop insulin resistance, diabetes and associated complications. However, about 20 percent of patients develop membranoproliferative glomerulonephritis within 10 years of APL onset. Others have developed various autoimmune disorders[50,51].

The majority of APL patients have low serum C3 levels with concomitant elevation of C3 nephritic factor, a polyclonal IgG[52-54]. Other complement factors are normal. It is thought that C3 nephritic factor acts via adipsin (complement D) to cause adipocytes to lyse with subsequent development of APL. However, it is unknown what triggers the autoimmune reaction or why the APL does not affect the lower extremities.

3.3 Acquired Generalized Lipodystrophy

Similar to APL, patients who develop acquired generalized lipodystrophy (AGL) begin to lose subcutaneous adipose tissue during childhood and adolescence in the face and all extremities with sparing of retro-orbital and bone marrow fat[55]. However, some individuals lose fat from their palms and soles. Many patients develop herald panniculitis characterized histologically by infiltration of adipocytes by histiocytes, mononucleated giant cells and lymphocytes[56]. The healing of these lesions is associated with localized loss of adipocytes prior to more extensive losses, leading eventually to the AGL lipodystrophic phenotype. Curiously, panniculitis decreases the occurrence of diabetes and hypertriglyceridemia[55]. Another subset of AGL patients have associated autoimmune diseases, e.g., juvenile dematomyositis[57]. Unlike APL, affected children may develop an increased appetite, acanthosis nigricans and hepatic steatosis. Cirrhosis has been reported as a late complication of steatohepatitis or autoimmune hepatitis in about 20 percent of patients[55].

4. LESSONS FROM MURINE LIPODYSTROPHY

4.1 Congenital Murine Lipodystrophy

Mouse models have been used to better characterize the metabolic derangements seen in human lipodystrophy, and further our understanding of the mechanisms that lead to its development. SREBP1c, is a member of the family of SREBPs that control transcription of enzymes involved in lipid biosynthesis[2-4]. SREBPs are bound to membranes of nuclear envelope and endoplasmic reticulum, released by proteolysis in cholesterol deficient states, enter the nucleus and activate genes encoding enzymes that mediate synthesis of cholesterol and unsaturated fatty acids[58]. Conversely, proteolysis of SREBPs is blocked and transcription of target genes declines when cells are filled with sterols[58]. SREBP1c overexpression in 3T3-L1 cells enhances triglyceride accumulation and increases production of PPARγ[58]. In mice, expression of a truncated dominant-positive nSREBP1a whose transport is no longer regulated by nascent levels of cholesterol, results in free entry of SREBP1a into the nucleus and tremendous amount of hepatic lipid accumulation secondary to overproduction of cholesterol and triglycerides[58].

The laboratory of Brown and Goldstein developed mice that expressed a truncated nuclear form of SREBP (nSREBP1c) under control of the adipocyte-specific aP2 promoter[2]. The mutant protein lacked the membrane attachment domain, and hence entered the nucleus unregulated[2]. Adipocytes failed to develop normally in nSREBP1c transgenic mice[2]. These mutant mice demonstrated a phenotype similar to CGL early during postnatal development, with severe loss of adipocytes, runted appearance, enlarged abdomen and hyperinsulinemia[2]. Between 7 and 12 weeks of age, the nSREBP1c transgenic mice had marked organomegaly involving the liver, spleen, pancreas and abdominal lymph nodes. Linear growth was normal. Grossly, the transgenic livers appeared pale and weighed twice that of the wild-type controls. White adipose tissue (WAT) was deficient and intrascapular brown adipose tissue (BAT) appeared enlarged, was infiltrated by WAT and weighed slightly more than wild-type animals[2]. Histologic examination of nSREBP1c transgenic livers revealed infiltration by neutral lipids[2]. Epididymal adipocytes from the transgenic mice were small with eosinophilic cytoplasm and a single unilocular vacuole. Furthermore, there was significant reduction in expression of genes involved in adipocyte differentiation, e.g. C/EBPα, PPARγ, adipsin and leptin, while the preadipocyte marker Pref-1, as well as TNFα, was increased[2].

The nSREBP1c transgenic mice had approximately 60 times higher insulin levels than wild-type, profound insulin resistance and hyperglycemia (glucose >300 mg/dl) that was not reversed by insulin treatment. Since insulin-mediated glucose uptake was apparently normal in isolated soleus muscles, they proposed that the in vivo insulin resistance may be due to deficiency of a circulating factor involved in glucose uptake. Leptin was a candidate since the expression in adipose tissue was reduced by 90% and circulating levels were 6 times lower than wild-type[2]. Thus, as had been reported in congenital leptin deficiency, they investigated whether leptin replacement would reverse the metabolic derangements in nSREBP1c transgenic mice[2]. As predicted, restoration of leptin via chronic subcutaneous infusion for 12 days reversed the hyperlipidemia, hyperglycemia and insulin resistance in nSREBP1c transgenic mice[2]. Although leptin decreased food intake resulting in a modest decrease in weight, the effect on glucose and lipids was independent, since food restriction could not reproduce the same effect on glucose and lipids[2].

Moitra et al.[59] expressed a dominant-negative protein, termed A-ZIP/F, under the control of the aP2 enhancer/promoter, resulting in prevention of the DNA binding of B-ZIP transcription factors of both the C/EBP and Jun families. A-ZIP/F-1 transgenic mice had no WAT and drastically reduced BAT[59]. Although there was initial growth delay, the weight was normal by 12 weeks[59]. The liver was severely steatotic in A-ZIP/F-1 transgenic mice, and they were hyperinsulinemic, diabetic and had elevated free fatty acids and triglycerides. Leptin was also decreased[59]. Transplantation of wild-type fat reversed the hyperglycemia, lowered insulin levels, and improved muscle insulin sensitivity in A-ZIP/F-1 mice. Moreover, hyperphagia, hepatic steatosis, organomegaly and elevated triglyceride and fatty acid levels were either partially or completely reversed by transplantation of wild-type WAT[59]. In contrast, adipose tissue transplantation using $Lep^{ob/ob}$ fat had no effect on the phenotype of lipoatrophic A-ZIP/F-1 mice, suggesting that a secreted factor, likely leptin, was responsible for the improvement in metabolic profile[59]. In support of this idea, leptin infusion lowered insulin and glucose, and reversed lipid accumulation in the liver and various organs[59].

Adiponectin is an adipose-specific protein whose expression is decreased in insulin resistance and obesity[60]. Adiponectin production is stimulated by insulin sensitizing thiazolidinediones. Administration of adiponectin in rodents improves lipids by stimulating fatty acid oxidation and decreases insulin resistance by reducing triglyceride content in muscle and liver. Since adiponectin is decreased as a result of adipocyte loss in A-ZIP/F-1 mice, it was proposed that this may contribute to the observed metabolic derangement[61]. Administration of adiponectin in A-ZIP/F-1 mice reversed hyperglycemia, hyperinsulimia, hyperlipidemia and diabetes[61]. Importantly, the combination of physiological doses of adiponectin and leptin was more effective than either adiponectin or leptin alone[61].

Interestingly, a low-dose of leptin administered via the lateral cerebral ventricle corrected the insulin resistance, hyperlipidemia and steatosis in lipodystrophic aP2-nSREBP-1c mice, while the same dose given peripherally did not[62]. Central leptin suppressed stearoyl-CoA desaturase-1 (SCD-1) RNA and enzymatic activity, in parallel with reduction in lipid levels and hepatic steatosis[62]. Furthermore, central leptin treatment improved insulin-stimulated phosphorylation of the insulin receptor, insulin receptor substrate 2 (IRS-2), IRS-2-associated PI-3-kinase and Akt activities in liver, suggesting that the effects of leptin on glucose and lipid metabolism occurred through a central neuronal, likely hypothalamic, mechanism[62].

4.2 Acquired Murine Lipodystrophy

The mechanisms of antiretroviral drug-induced lipodystrophy and its adverse effects have been explored in mice[63-65]. In rodents, ritonavir treatment increases triglyceride and cholesterol levels through increased fatty acid and cholesterol biosynthesis in adipose and liver. Ritonavir treatment also results in hepatic steatosis and hepatomegaly, and reduction in leptin[63,64]. These abnormalities, which are profound after feeding a high fat (Western) diet, are due at least in part to accumulation of the activated forms of SREBP-1 and -2 in the nucleus of hepatocytes and adipocytes, and enhanced expression of lipogenic genes[63,64]. This murine model has been used to investigate whether leptin replacement therapy alleviates the ritonavir-induced metabolic abnormalities[66]. As predicted, chronic intraperitoneal injection of leptin significantly reversed the elevated plasma cholesterol level induced by ritonavir, and decreased hepatic steatosis, in part by reducing activation of SREBP1[66].

Chronic treatment with ritonavir in mice decreases adiponectin and increases plasma triglyceride, fatty acids and cholesterol[65]. Importantly, adiponectin replacement therapy ameliorates these ritonavir-induced metabolic abnormalities, partly by reducing the synthesis of fatty acids and triglyceride, and stimulating fatty acid oxidation in liver[65]. However, adiponectin had no effect on ritonavir-induced hypercholesterolemia and hepatic cholesterol synthesis[65].

In contrast to previous studies that found no effect of ritonavir on body fat, chronic ritonavir treatment has been shown to induce whole body lipoatrophy in male mice, loss of gonadal fat depot in females, and increased triglyceride levels in both genders[64]. Interestingly, this model was not associated with liver abnormalities. In contrast to leptin and adiponectin in the preceding studies, treatment with the PPARα agonist gemfibrozil and PPARγ agonist rosiglitazone, did not alleviate the hypertriglyceridemia or lipoatrophy in ritonavir-treated male mice[64].

The Scherer laboratory has recently described a lipoatrophic mouse model, FAT-ATTAC, where apoptotic death of adipocytes is induced through targeted activation of caspase 8[67]. The transgenic mouse develops normally, but death of adipocytes can be induced at any developmental stage by administration of a FK1012 analog that leads to the dimerization of a membrane-bound, adipocyte-specific caspase 8-FKBP fusion protein[67]. Within 2 weeks of dimerizer administration, FAT-ATTAC mice show a near depletion of adipocytes, and profound reduction in leptin, adiponectin, resistin and various adipokines. FAT-ATTAC mice become glucose intolerant, have diminished basal and endotoxin-induced inflammation, and are less responsive to glucose-stimulated insulin secretion[67]. The FAT-ATTAC mice are hyperphagic, consistent with leptin deficiency. Importantly, adipocyte can be recovered upon cessation of treatment, thus providing a unique reversible model for studying lipoatrophy[67].

5. LEPTIN AND HUMAN LIPODYSTROPHY

Based on the murine lipodystrophic studies described earlier, Oral et al.[5] examined the effect of leptin replacement in lipodystrophic patients. In the initial study, nine female patients (age range, 15 to 42 years; eight with diabetes mellitus) who had lipodystrophy and leptin concentrations less than 4 ng/ml, received recombinant methionyl-human leptin subcutaneously twice a day for four months at escalating doses to achieve physiologic replacement[5]. During treatment, the serum leptin increased from a mean of 1.3 ± 0.3 to 11.1 ± 2.5 ng/ml. The glycosylated hemoglobin value decreased significantly in the eight patients with diabetes. Moreover, triglyceride levels decreased by 60% over four months, and the liver volume by 28%. All nine patients were able to discontinue or decrease their antidiabetic treatment. Importantly, leptin was more effective than plasmapheresis, which was the standard care.

In a subsequent study, Petersen et al.[6] showed that chronic leptin treatment improved insulin-stimulated hepatic and peripheral glucose metabolism in lipodystrophic patients. This improvement in insulin action was the result of reduced hepatic and muscle triglyceride content. As is the case with congenital leptin deficiency, the low leptin level in lipodystrophy is also associated with abnormalities of the neuroendocrine axis. Thus, Oral et al.[68] inquired whether hormonal abnormalities seen in lipodystrophic patients could be reversed by replacement of leptin[68]. Seven lipodystrophic female patients (ages 15-42 years), all diabetic and with serum leptin levels less than 4 ng/ml were treated with recombinant methionyl-human leptin in physiological doses in an open-labeled study. While on recombinant leptin, the mean serum leptin concentration increased from 1.3 ± 0.3 to 11.1 ± 2.5 ng/ml. Four of five patients who had intact reproductive systems had irregular menstrual cycles before leptin therapy, which were restored by the fourth month of leptin therapy. Estradiol concentrations increased 3-fold on leptin therapy[68]. Moreover, leptin replacement attenuated the gonadotropin response to LHRH, suggesting a central action[68]. In this particular study, leptin had no significant effects on the thyroid or adrenal axes[68].

A longer term study on the effects of leptin replacement on pituitary hormones was conducted[69]. Ten females and 4 males with generalized lipodystrophy were treated with human leptin in physiologic doses in an open-labeled study for 8 to 12 months[69]. In the females, serum free testosterone decreased, sex hormone binding globulin increased, and luteinizing hormone responses to LHRH were more robust after therapy, especially in the youngest patients[69]. Eight of ten patients had amenorrhea prior to therapy and developed normal menstrual cycles after leptin therapy. Among the males, serum testosterone tended to increase although not significantly, and the LH response to LHRH did not show significant changes. Importantly, five additional hypoleptinemic male subjects underwent spontaneous pubertal development without leptin therapy. In both genders, insulin-like growth factor increased but there were no differences in growth hormone, thyroid, or pituitary-adrenal axis following leptin therapy. As expected, glycemic parameters and lipids improved in response to leptin[69]. Together, these data indicate that leptin is not absolutely required for pubertal development in lipodystrophy, but exerts a permissive effect on menstrual cycles by restoring LH pulsatility.

There have been recent reports on the long-term (6-12 months) effects of leptin on energy balance in generalized lipodystrophy[7,9,69-72]. Leptin significantly decreased glucose and glycosylated hemoglobin, triglycerides, total and LDL cholesterol. HDL was unchanged. Liver volumes were significantly reduced, indicating reduction in steatosis. Importantly, leptin significantly reduces transaminases and hepatocellular ballooning injury seen in non-alcoholic steatohepatitis[70]. Decreases in appetite, increased satiety and reduction in total body weight and fat content, have been seen with chronic leptin treatment[72]. However, in contrast to rodents, leptin decreases resting energy expenditure[7].

6. LIPODYSTROPHY AND OBESITY: METABOLIC PARADOX LINKED TO LEPTIN?

The survival of mammals requires an ability to maintain energy balance in the face of an unpredictable food supply[73]. We consume more calories per meal than is required for immediate metabolic needs, and the excess is stored for use during fasting[73]. Adipose tissue plays a crucial role in survival by providing an almost limitless capacity for energy storage in the form of triglyceride. The fall in leptin during fasting acts as a critical starvation signal by stimulating hyperphagia and reducing energy expenditure, mainly through the suppression of thyroid thermogenesis, reproduction and immunity[74]. In its most extreme form, total leptin deficiency in $Lep^{ob/ob}$ mice or leptin insensitivity in $Lepr^{db/db}$ mice, results in voracious feeding, morbid obesity, hypothalamic hypogonadism, and suppression of thyroid and growth hormones, and the immune system[75]. Similarly, the loss of adipocytes in lipodystrophy is associated with varying degrees of hyperphagia, central hypogonadism and immunodeficiency[1]. In both cases, leptin treatment reverses these abnormalities, mainly by binding to the long receptor (LRb) in hypothalamic and other CNS regions, activating the Jak-STAT signal transduction pathway, and inhibiting the expression of orexigenic neuropeptides, e.g., neuroeptide Y (NPY) and agouti-related peptide (AGRP). In contrast, anorexigenic peptides, e.g. α-melanocyte stimulating hormone (MSH), derived from proopiomelanocortin (POMC) and cocaine and amphetamine-regulated transcript (CART), are increased by leptin[76]. Additionally, leptin exerts a permissive effect on reproduction by acting at all levels of the hypothalamic-pituitary-gonadal axis[76].

Studies in rodents have shown that leptin-replete normal and especially DIO animals are relatively insensitive to leptin[77]. Hyperleptinemia and resistance to exogenous leptin treatment in DIO is not due to leptin receptor defects, but may involve impairment of leptin transport across the blood-brain barrier or leptin signaling, e.g. through the induction of suppressors of cytokine signaling (SOCS)-3[77]. Importantly, there are similarities between the metabolic derangements of "common" diet-induced obesity and those associated with lipodystrophy and congenital leptin deficiency, such as insulin resistance that may progress to diabetes, hyperlipidemia and steatosis, i.e. an increase in lipid accumulation in liver, muscle and other organs[77]. The latter may induce lipotoxicity through oxidative damage, and has been implicated in cardiovascular complications and pancreatic islet failure[78]. Lipotoxicity in the pancreas and cardiomyocytes results from an increase in ceramide formation via condensation of unoxidized palmitoyl CoA and serine, catalyzed by the enzyme serine palmitoyl transferase. In rodents, the increased ceramide is associated with upregulation of inducible nitric oxide synthase, leading to increased nitric oxide and peroxynitrite formation, generation of reactive oxygen species and apoptotic death[78].

This paradox of metabolic similarities between extremes of adiposity phenotypes, i.e. lipodystrophy and obesity, has led to the idea that a major function of leptin is to induce compensatory oxidation of surplus fatty acids in non-adipose tissues[79]. Leptin stimulates the oxidation of fatty acids through activation of 5'-AMP-activated protein kinase (AMPK), a sensor of cellular energy status[79] (Fig. 1). The fall in ATP:ADP ratio during fasting or stress leads to an increase in AMP, which activates AMPK by binding to two tandem domains on the gamma subunits of AMPK, causing phosphorylation of AMPK by the tumor suppressor LKB1. Once activated, AMPK switches on catabolic pathways that generate ATP, while switching off ATP consumption[80]. Activation of AMPK potently stimulates fatty-acid oxidation in liver and muscle by inhibiting the activity of acetyl coenzyme A carboxylase (ACC). Leptin selectively stimulates phosphorylation and activation of the α2 catalytic subunit of AMPK leading to inhibition of ACC activity, thereby stimulating the oxidation of fatty acid[81] (Fig. 1). The latter is also augmented by leptin's ability to increase sympathetic nervous activity through regulation of AMPK in the hypothalamus[82]. Likewise, adiponectin has been demonstrated to stimulate fatty acid oxidation and reduce glucose through activation of AMPK and subsequent inhibition of ACC[61].

The severe lipid and glucose abnormalities in lipodystrophy may be attributed to three factors: (i) loss of adipocytes and hence normal lipid storage capacity, (ii) diminished fatty acid oxidation as a result of deficiency of leptin, adiponectin and as yet unknown insulin-sensitizing adipocyte hormones, and (iii) increased nutrient load from overeating as a failure of the satiety effect of leptin. Ectopic lipid deposition in muscle and liver is well known to reduce insulin signaling, as well as attenuate insulin secretion from β-cells[78]. The critical role of leptin has been confirmed by its ability to inhibit feeding, stimulate lipid oxidation and enhance insulin sensitivity. On the other hand, the fact that transplantation of adipose tissue from $Lep^{ob/ob}$ mice does not reverse the metabolic phenotype in lipodystrophic mice suggests that the diminished lipid storage capacity *per se* is not a critical determinant of lipid and glucose dysregulation[4].

As with lipodystrophy, the liver in DIO is exposed to a high nutrient load, and the hyperinsulinemia induced by the high carbohydrate and lipid content of food upregulates lipogenic transcription factors in the liver, increasing the expression of their lipogenic target enzymes. This raises the hepatic production of very low-density lipoproteins (VLDL), which deliver fatty acids throughout the body. The mechanisms for decompensation of antilipotoxic protection in DIO appear to involve decreasing leptin sensitivity, perhaps in combination with insufficient leptin production[79]. Ultimately, leptin resistance and relative hypoleptinemia in DIO culminate in a reduction in fatty acid oxidation, increased lipid deposition, insulin resistance and diabetes[79]. Although the precise pathways are poorly understood, aging and DIO in rodents provide some clues[83]. For example, aging rats are less sensitive to leptin action in the brain and peripheral tissues, which results in increased visceral fat deposition[83]. SOCS-3 is increased in the leptin-unresponsive adipocytes of aged rats, and may mediate the age-related obesity, lipotoxicity, insulin resistance and diabetes. However, in contrast to total leptin deficiency in $Lep^{ob/ob}$ and leptin resistance in $Lepr^{db/db}$, some response to leptin is maintained even in long-standing DIO. Thus, the degree of lipid and glucose elevation and steatosis in DIO is never as severe as $Lep^{ob/ob}$ or $Lepr^{db/db}$ [79] (Figure 1).

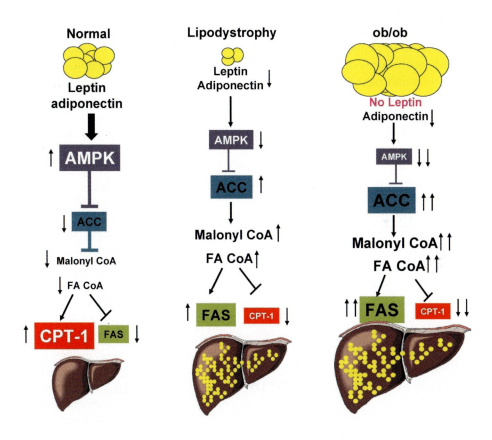

Figure 1. Regulation of lipids by leptin in normal, lipodystrophic and congenital leptin-deficient (ob/ob) states. Leptin activates AMPK, leading to reduced activity of ACC, which blocks the formation of malonyl CoA. Malonyl Co A is critical substrate for fatty acid synthesis, as well as an allosteric inhibitor of carnitine palmitoyltransferase (CPT)-1, which mediates mitochondrial oxidation of fatty acids. By lowering malonyl CoA, leptin maintains appropriate fatty acid oxidation, preventing lipid accumulation in liver and other peripheral tissues, hence lipotoxicity and organ dysfunction is prevented. When leptin action is lacking in lipodystrophy and particularly congenital leptin deficiency, AMPK activity is diminished, leading to high level of ACC activity, and generation of malonyl CoA. Fatty acid synthase (FAS) levels and activity are enhanced, CPT-1 activity is reduced, and more triglyceride is formed than oxidized, thus raising the levels of fatty acyl CoA (FA CoA) and triglyceride in liver, muscle, pancreatic islets and other tissues. Steatosis results in lipotoxicity, insulin resistance and diabetes.

7. CONCLUDING REMARKS AND MAJOR ISSUES TO BE ADDRESSED IN THE FUTURE

Leptin clearly has dramatic effects on appetite, glucose, lipids and reproductive function in lipodystrophy. A large body of evidence is emerging to support the hypothesis that leptin functions as an anti-steatotic and insulin-sensitizing hormone, by acting through hypothalamic neuronal circuits and mediating the activation of AMPK in peripheral tissues. While the metabolic consequences of generalized lipodystrophy are unlikely to be entirely attributable to low levels of leptin, the clinical response to leptin therapy has been most effective so far. Future studies must determine whether leptin can act in concert with adiponectin to increase lipid catabolism and enhance insulin response, as is the case in mice. Leptin replacement also deserves to be tested in patients with HIV lipodystrophy, to determine whether the abnormalities of fat distribution and metabolism can be prevented or reversed. Finally, lipodystrophy offers a unique model for understanding the role of adipose tissue as an endocrine organ. Similarities with the "metabolic syndrome" associated with obesity could be explored to better understand how adipocyte hormones and other secreted factors act on adipose tissue, the brain and other organs, leading to a coordinated regulation of energy balance, neuroendocrine and immune function.

ACKNOWLEDGEMENTS

This work was partially supported with grants from: The National Institutes of Health NIDDK PO1 DK49250, RO1 DK62348, T32 DK63688.

REFERENCES

1. A. Garg, Acquired and inherited lipodystrophies. *N Engl J Med*, **350,** 1220-1234 (2004).
2. I. Shimomura, R.E. Hammer, S. Ikemoto, M.S. Brown, J.L. Goldstein, Leptin reverses insulin resistance and diabetes mellitus in mice with congenital lipodystrophy. *Nature*, **401,** 73-76 (1999).
3. O. Gavrilova, B. Marcus-Samuels, D. Graham, J.K. Kim, G.I. Shulman, A.L. Castle, C. Vinson, M. Eckhaus, M.L. Reitman, Surgical implantation of adipose tissue reverses diabetes in lipoatrophic mice. *J Clin Invest*, **105,** 271-278 (2000).
4. C. Colombo, J.J. Cutson, T. Yamauchi, C. Vinson, T. Kadowaki, O. Gavrilova, M.L.Reitman, Transplantation of adipose tissue lacking leptin is unable to reverse the metabolic abnormalities associated with lipoatrophy. *Diabetes*, **51,** 2727-2733 (2002).
5. E.A. Oral, V. Simha, E. Ruiz, A. Andewelt, A. Premkumar, P. Snell, A.J. Wagner, A.M. DePaoli, M.L. Reitman, S.I. Taylor, P. Gorden, A. Garg, Leptin-replacement therapy for lipodystrophy. *N Engl J Med*, **346,** 570-578 (2002).
6. K.F. Petersen, E.A. Oral, S. Dufour, D. Befroy, C. Ariyan, C. Yu, G.W. Cline, A.M. DePaoli, S.I. Taylor, P. Gorden, G.I. Shulman, Leptin reverses insulin resistance and

hepatic steatosis in patients with severe lipodystrophy. *J Clin Invest*, **109**, 1345-1350 (2002).
7. S.A. Moran, N. Patten, J.R. Young, E. Cochran, N. Sebring, J. Reynolds, A. Premkumar, A.M. Depaoli, M.C. Skarulis, E.A. Oral, P. Gorden, Changes in body composition in patients with severe lipodystrophy after leptin replacement therapy. *Metabolism*, **53**, 513-519 (2004).
8. E. Cochran, J.R. Young, N. Sebring, A.M. DePaoli, E.A. Oral, P. Gorden, Efficacy of recombinant methionyl human leptin therapy for the extreme insulin resistance of the Rabson-Mendenhall syndrome. *J Clin Endocrinol Metab*, **89**, 1548-1554 (2004).
9. V. Simha, L.S. Szczepaniak, A.J. Wagner, A.M. DePaoli, A. Garg, Effect of leptin replacement on intrahepatic and intramyocellular lipid content in patients with generalized lipodystrophy. *Diabetes Care*, **26**, 30-35 (2003).
10. M. Seip, Lipodystrophy and gigantism with associated endocrine manifestations: a new diencephalic syndrome? *Acta Paediatr*, **48**, 555-574 (1959).
11. L. Van Maldergem, J. Magre, T.E. Khallouf, T. Gedde-Dahl Jr., M. Delepine, O. Trygstad, E. Seemanova, T. Stephenson, C.S. Albott, F. Bonnici, V.R. Panz, J.L. Medina, P. Bogalho, F. Huet, S. Savasta, A. Verloes, J.J. Robert, H. Loret, M. De Kerdanet, N. Tubiana-Rufi, A. Megarbane, J. Maassen, M. Polak, D. Lacombe, C.R. Kahn, E.L. Silveira, F.H. D'Abronzo, F. Grigorescu, M. Lathrop, J. Capeau, S. O'Rahilly, Genotype-phenotype relationships in Berardinelli-Seip congenital lipodystrophy. *J Med Genet*, **39**, 722-733 (2002).
12. A. Garg, R. Wilson, R. Barnes, E. Arioglu, Z. Zaidi, F. Gurakan, N. Kocak, S. O'Rahilly, S.I. Taylor, S.B. Patel, A.M. Bowcock, A gene for congenital generalized lipodystrophy maps to human chromosome 9q34. *J Clin Endocrinol Metab*, **84**, 3390-3394 (1999).
13. A.K. Agarwal, E. Arioglu, S. de Almeida, N. Akkoc, S.I. Taylor, A.M. Bowcock, R.I. Barnes, A. Garg, AGPAT2 is mutated in congenital generalized lipodystrophy linked to chromosome 9q34. *Nat Genet*, **31**, 21-23 (2002).
14. V. Simha, A. Garg, Phenotypic heterogeneity in body fat distribution in patients with congenital generalized lipodystrophy caused by mutations in the AGPAT2 or Seipin genes. *J Clin Endocrinol Metab*, **88**, 5433-5437 (2003).
15. J. Magre, M. Delepine, E. Khallouf, et al. Identification of the gene altered in Berardinelli-Seip congenital lipodystrophy on chromosome 11q13. *Nat Genet*, **28**, 365-370 (2001).
16. K. Heathcote, A. Rajab, J. Magre, et al, Molecular analysis of Berardinelli-Seip congenital lipodystrophy in Oman: evidence for multiple loci. *Diabetes*, **51**, 1291-1293 (2002).
17. A.K. Agarwal, V. Simha, E.A. Oral, S.A. Moran, P. Gorden, S. O'Rahilly, Z. Zaidi, F. Gurakan, S.A. Arslanian, A. Klar, A. Ricker, N.H. White, L. Bindl, K. Herbst, K. Kennel, S.B. Patel, L. Al-Gazali, A. Garg, Phenotypic and genetic heterogeneity in congenital generalized lipodystrophy. *J Clin Endocrinol Metab*, **88**, 4840-4847 (2003).
18. M.G. Dunnigan, M.A. Cochrane, A. Kelly, J.W. Scott, Familial lipoatrophic diabetes with dominant transmission: a new syndrome. *Q J Med*, **43**, 33-48 (1974).
19. A. Garg, R.M. Peshock, J.L. Fleckenstein, Adipose tissue distribution pattern in patients with familial partial lipodystrophy (Dunnigan variety). *J Clin Endocrinol Metab*, **84**, 170-174 (1999).
20. A. Garg, Gender differences in the prevalence of metabolic complications in familial partial lipodystrophy (Dunnigan variety). *J Clin Endocrinol Metab*, **85**, 1776-1782 (2000).
21. W.A. Haque, E.A. Oral, K. Dietz, A.M. Bowcock, A.K. Agarwal, A. Garg, Risk factors for diabetes in familial partial lipodystrophy, Dunnigan variety. *Diabetes Care*, **26**, 1350-1355 (2003).

22. J.M. Peters, R. Barnes, L. Bennett, W.M. Gitomer, A.M. Bowcock, A. Garg, Localization for the gene for familial partial lipodystrophy (Dunnigan variety) to chromosome 1q21. *Nat Genet*, **18,** 292-295 (1998).
23. H. Cao, R.A. Hegele, Nuclear lamin A/C R482Q mutation in Canadian kindreds with Dunnigan-type familial partial lipodystrophy. *Hum Mol Genet*, **9,** 109-112 (2000).
24. R.A. Speckman, A. Garg, F. Du, et al, Mutational and haplotype analyses of families with familial partial lipodystrophy (Dunnigan variety) reveal recurrent missense mutations in the globular C-terminal domain of lamin A/C. *Am J Hum Genet*, **66,** 1192-1198 (2000). Erratum, *Am J Hum Genet*, **67,** 775 (2000).
25. S. Shackleton, D.J. Lloyd, S.N. Jackson, et al, LMNA, encoding lamin A/C, is mutated in partial lipodystrophy. *Nat Genet*, **24,** 153-156 (2000).
26. C. Vigouroux, J. Magre, M.C. Vantyghem, et al, Lamin A/C gene: sex-determined expression of mutations in Dunnigan-type familial partial lipodystrophy and absence of coding mutations in congenital and acquired generalized lipoatrophy. *Diabetes*, **49,** 1958-1962 (2000).
27. A, Garg, R.A. Speckman, A.M. Bowcock, Multisystem dystrophy syndrome due to novel missense mutations in the amino-terminal head and alpha-helical rod domain of the lamin A/C gene. *Am J Med*, **112,** 549-555 (2002).
28. A.J. van der Kooi, G. Bonne, B. Eymard, et al, Lamin A/C mutations with lipodystrophy, cardiac abnormalities, and muscular dystrophy. *Neurology*, **59,** 620-623 (2002).
29. F. Lin, H.J. Worman, Structural organization of the human gene encoding nuclear lamin A and nuclear lamin C. *J Biol Chem*, **268,** 16321-16326 (1993).
30. C. Vigouroux, M. Auclair, E. Dubosclard, et al, Nuclear envelope disorganization in fibroblasts from lipodystrophic patients with heterozygous R482Q/W mutations in the lamin A/C gene. *J Cell Sci*, **114,** 4459-4468 (2001).
31. A. Garg, M. Vinaitheerthan, P.T. Weatherall, A.M. Bowcock, Phenotypic heterogeneity in patients with familial partial lipodystrophy (Dunnigan variety) related to the site of missense mutations in lamin A/C gene. *J Clin Endocrinol Metab*, **86,** 59-65 (2001).
32. I. Barroso, M. Gurnell, V.E. Crowley, et al, Dominant negative mutations in human PPARgamma associated with severe insulin resistance, diabetes mellitus and hypertension. *Nature*, **402,** 880-883 (1999).
33. R.A. Hegele, H. Cao, C. Frankowski, S.T. Mathews, T. Leff, PPARG F388L, a transactivation-deficient mutant, in familial partial lipodystrophy. *Diabetes*, **51,** 3586-3590 (2002).
34. A.K. Agarwal, A. Garg. A novel heterozygous mutation in peroxisome proliferator-activated receptor-gamma gene in a patient with familial partial lipodystrophy. *J Clin Endocrinol Metab*, **87,** 408-411 (2002).
35. D.B. Savage, G.D. Tan, C.L. Acerini, et al, Human metabolic syndrome resulting from dominant-negative mutations in the nuclear receptor peroxisome proliferator-activated receptor-gamma. *Diabetes*, **52,** 910-917 (2003).
36. L.W. Young, J.F. Radebaugh, P. Rubin, J.A. Sensenbrenner, G. Fiorelli, V.A. McKusick, New syndrome manifested by mandibular hypoplasia, acroosteolysis, stiff joints and cutaneous atrophy (mandibuloacral dysplasia) in two unrelated boys. *Birth Defects Orig Artic Ser*, **7,** 291-297 (1971).
37. V. Simha, A. Garg, Body fat distribution and metabolic derangements in patients with familial partial lipodystrophy associated with mandibuloacral dysplasia. *J Clin Endocrinol Metab*, **87,** 776-785 (2002).
38. D.L. Cutler, S. Kaufmann, G.R. Freidenberg. Insulin-resistant diabetes mellitus and hypermetabolism in mandibuloacral dysplasia: a newly recognized form of partial lipodystrophy. *J Clin Endocrinol Metab*, **73,** 1056-1061 (1991).

39. G. Novelli, A. Muchir, F. Sangiuolo, et al, Mandibuloacral dysplasia is caused by a mutation in LMNA-encoding lamin A/C. *Am J Hum Genet*, **71**, 426-431 (2002).
40. V. Simha, A.K. Agarwal, E.A. Oral, J.P. Fryns, A. Garg, Genetic and phenotypic heterogeneity in patients wtih mandibuloacral dysplasia-associated lipodystrophy. *J Clin Endocrinol Metab*, **88**, 2821-2824 (2003).
41. A.K. Agarwal, J.P. Fryns, R.J. Auchus, A. Garg, Zinc metalloproteinase, ZMPSTE24, is mutated in mandibuloacral dysplasia. *Hum Mol Genet*, **12**, 1995-2001 (2003).
42. J. Kobberling, M.G. Dunnigan, Familial partial lipodystrophy: two types of an X linked dominant syndrome, lethal in the hemizygous state. *J Med Genet*, **23**,120-127 (1986).
43. E.K. Pivnick, B. Angle, R.A. Kaufman, et al, Neonatal progeroid (Wiedemann-Rautenstrauch) syndrome: report of five new cases and review. *Am J Med Genet*, **90**, 131-140 (2000).
44. A. Carr, K. Samaras, S. Burton, et al, A syndrome of peripheral lipodystrophy, hyperlipidaemia and insulin resistance in patients receiving HIV protease inhibitors. *AIDS*, **12**, F51-F58 (1998).
45. S. Grinspoon, A. Carr, Cardiovascular risk and body-fat abnormalities in HIV-infected adults. *N Engl J Med*, **352**, 48-62 (2005).
46. A. Carr, K. Samaras, A. Thorisdottir, G.R. Kaufmann, D.J. Chisholm, D.A. Cooper, Diagnosis, prediction, and natural course of HIV-1 protease-inhibitor-associated lipodystrophy, hyperlipidaemia, and diabetes mellitus: a cohort study. *Lancet*, **353**, 2093-2099 (1999).
47. H. Murata, P.W. Hruz, M. Mueckler, The mechanism of insulin resistance caused by HIV protease inhibitor therapy. *J Biol Chem*, **275**, 20251-20254 (2000).
48. P. Dowell, C. Flexner, P.O. Kwiterovich, M.D. Lanes, Suppression of preadipocyte differentiation and promotion of adipocyte death by HIV protease inhibitors. *J Biol Chem*, **275**, 41325-41332 (2000).
49. A. Carr, J. Miller, M. Law, D.A. Cooper. A syndrome of lipoatrophy, lactic acidaemia and liver dysfunction associated with HIV nucleoside analogue therapy: contribution to protease inhibitor-related lipodystrophy syndrome. *AIDS*, **14**, F25-F32 (2000).
50. H.E. Jasin, Systemic lupus erythematosus, partial lipodystrophy and hypocomplementemia. *J Rheumatol* **6**, 43-50 (1979).
51. A. Torrelo, A. Espana, P. Boixeda, A. Ledo, Partial lipodystrophy and dermatomyositis. *Arch Dermatol*, **127**, 1846-1847 (1991).
52. D.G. Williams, A. Bartlett, P. Duffus, Identification of nephritic factor as an immunoglobulin. *Clin Exp Immunol*, **33**, 425-429 (1978).
53. C.D. West, A.J. McAdams, The alternative pathway C3 convertase and glomerular deposits. *Pediatr Nephrol* **13**, 448-453 (1999).
54. P.W. Mathieson, R. Wurzner, D.B. Oliveria, P.J. Lachmann, D.K. Peters, Complement-mediated adipocyte lysis by nephritic factor sera. *J Exp Med*, **177**, 1827-1831 (1993).
55. A. Misra, A. Garg, Clinical features and metabolic derangements in acquired generalized lipodystrophy: case reports and review of the literature. *Medicine (Baltimore)*, **82**, 129-146 (2003).
56. J.K. Billings, S.S. Milgraum, A.K. Gupta, J.T. Headington, J.E. Rasmussen, Lipoatrophic panniculitis: a possible autoimmune inflammatory disease of fat: report of three cases. *Arch Dermatol*, **123**, 1662-1666 (1987).
57. C. Huemer, H. Kitson, P.N. Malleson, et al, Lipodystrophy in patients with juvenile dermatomyositis -- evaluation of clinical and metabolic abnormalities. *J Rheumatol*, **28**, 610-615 (2001).

58. I. Shimomura, R.E. Hammer, J.A. Richardson, et al, Insulin resistance and diabetes mellitus in transgenic mice expressing nuclear SREBP-1c in adipose tissue: model for congenital generalized lipodystrophy. *Genes Dev*, **12,** 3182-3194 (1998).
59. J. Moitra, M.M. Mason, M. Olive, D. Krylov, O. Gavrilova, B. Marcus-Samuels, L. Feigenbaum, E. Lee, T. Aoyama, M. Eckhaus, M.L. Reitman, C. Vinson, Life without white fat: a transgenic mouse. *Genes Dev*, **12,** 3168-3181 (1998).
60. T. Kadowaki, T. Yamauchi, Adiponectin and adiponectin receptors. *Endocr Rev*, **26,** 439-451 (2005).
61. T. Yamauchi, J. Kamon, H. Waki, Y. Terauchi, N. Kubota, K. Hara, Y. Mori, T. Ide, K. Murakami, N. Tsuboyama-Kasaoka, O. Ezaki, Y. Akanuma, O. Gavrilova, C. Vinson, M.L. Reitman, H. Kagechika, K. Shudo, M. Yoda, Y. Nakano, K. Tobe, R. Nagai, S. Kimura, M. Tomita, P. Froguel, T. Kadowaki, The fat-derived hormone adiponectin reverses insulin resistance associated with both lipoatrophy and obesity. *Nat Med*, **7,** 941-946 (2001).
62. E. Asilmaz, P. Cohen, M. Miyazaki, P. Dobrzyn, K. Ueki, G. Fayzikhodjaeva, A.A Soukas, C.R. Kahn, J.M Ntambi, N.D. Socci, J.M. Friedman, Site and mechanism of leptin action in a rodent form of congenital lipodystrophy. *J Clin Invest*, **113,** 414-424 (2004).
63. T.M. Riddle, D.G. Kuhel, L.A. Woollett, C.J. Fichtenbaum, D.Y. Hui, HIV protease inhibitor induces fatty acid and sterol biosynthesis in liver and adipose tissues due to the accumulation of activated sterol regulatory element-binding proteins in the nucleus. *J Biol Chem*, **276,** 37514-37519 (2001).
64. E.S. Goetzman, L. Tian, T.R. Nagy, B.A. Gower, T.R. Schoeb, A. Elgavish, E.P. Acosta, M.S. Saag, P.A. Wood, HIV protease inhibitor ritonavir induces lipoatrophy in male mice. *AIDS Res Hum Retroviruses*, **19,** 1141-1150 (2003).
65. A. Xu, S. Yin, L. Wong, K.W. Chan, K.S. Lam, Adiponectin ameliorates dyslipidemia induced by the human immunodeficiency virus protease inhibitor ritonavir in mice. *Endocrinology*, **145,** 487-494 (2004).
66. T.M. Riddle, C.J. Fichtenbaum, D.Y. Hui, Leptin replacement therapy but not dietary polyunsaturated fatty acid alleviates HIV protease inhibitor-induced dyslipidemia and lipodystrophy in mice. *J Acquir Immune Defic Syndr*, **33,** 564-570 (2003).
67. U.B. Pajvani, M.E. Trujillo, T.P. Combs, P. Iyengar, L. Jelicks, K.A. Roth, R.N. Kitsis, P.E. Scherer, Fat apoptosis through targeted activation of caspase 8: a new mouse model of inducible and reversible lipoatrophy. *Nat Med*, **11,** 797-803 (2005).
68. E.A. Oral, E. Ruiz, A. Andewelt, N. Sebring, A.J.Wagner, A.M. Depaoli, P. Gorden, Effect of leptin replacement on pituitary hormone regulation in patients with severe lipodystrophy. *J Clin Endocrinol Metab*, **87,** 3110-3117 (2002).
69. C. Musso, E. Cochran, E. Javor, J. Young, A.M. Depaoli, P. Gorden, The long-term effect of recombinant methionyl human leptin therapy on hyperandrogenism and menstrual function in female and pituitary function in male and female hypoleptinemic lipodystrophic patients. *Metabolism*, **54,** 255-263 (2005).
70. E.D. Javor, M.G. Ghany, E.K. Cochran, E.A. Oral, A.M. DePaoli, A. Premkumar, D.E. Kleiner, P. Gorden, Leptin reverses nonalcoholic steatohepatitis in patients with severe lipodystrophy. *Hepatology*, **41,** 753-760 (2005).
71. E.D. Javor, E.K. Cochran, C. Musso, J.R. Young, A.M. Depaoli, P. Gorden, Long-term efficacy of leptin replacement in patients with generalized lipodystrophy. *Diabetes*, **54,** 1994-2002 (2005).
72. J.R. McDuffie, P.A. Riggs, K.A. Calis, R.J. Freedman, E.A. Oral, A.M. DePaoli, J.A. Yanovski, Effects of exogenous leptin on satiety and satiation in patients with lipodystrophy and leptin insufficiency. *J Clin Endocrinol Metab*, **89,** 4258-4263 (2004).
73. R.S. Ahima, Leptin and the neuroendocrinology of fasting. *Front Horm Res*, **26,** 42-56 (2000).

74. R.S. Ahima, D. Prabakaran, C. Mantzoros, D. Qu, B. Lowell, E. Maratos-Flier, J.S. Flier, Role of leptin in the neuroendocrine response to fasting. *Nature*, **382,** 250-252 (1996).
75. R.S. Ahima, J.S. Flier, Leptin. *Annu Rev Physiol*, **62,** 413-437 (2000).
76. R.S. Ahima, S.Y. Osei, Leptin signaling. *Physiol Behav*, **81,** 223-241 (2004).
77. J.S. Flier, Obesity wars: molecular progress confronts an expanding epidemic. *Cell*, **116,** 337-350 (2004).
78. R.H. Unger, The hyperleptinemia of obesity-regulator of caloric surpluses. *Cell*, **117,** 145-146 (2004).
79. R.H. Unger, Longevity, lipotoxicity and leptin: the adipocyte defense against feasting and famine. *Biochimie*, **87,** 57-64 (2005).
80. D.G. Hardie, Minireview: the AMP-activated protein kinase cascade: the key sensor of cellular energy status. *Endocrinology*, **144,** 5179-5183 (2003).
81. Y. Minokoshi, Y.B. Kim, O.D. Peroni, L.G. Fryer, C. Muller, D. Carling, B.B. Kahn, Leptin stimulates fatty-acid oxidation by activating AMP-activated protein kinase. *Nature*, **415,** 339-343 (2002).
82. Y. Minokoshi, T. Alquier, N. Furukawa, Y.B. Kim, A. Lee, B. Xue, J. Mu, F. Foufelle, P. Ferre, M.J. Birnbaum, B.J. Stuck, B.B. Kahn, AMP-kinase regulates food intake by responding to hormonal and nutrient signals in the hypothalamus. *Nature*, **428,** 569-574 (2004).
83. Z.W. Wang, W.T. Pan, Y. Lee, T. Kakuma, Y.T. Zhou, R.H. Unger, The role of leptin resistance in the lipid abnormalities of aging. *FASEB J*, **15,** 108-114 (2001).

Chapter 13

PULSATILE AND DIURNAL LEPTIN RHYTHMS

Luciana Ribeiro[1], João Vicente Busnello[1], Ma-Li Wong[1] and Julio Licínio[1]
[1] *Center for Pharmacogenomics and Clinical Pharmacology. Semel Institute for Neuroscience & Human Behavior, David Geffen School of Medicine at University of California, Los Angeles – UCLA, Los Angeles, CA*

Abstract: Soon after the discovery of the mouse *ob* gene and the characterization of leptin as its hormonal product, intensive research has defined many of the molecules physiological properties. Early research indicated that the molecule exhibited a rhythmic variation akin to that of other hormones. More detailed investigation revealed pulsatility as a key feature of this hormone's rhythm. The pattern of secretion is very closely tied to that of other hormones in a manner that is highly indicative of mechanistic interactions. The rhythms of leptin are altered in disease states or physiological imbalances. Gender and body weight may alter the quantities of hormonal secretion, but do not seem capable of disrupting the intrinsic nicto-hemeral rhythm, which is surprisingly stable across wide ranges of subjects and body weight. This chapter reviews the dynamics of daily variations in leptin levels.

Key words: leptin, circadian, rhythm, pulsatile, ultradian, diurnal

1. INTRODUCTION

Plasma leptin levels are highly organized and pulsatile, with significant ultradian and diurnal variation in spite of the fact that leptin is secreted by widely dispersed adipocytes. Such fluctuations of plasma leptin concentrations are biologically relevant.[1-6] At first glance, it may be difficult to conceptualize adipose tissue as an endocrine gland. Unlike other tissues, which are regulated by finely orchestrated feedback mechanisms; fat deposits are not under the influence of any single predominant control. Circulating leptin levels have been shown to suffer the influence of diverse physiological, experimental and pathological conditions.[7-10] Soon after the isolation of the mouse *ob* gene and the characterization of leptin as its protein product, different groups proposed a rhythmic pattern of secretion for the hormone. This was rapidly characterized and particularities in its circadian rhythm were further explored. Today much is known about the diurnal rhythm of the hormone's secretion and its pulsatility.

Circulating leptin concentrations exhibit a diurnal pattern, with a mid-morning nadir and a nocturnal peak that typically occurs between midnight and 2 am in subjects consuming meals on a regular schedule.[4] The largest increase of leptin is observed approximately 4 to 6 hours after each meal. Pulses of secretion are observed throughout the day provided adequate sampling techniques are used. Mechanisms regulating endogenous leptin secretion are the subject of considerable research efforts. Alterations in the secretion pattern of the hormone have emerged as a promising field of study and may translate into a more thorough understanding of the pathophysiology of illnesses such as obesity and its metabolic complications. This chapter aims to review the scientific advances achieved over this topic.

2. DIURNAL AND ULTRADIAN OSCILLATIONS

Most hormones have diurnal and ultradian oscillations, which are distinctive characteristics. Several mechanisms that modulate the amplitude and frequency of pulsatile and oscillatory hormonal release have been described.[11] Leptin secretion has a periodicity similar to those previously reported for other hormones. The most important ones include modulation by feedback of peripheral signals and modulation by the central nervous system.

Circulating leptin concentrations normally exhibit a diurnal pattern, with a mid-morning nadir and a nocturnal peak that typically occurs between midnight and 2 am in subjects consuming meals on a regular schedule.[4] The diurnal pattern is not present in fasting subjects and, in fact, leptin concentrations will decrease and remain low until food is ingested.[12] The diurnal pattern of leptin secretion does not appear to be directly related to the circadian rhythm of the hypothalamic-pituitary-adrenal axis because the timing of the nocturnal leptin peak is shifted by the timing of meal consumption, independently of any effects on circulating cortisol concentrations.[13] The largest increase of leptin is observed approximately 4 to 6 hours after each meal, and the consumption of high-carbohydrate meals increases the entire 24-hour leptin profile relative to consumption of high-fat meals.[14]

Because leptin is secreted by widely dispersed fat cells, it was not initially apparent that such secretion would be highly pulsatile with ultradian and diurnal rhythms organized like those of any other hormone. We hypothesized that the fat cell was an endocrine organ just like other endocrine glands such as the pituitary, thyroid, and adrenals, and if that was indeed the case, leptin secretion would be highly organized.

To test that hypothesis, we developed a highly intensive 24-h sampling paradigm with blood collections at every seven minutes resulting in 207 data points through the 24-h period. Using this approach our group[2] discovered leptin pulsatility and also demonstrated that minute-to-minute variations in plasma leptin concentrations are in inverse relation to pituitary-adrenal function. Analysis of the pulse parameters of total circulating leptin with Cluster, a well-validated, computerized pulse-detection algorithm developed by Johnson & Veldhuis,[16] showed a mean pulse frequency of 32 pulses/24hours. Pulse duration was 32.8 minutes, with an average interpeak interval of 43.8 minutes. The average pulse height was 5.94 ng/ml, representing a 133% increase over baseline. We also analyzed the same data using the program Detect, an independently derived peak-detection algorithm.[15] The Detect algorithm identified 39.4 pulses/24hours, which agrees with the mean Cluster estimate of 32.0 pulses/24hours (Fig. 1a); Detect identified a pulse height of 6.69, which also agrees with the mean Cluster estimate. The Pearson correlation of individual pulse height estimated by Cluster and independently by Detect was highly significant. (Fig. 1)

Using a less intense sampling protocol, Sinha and colleagues independently confirmed the diurnal and/or ultradian oscillations of plasma leptin concentrations.[4] Previously, their group had demonstrated a nocturnal rise of leptin secretion in humans that could be related to appetite suppression during sleep.[3] In that study it was demonstrated that in addition to nightly rhythms of leptin secretion, ultradian oscillations of leptin secretion exist. Even with the less than optimal blood sampling protocol used, leptin pulses were detected during 24 hour periods (number of pulses: 3.25). Subsequently, they utilized blood samples, which were obtained every 15 minutes over a 12-hour period during oscillatory glucose infusion following an overnight fast. With this blood sampling protocol, additional evidence about the pulsatile nature of leptin secretion in humans was evidenced. During 12-hours, the number of leptin pulses was 4.2, which clearly underestimates true leptin pulsatility, due to insufficient sampling.

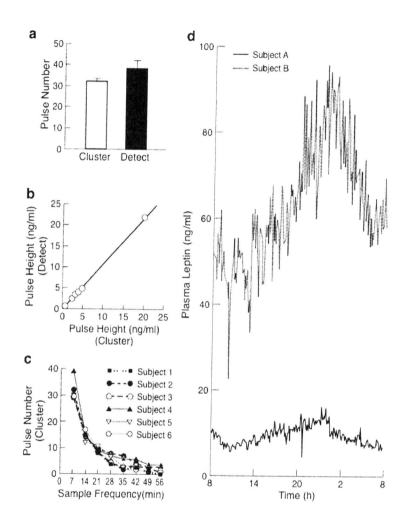

Figure 1. a, Number of leptin pulses assessed with Cluster (white) [16] and Detect (black) [15]. b, Pulse height assessed with cluster (x-axis) and Detect (y-axis) (r=0.9998; p< 8 x 10-8, Pearson correlation). c, Assessment of leptin pulse numbers in data sets corresponding to sampling every 7, 14, 21, 28, 35, 49 and 56 min, assessed by Cluster. d, Comparison of leptin levels and pulse parameters in two Caucasian women. Subject A is a normal-weight control and subject B is obese. Figure is from ref. [2], with permission.

We demonstrated that leptin pulse parameters may be accurately ascertained only with frequent sampling. To examine the extent to which sample interval affected our ability to accurately estimate leptin pulse parameters, we created surrogate data sets in which leptin levels were listed every 7, 14, 21, 28, 35, 42, 49 and 56 minutes. Cluster analysis was applied to each surrogate data set. We showed a dramatic loss in the detection of pulsatility with each increasing sampling interval (Fig. 1c, above). When samples are taken every 28 minutes, we observed an 81.8% loss in the ability to ascertain the number of pulses as compared with sampling every 7 minutes. We concluded that because leptin pulses are short, lasting 32.8 minutes, rapid sampling is required to characterize the true pulsatile parameters of leptin in humans. It is possible that by sampling more frequently than every 7 minutes we might have detected additional, short pulses. Our data reflects true pulsatility of endogenous leptin levels: however, one should bear in mind that pulse parameters are dependent not only on the intrinsic pulsatility of leptin, but are also limited by the sensitivity of the sampling protocol and by the detection limit and the coefficient of variation of the assays.

Because the pulse duration of leptin is relatively short (32.8 min), we could only determine that leptin levels in humans were highly pulsatile by using rapid plasma sampling (Fig. 1c). Sinha reported ultradian fluctuations in leptin levels.[4] However, their less frequent sampling, as predicted in our surrogate data sets (Fig. 1c), lead to the observation of far fewer pulses. Moreover, their correlations between number of oscillations, BMI, fasting leptin levels, and absolute amplitude might be secondary to infrequent sampling. Frequent sampling is required to fully characterize leptin pulsatility in humans. In our sample of healthy men there was no association between ages, BMI, mean 24-hour leptin concentrations, and pulse numbers/24-hours. These findings opened the door to a new area of investigation aimed at the identification of humoral and neuronal signals that regulate rapid fluctuations in leptin secretion or clearance. Leptin seems to have the capacity to regulate highly pulsatile systems, such as the hypothalamic-pituitary-gonadal (HPG) and hypothalamic-pituitary-adrenal (HPA) axis. The pulsatility of leptin might not be as profound as that of other hormonal systems; nevertheless, pulsatility can affect hormonal bioactivity. The maximal biologic activity of exogenous luteinizing hormone-releasing hormone (LHRH) has been shown to require pulsatile secretion. Women who fail to ovulate due to idiopathic hypogonadotrophic hypogonadism, amenorrhea related to low weight, organic pituitary disease or polycystic ovaries can ovulate and become pregnant provided this hormone is exogenously administered in a pulsatile pattern.[17] Infertility in men with oligospermia can also be treated by Pulsatile LHRH Therapy.[18]

These can be explained by the fact that to increase transcription of the LHRH receptor and gonadotropin subunits genes in vitro and in vivo a pulsatile gonadotropin-releasing hormone stimulus is required[19,20]; for such reasons the hypothalamic LHRH pulse generator is recognized as the reproductive core.[21] For growth hormone (GH), there are differential effects after pulsatile and continuous administrations. Pulsatility is essential for the maximal stimulation of somatomedine-C/insulin-like growth factor 1 and subsequent growth, but continuous exposure to GH is required for the upregulation of hepatic GH receptors.[22,23]

To access specific alteration in leptin pulsatility in obesity, we conducted a pilot study comparing leptin pulsatility in two Caucasian women, one obese [body mass index (BMI) = 43.6 kg/m^2] and one with normal body weight (BMI=20.5 kg/m^2). Both subjects were studied at the same phase of the menstrual cycle. The 24-hour average leptin level was seven times higher in the obese individual (63.03 vs. 9.34 ng/ml) (Fig. 1d). Concentration-independent pulsatility parameters, such as pulse number/24 hours, pulse duration, inter-peak interval, and pulse height, expressed as the percent increase from baseline, were almost identical in the two women. Both also exhibited statistically significant diurnal variation in circulating leptin levels. Using the 8:00-12:00 period as baseline, we found that leptin levels increased significantly during the 20:00-00:00 and 00:00-00:4:00 time periods in the two women. These results show that, in obesity, the diurnal architecture of leptin was maintained (albeit in higher concentrations)[24] (Fig. 2)

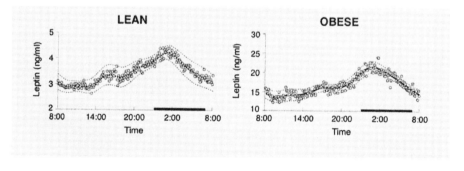

Figure 2. Estimated 24-h profiles of plasma and leptin in lean and obese subjects. Mean hormone levels are plotted as circles. The semiparametric linear mixed-effects model, across-subject prediction is drawn as a solid line. Dashed lines trace out the prediction's approximate 95% confidence interval. Sleep period is noted by a black strip. Figure is from ref. 24, with permission.

3. RHYTHM CONTROL

The mechanisms that regulate endogenous leptin secretion are the subject of considerable research efforts. Diurnal leptin rhythmicity does not seem to be controlled by the endogenous circadian clock. Schoeller and colleagues[13] have shown that day/night reversal produced a rapid phase shift that was dissociated from the change in cortisol. Meal time and insulin seem to play a major role, because delaying meals for 6.5 h caused peak leptin levels to move forward by 4–7.[13] Other hormones that show diurnal changes and can influence plasma leptin, such as neuropeptide Y[25], corticosteroids[26], and catecholamines[27], could also modulate its diurnal rhythm. In addition, circulating leptin is bound to one or more binding proteins[28,29] that may modulate its plasma pattern.

Insulin may be the major determinant of leptin secretory pattern. Although several studies showed that insulin infusions for 2–10 h had no effect on plasma leptin concentration[8,30-32], Saad et al.[33] showed that physiologic insulin concentrations can increase plasma leptin by approximately 50% and that such an effect takes 2–3 h to become evident. Other studies showed that insulin or glucose are capable of increasing leptin concentrations 4–6 hours after infusion.[34] Therefore, it is plausible, that increases in leptinemia that become apparent in the afternoon and during the night are caused by postprandial insulin increases. Conversely, the nocturnal post-absorptive diminution in insulinemia could cause a decline in leptinemia that becomes manifest in the early morning hours. In this manner, insulin could influence the nicto-hemeral tidal magnitude of serum leptin. Meanwhile, postprandial insulin excursions could cause fluctuations in plasma leptin, which are reflected as episodic pulsations. This is supported by the occurrence of prominent leptin pulsatility 2–3 h after meals. Thus, the insulin secretory pattern seems to modulate the 24-h leptin profile. However, the hypothesis that such an association might be an artifact of infrequent sampling cannot be ruled out. Future studies employing intensive sampling methods have to be undertaken to confirm the association among insulinemia, obesity, and patterns of leptin pulsatility.

Endogenous glucocorticoids do not seem significantly related to circulating leptin levels. A study measured plasma leptin levels in ten patients with Cushing's disease both before and after curative surgery. Serum leptin levels remained unchanged 10 days after the resection of the ACTH-secreting adenoma. Plasma ACTH levels were reduced to $1/15^{th}$ of their preoperative values and cortisol to $1/10^{th}$. Administration of exogenous corticotropin-releasing hormone (CRH) before surgery and 10 days after surgery resulted in no changes of plasma leptin levels when measured up to

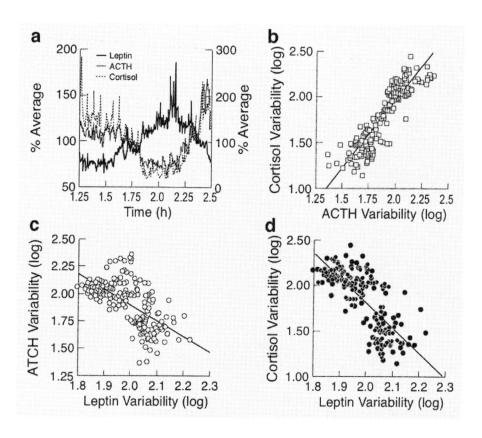

Figure 3. Simultaneous fluctuations in leptin, ACTH and cortisol levels (a). Each measurement is expressed as variability, defined as a percentage of individual 24-h averages, using the formula: variability at time t= (hormone level at time t/24-h individual average level) x 100. Lines show averages for the six male subjects at each time point; black, leptin; gray, ACTH; and dashed, cortisol. The left-hand y-axis shows leptin levels expressed as variability or percent of average, and the right-hand y-axis shows ACTH and cortisol levels expressed as variability or percent of average. Pearson correlations of simultaneous fluctuations in leptin, ACTH and cortisol collected from the six men at 7-min intervals for 24 h are expressed as log of variability (b, c and d). There is a highly significant positive correlation between the instantaneous variability in plasma ACTH and cortisol levels (b), indicating that an increase or decrease in ACTH levels is accompanied by similar changes in cortisol levels (r=0.906; p< 10^{-9}). There is a highly significant correlation between simultaneous leptin and ACTH (c), indicating that an increase or decrease in leptin levels is accompanied by opposite changes in ACTH levels (r=0.651; p< 10^{-9}). Likewise, there is a highly significant negative correlation between the simultaneous variability in plasma leptin and cortisol (r= 0.764; p< 10^{-9}). Figure is from ref. 2, with permission.

2-hours after intravenous CRH injection. Thus, severe changes in the levels of ACTH and cortisol have no impact on basal leptin levels.[10]

In animal models, exogenous leptin administration has been shown to suppress starvation-induced HPA activation. This effect establishes hypothalamic neuro-endocrine regulation as a component of leptin-mediated adaptive changes during the stress of starvation.[35] In a protocol taking frequent samples of ACTH, cortisol and leptin we showed that fluctuations in the 24-hour patterns of circulating human leptin are the inverse that of ACTH and cortisol (Fig. 3a). We have shown a strong positive Pearson correlation between the 24-hour patterns of variability in ACTH and cortisol levels (r= 0.906; $p<10^{-9}$, Fig. 3b) and a highly significant negative Pearson correlation between the variability in leptin and ACTH levels (r=0.651; $p<10^{-9}$, Fig. 3c) and cortisol levels (r=0.764; $p<10^{-9}$, Fig. 3d). The absence of a suppressive effect of glucocorticoids on the levels of circulating leptin leads us to suggest that one of the CNS effects of leptin might be the acute suppression of HPA function.

4. SEX DIFFERENCES IN CIRCULATING HUMAN LEPTIN

Sex differences in fasting basal plasma levels of leptin have been identified across a broad spectrum of age, body mass indexes (BMIs), and body fat composition in both rodents and men.[36-42]

Approximate entropy (ApEn), a statistic that distinguishes random variation from orderly structure, shows that certain hormones have a strong sex contrast in the orderliness or regularity of their release processes.[43] ApEn is a model-independent regularity statistic developed to quantify the orderliness of sequential measures[44], such as hormonal time series. To assess sex-related differences in ApEn of leptin levels our group conducted a 24-h blood collection study in women and men. The respective profiles are shown in Fig. 4.

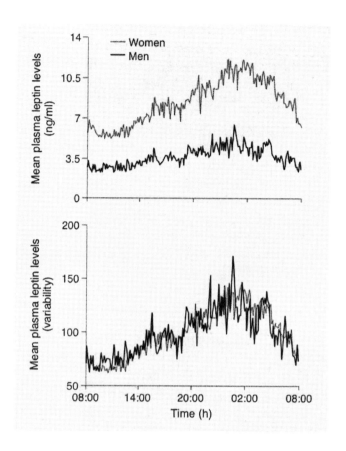

Figure 4. Frequently sampled 24-h profiles of total plasma leptin concentrations in men and women. The *top panel* shows absolute levels, which are higher in women throughout the 24-h period. The *bottom panel* shows leptin levels normalized and expressed as variability, defined as a percentage of the individual 24-h averages, using the formula: variability at time t = (hormone level at time t/24 h individual average level) x 100. Figure is from ref. 51 with permission.

Women and men had 24-h leptin levels with both ultradian and 24-h variability. Raw leptin levels were consistently higher in women than in men throughout the 24-h period; however, were expressed as variability over 24-h averages, the 24-h leptin profiles of women and men showed no significant difference. All subjects showed evidence of diurnal periodicity in 24-h leptin levels as assessed by two different procedures. Periodicities in the two sexes were similar and approximated 4–10 h in women and 4–12 h in men. Ultradian rhythms had amplitudes greater than randomly shuffled leptin time series at $P < 0.05$. Moreover, when leptin levels were normalized, expressed as percent variability, and averaged in women and men by 4-h intervals starting at 08:00 h, we showed a clear and statistically significant 24-h pattern in both sexes, with no significant differences at each 4-h interval. Both women and men had a nadir of leptin levels during the 08:00–12:00 h period and highest levels during the 00:00–04:00 h period.

As the leptin gene is expressed in fat cells, leptin levels vary as a function of body fat. However, female sex is associated with higher leptin levels, independent of adiposity. The studies conducted to date have used far fewer measures of leptin dynamics and are limited by infrequent sampling. Several studies, however, have indicated that for equivalent levels of adiposity, serum leptin is higher in females, both in rodents as well as in humans. Leptin levels have been shown to reflect total body lipid content, as assessed by carcass analysis, in normal and transgenic mice across a broad range of body lipid content; importantly, at any body fat content, female mice have higher leptin levels than males.[36] Similarly, in humans, leptin levels are a direct function of adiposity, but with considerable individual variation. Four large studies combining a total of 654 individuals reported that women have higher fasting leptin levels than men regardless of BMI, adiposity, and body fat composition.[38-40,45] Likewise, studies in 1691 children have shown sex dimorphism of fasting plasma leptin concentrations independent of body fat distribution. In a study with 112 lean and obese children and adolescents, Lahlou and colleagues[41] observed a strong correlation between leptin levels and BMI, but for any level of normal or elevated BMI, leptin concentrations were higher in girls than in boys. Likewise, the study by Hassink et al. of 77 normal weight and obese children (mean age, 11.3 yr)[46], the study by Blum et al. of 713 children (312 boys and 401 girls; age range, 5.8–19.9 yr)[47], and the study by Garcia-Mayor et al. of 789 children (343 girls and 446 boys; age range, 5–15 yr)[48] showed that girls have increased leptin concentrations when compared to boys, independent of adiposity.

Interestingly, this pattern is already evident in newborns. Leptin levels measured in cord blood are 63–90% higher in girls than in boys despite similar leptin concentrations in the plasma of their mothers[42,49]: such sex differences in fetal leptin levels are very likely to reflect genetic differences between females rather than body fat content or distribution or reproductive hormone status. However, it must be noted that an independent study could not replicate the observed sex dimorphism in leptin levels in newborns.[21]

Saad et al. conducted a 24-h study with sampling every 20 min for measurements of glucose, insulin, and leptin in lean and obese males and females.[33] In that study, plasma leptin profiles were higher in obese than in lean subjects and higher in women than in men regardless of fat mass. Leptin showed diurnal rhythmicity, with peaks between 2200–0300 h (median, 01:20 h) and nadirs between 0800–1740 h (median, 10:33 h). The relative diurnal amplitude also was higher in men than in women, controlling for adiposity.

Within a normal range of BMI, women have higher leptin levels than men[33,36-42,45,47-49], and we find that this difference is due solely to higher leptin pulse amplitude. All other concentration-independent and frequency-related pulsatility parameters, as well as diurnal variation and ApEn have been repeatedly found to be the same in women as well as in men.[51] Elevations in circulating levels of leptin have been reported to result from accelerated secretion rates of the peptide from adipose tissue due to increased leptin gene expression.[52] Those findings would lead us to suggest that individual bursts of leptin may contain more leptin molecules in women than in men. Assuming similar plasma leptin half-lives are the same in both sexes, we infer that there may be sex dimorphism in the production of leptin; to maintain normal body weight women appear to require a higher leptin output per pulse. This would indicate that women may be more resistant to the actions of leptin than men. Interestingly, all diseases that affect body weight (obesity, major depression, anorexia nervosa, bulimia nervosa, and binge eating disorder) are more common in women than in men. Does women's increased resistance to leptin in comparison to men predispose then to disorders characterized by disruption of mechanisms that regulate body weight? Future work should address this important clinical research question. A careful review of all existing data on sex dimorphism in leptin concentrations indicates that genetic factors may be of importance, independent of body fat composition and hormonal milieu[39, 41, 53] Thus, the sex differences in circulating plasma leptin pulse amplitude, resulting in higher 24-h leptin concentrations in women than in men without alterations in oscillator mechanisms and the orderliness (ApEn) of the leptin secretion process could be attributed to the combined effects of genetics, body fat distribution, and sex steroid levels.

5. EXAMPLES OF LOSS OF PATTERN

Dramatically increased fasting leptin concentrations as well as increased plasma levels of a number of other hormones and inflammatory mediators, including cortisol and interleukin-6 have been reported in studies of patients with sepsis.[54-56] Increased leptin levels in some of these patients were accompanied by a complete loss of the typical diurnal pattern of leptin secretion.[54] There is some evidence that the administration of cytokines, such as tumor necrosis factor-alpha[57] and interleukins[58] or glucocorticoids[59,60] can increase circulating leptin levels.

Individuals with severe burns have features typically observed with the administration of leptin in animals, including anorexia and an increased metabolic rate. In contrast to septic patients, leptin levels in burn injury individuals are in the normal to low range. However, septic patients as well as burn victims lose the normal diurnal pattern of circulating leptin levels. Although the implications of these findings are not clear, they suggest that factors other than leptin control the anorexia related to burn injury. The loss of the diurnal leptin pattern most likely results from a combination of the continuous nutritional supplementation and the significant degree of insulin resistance observed in burned patients. There is a chance that changes in the timing of the feeding regimen, in order to better approximate to normal meal times, could reproduce meal-induced insulin and glucose excursions and therefore normalize the diurnal pattern of circulating leptin concentrations.[61]

Spiegel et al, in a recent study demonstrate that sleep duration plays an important role in the regulation of human leptin levels and diurnal variation. The comparison of leptin profiles in the same subjects studied with 4-h, 8-h, and 12-h bedtimes revealed that daytime and nighttime leptin levels and the amplitude of the diurnal variation decrease when sleep duration is restricted in the absence of changes in body weight. Relative to a fully rested condition (12-h bedtimes), 6 days of 4-h bedtimes in healthy young subjects were associated with a 26% decrease in maximal leptin levels.[62]

6. CONCLUSION

The pulsatile and rhythmic pattern of leptin secretion has already been well characterized. Our group and others have provided strong evidence indicating that plasma concentrations peak at approximately two times the values observed at nadir measurements, and that the endogenous rhythmicity of leptin is dependent on secretion pulses. Frequent sampling techniques are crucial for the appropriate determination of these pulses. Inconsistent results are most commonly the result of improper sampling protocols, and better data can be obtained once this common study limitation is overcome by frequent sampling, as the quality of data seems to increase exponentially with the frequency samples are taken. Future research in this area should be built on past advances, including optimal sampling.

ACKNOWLEDGEMENTS

The authors have been supported by NIH grants DK58851, DK063240, RR16996, RR017365, RR000865, HL04526, MH062777, and HG002500, and by awards from the Dana Foundation and the Diana, Princess of Wales Memorial Fund.

REFERENCES

1. J. Licínio, Longitudinally sampled human plasma leptin and cortisol concentrations are inversely correlated. *J Clin Endocrinol Metab*, 1998. **83**(3): p. 1042.
2. J. Licínio, et al., Human leptin levels are pulsatile and inversely related to pituitary-adrenal function. *Nat Med*, 1997. **3**(5): p. 575-9.
3. M.K. Sinha, et al., Nocturnal rise of leptin in lean, obese, and non-insulin-dependent diabetes mellitus subjects. *J Clin Invest*, 1996. **97**(5): p. 1344-7.
4. M.K. Sinha, et al., Ultradian oscillations of leptin secretion in humans. *Biochem Biophys Res Commun*, 1996. **228**(3): p. 733-8.
5. P. Prolo, M.L. Wong, and J. Licinio, Leptin. *Int J Biochem Cell Biol*, 1998. **30**(12): p. 1285-90.
6. J. Licínio, et al., Synchronicity of frequently sampled, 24-h concentrations of circulating leptin, luteinizing hormone, and estradiol in healthy women. *Proc Natl Acad Sci U S A*, 1998. **95**(5): p. 2541-6.
7. L.J Slieker, et al., Regulation of expression of ob mRNA and protein by glucocorticoids and cAMP. *J Biol Chem*, 1996. **271**(10): p. 5301-4.
8. J.W. Kolaczynski, et al., Acute and chronic effects of insulin on leptin production in humans: Studies in vivo and in vitro. *Diabetes*, 1996. **45**(5): p. 699-701.
9. R.V. Considine and J.F. Caro, Leptin: genes, concepts and clinical perspective. *Horm Res*, 1996. **46**(6): p. 249-56.
10. G. Cizza, et al., Plasma leptin levels do not change in patients with Cushing's disease shortly after correction of hypercortisolism. *J Clin Endocrinol Metab*, 1997. **82**(8): p. 2747-50.
11. E. Van Cauter and S. Refetoff, Multifactorial control of the 24-hour secretory profiles of pituitary hormones. *J Endocrinol Invest*, 1985. **8**(4): p. 381-91.
12. G. Boden, et al., Effect of fasting on serum leptin in normal human subjects. *J Clin Endocrinol Metab*, 1996. **81**(9): p. 3419-23.
13. D.A. Schoeller, et al., Entrainment of the diurnal rhythm of plasma leptin to meal timing. *J Clin Invest*, 1997. **100**(7): p. 1882-7.
14. P.J. Havel, et al., High-fat meals reduce 24-h circulating leptin concentrations in women. *Diabetes*, 1999. **48**(2): p. 334-41.
15. K.E. Oerter, V. Guardabasso, and D. Rodbard, Detection and characterization of peaks and estimation of instantaneous secretory rate for episodic pulsatile hormone secretion. *Comput Biomed Res*, 1986. **19**(2): p. 170-91.
16. J.D. Veldhuis and M.L. Johnson, Cluster analysis: a simple, versatile, and robust algorithm for endocrine pulse detection. *Am J Physiol*, 1986. **250**(4 Pt 1): p. E486-93.
17. R. Homburg, et al., One hundred pregnancies after treatment with pulsatile luteinising hormone releasing hormone to induce ovulation. *Bmj*, 1989. **298**(6676): p. 809-12.
18. W. Aulitzky, J. Frick, and F. Hadziselimovic, Pulsatile LHRH therapy in patients with oligozoospermia and disturbed LH pulsatility. *Int J Androl*, 1989. **12**(4): p. 265-72.
19. D.J. Haisenleder, et al., A pulsatile gonadotropin-releasing hormone stimulus is required to increase transcription of the gonadotropin subunit genes: evidence for differential

regulation of transcription by pulse frequency in vivo. *Endocrinology*, 1991. **128**(1): p. 509-17.

20. D.J. Haisenleder, et al., Regulation of gonadotropin subunit messenger ribonucleic acid expression by gonadotropin-releasing hormone pulse amplitude in vitro. *Endocrinology*, 1993. **132**(3): p. 1292-6.

21. J.D. Veldhuis, The hypothalamic pulse generator: the reproductive core. *Clin Obstet Gynecol*, 1990. **33**(3): p. 538-50.

22. D. Maiter, et al., Different effects of intermittent and continuous growth hormone (GH) administration on serum somatomedin-C/insulin-like growth factor I and liver GH receptors in hypophysectomized rats. *Endocrinology*, 1988. **123**(2): p. 1053-9.

23. J. Lopez-Fernandez, et al., Growth hormone induces somatostatin and insulin-like growth factor I gene expression in the cerebral hemispheres of aging rats. *Endocrinology*, 1996. **137**(10): p. 4384-91.

24. B.O. Yildiz, et al., Alterations in the dynamics of circulating ghrelin, adiponectin, and leptin in human obesity. *Proc Natl Acad Sci U S A*, 2004. **101**(28): p. 10434-9.

25. A. Sainsbury, et al., Intracerebroventricular administration of neuropeptide Y to normal rats increases obese gene expression in white adipose tissue. *Diabetologia*, 1996. **39**(3): p. 353-6.

26. K. Berneis, S. Vosmeer, and U. Keller, Effects of glucocorticoids and of growth hormone on serum leptin concentrations in man. *Eur J Endocrinol*, 1996. **135**(6): p. 663-5.

27. P. Trayhurn, J.S. Duncan, and D.V. Rayner, Acute cold-induced suppression of ob (obese) gene expression in white adipose tissue of mice: mediation by the sympathetic system. *Biochem J*, 1995. **311** (Pt 3): p. 729-33.

28. M.K. Sinha, et al., Evidence of free and bound leptin in human circulation. Studies in lean and obese subjects and during short-term fasting. *J Clin Invest*, 1996. **98**(6): p. 1277-82.

29. K.L. Houseknecht, et al., Evidence for leptin binding to proteins in serum of rodents and humans: modulation with obesity. *Diabetes*, 1996. **45**(11): p. 1638-43.

30. S. Dagogo-Jack, et al., Plasma leptin and insulin relationships in obese and nonobese humans. *Diabetes*, 1996. **45**(5): p. 695-8.

31. E. Muscelli, et al., Acute insulin administration does not affect plasma leptin levels in lean or obese subjects. *Eur J Clin Invest*, 1996. **26**(10): p. 940-3.

32. G. Boden, et al., Effects of prolonged hyperinsulinemia on serum leptin in normal human subjects. *J Clin Invest*, 1997. **100**(5): p. 1107-13.

33. M.F. Saad, et al., Diurnal and ultradian rhythmicity of plasma leptin: effects of gender and adiposity. *J Clin Endocrinol Metab*, 1998. **83**(2): p. 453-9.

34. T. Utriainen, et al., Supraphysiological hyperinsulinemia increases plasma leptin concentrations after 4 h in normal subjects. *Diabetes*, 1996. **45**(10): p. 1364-6.

35. R.S. Ahima, et al., Role of leptin in the neuroendocrine response to fasting. *Nature*, 1996. **382**(6588): p. 250-2.

36. R.C. Frederich, et al., Leptin levels reflect body lipid content in mice: evidence for diet-induced resistance to leptin action. *Nat Med*, 1995. **1**(12): p. 1311-4.

37. P.J. Havel, et al., Gender differences in plasma leptin concentrations. *Nat Med*, 1996. **2**(9): p. 949-50.

38. R.E. Ostlund, Jr., et al., Relation between plasma leptin concentration and body fat, gender, diet, age, and metabolic covariates. *J Clin Endocrinol Metab*, 1996. **81**(11): p. 3909-13.

39. M. Rosenbaum, et al., Effects of gender, body composition, and menopause on plasma concentrations of leptin. *J Clin Endocrinol Metab*, 1996. **81**(9): p. 3424-7.

40. A. Kennedy, et al., The metabolic significance of leptin in humans: gender-based differences in relationship to adiposity, insulin sensitivity, and energy expenditure. *J Clin Endocrinol Metab*, 1997. **82**(4): p. 1293-300.

41. N. Lahlou, et al., Circulating leptin in normal children and during the dynamic phase of juvenile obesity: relation to body fatness, energy metabolism, caloric intake, and sexual dimorphism. *Diabetes*, 1997. **46**(6): p. 989-93.
42. J. Matsuda, et al., Serum leptin concentration in cord blood: relationship to birth weight and gender. *J Clin Endocrinol Metab*, 1997. **82**(5): p. 1642-4.
43. S.M. Pincus, et al., Females secrete growth hormone with more process irregularity than males in both humans and rats. *Am J Physiol*, 1996. **270**(1 Pt 1): p. E107-15.
44. S.M. Pincus, Approximate entropy as a measure of system complexity. *Proc Natl Acad Sci U S A*, 1991. **88**(6): p. 2297-301.
45. M.F. Saad, et al., Sexual dimorphism in plasma leptin concentration. *J Clin Endocrinol Metab*, 1997. **82**(2): p. 579-84.
46. S.G. Hassink, et al., Serum leptin in children with obesity: relationship to gender and development. *Pediatrics*, 1996. **98**(2 Pt 1): p. 201-3.
47. W.F. Blum, et al., Plasma leptin levels in healthy children and adolescents: dependence on body mass index, body fat mass, gender, pubertal stage, and testosterone. *J Clin Endocrinol Metab*, 1997. **82**(9): p. 2904-10.
48. R.V. Garcia-Mayor, et al., Serum leptin levels in normal children: relationship to age, gender, body mass index, pituitary-gonadal hormones, and pubertal stage. *J Clin Endocrinol Metab*, 1997. **82**(9): p. 2849-55.
49. M.A. Tome, et al., Sex-based differences in serum leptin concentrations from umbilical cord blood at delivery. *Eur J Endocrinol*, 1997. **137**(6): p. 655-8.
50. C.S. Mantzoros, et al., Effect of birth weight and maternal smoking on cord blood leptin concentrations of full-term and preterm newborns. *J Clin Endocrinol Metab*, 1997. **82**(9): p. 2856-61.
51. J. Licínio, et al., Sex differences in circulating human leptin pulse amplitude: clinical implications. *J Clin Endocrinol Metab*, 1998. **83**(11): p. 4140-7.
52. F. Lonnqvist, et al., Leptin secretion from adipose tissue in women. Relationship to plasma levels and gene expression. *J Clin Invest*, 1997. **99**(10): p. 2398-404.
53. N. Vahl, et al., Abdominal adiposity rather than age and sex predicts mass and regularity of GH secretion in healthy adults. *Am J Physiol*, 1997. **272**(6 Pt 1): p. E1108-16.
54. D.J. Torpy, S.R. Bornstein, and G.P. Chrousos, Leptin and interleukin-6 in sepsis. *Horm Metab Res*, 1998. **30**(12): p. 726-9.
55. S.R. Bornstein, et al., Plasma leptin levels are increased in survivors of acute sepsis: associated loss of diurnal rhythm, in cortisol and leptin secretion. *J Clin Endocrinol Metab*, 1998. **83**(1): p. 280-3.
56. F. Arnalich, et al., Relationship of plasma leptin to plasma cytokines and human survival in sepsis and septic shock. *J Infect Dis*, 1999. **180**(3): p. 908-11.
57. P. Sarraf, et al., Multiple cytokines and acute inflammation raise mouse leptin levels: potential role in inflammatory anorexia. *J Exp Med*, 1997. **185**(1): p. 171-5.
58. R. Faggioni, et al., IL-1 beta mediates leptin induction during inflammation. *Am J Physiol*, 1998. **274**(1 Pt 2): p. R204-8.
59. H. Larsson and B. Ahren, Short-term dexamethasone treatment increases plasma leptin independently of changes in insulin sensitivity in healthy women. *J Clin Endocrinol Metab*, 1996. **81**(12): p. 4428-32.
60. S. Dagogo-Jack, et al., Robust leptin secretory responses to dexamethasone in obese subjects. *J Clin Endocrinol Metab*, 1997. **82**(10): p. 3230-3.
61. K.G. Hobson, et al., Circulating leptin and cortisol after burn injury: loss of diurnal pattern. *J Burn Care Rehabil*, 2004. **25**(6): p. 491-9.
62. K. Spiegel, et al., Leptin levels are dependent on sleep duration: relationships with sympathovagal balance, carbohydrate regulation, cortisol, and thyrotropin. *J Clin Endocrinol Metab*, 2004. **89**(11): p. 5762-71.

Chapter 14

LEPTIN IN FARM ANIMALS

C. Richard Barb[1], Gary J. Hausman[1], and Timothy G. Ramsay[2]
[1]*Animal Physiology Research Unit, USDA-ARS, Russell Research Center, Athens, GA, USA*
[2]*Growth Biology Laboratory, USDA-ARS, BARC-East, Beltsville, MD, USA*

Abstract: The recently discovered protein, leptin, which is secreted by fat cells, has been implicated in regulation of feed intake, energy balance and the neuroendocrine axis in rodents, humans and large domestic animals. The leptin receptor which has been cloned and is a member of the class 1 cytokine family of receptors is found in the brain and pituitary and numerous peripheral tissues. The interaction of leptin in energy metabolism, feed intake regulation, growth and immune function in domestic animals is reviewed. Preadipocyte recruitment and subsequent fat cell size and leptin gene expression are regulated by such hormones as insulin and cortisol and its interactions. Leptin serves as a metabolic signal that acts on the hypothalamic-pituitary-ovarian axis to enhance GnRH and LH secretion and ovarian function.

Key words: leptin; reproduction; hormone; metabolism; nutrition; adipocyte

1. INTRODUCTION

The recently discovered protein, leptin, is a 16 kD protein consisting of 146 amino acids which is synthesized primarily by adipose tissue and is secreted into the bloodstream after cleavage of the 21 amino acid signal peptide. Leptin impacts feed intake, the neuroendocrine-axis, metabolism and immunological processes.[1,2,3] Leptin was first identified as the gene product found deficient in the obese *ob/ob* mouse.[4] The hypothalamus appears to be the primary site of action, since leptin receptors are located within hypothalamic areas associated with control of appetite, reproduction and growth.[5,6] Discovery of leptin has improved our understanding of the relationship between adipose tissue and energy homeostasis.[3,7] Increased leptin production by adipose tissue and rising levels of triglyceride stores in adipose tissue could serve as a signal to the brain, to decrease food intake and to increase energy expenditure and resistance to obesity.[3] Moreover, when energy intake and output are equal, leptin reflects the amount of stored triglycerides in adipose tissue. Thus, leptin may serve as a circulating signal of nutritional status or lipostat, first proposed by Kennedy in 1953.[8] Furthermore, leptin may act as an important regulator of appetite, energy metabolism, body composition and reproduction. The intent of this review is to examine the biological role of leptin in farm animals with reference to other species.

2. RELATIONSHIP OF LEPTIN WITH PERIPHERAL METABOLISM

In comparison to rodent or human leptin, our knowledge of the function of leptin in peripheral metabolism in domestic animals is limited by a lack of depth in the number of studies for each species. This review is confounded by an inability to perform comparative analyses across ruminant and non-ruminant mammals and birds due to the significant differences in physiology, endocrinology and metabolism. Therefore, this review is divided according to species.

2.1 Leptin Administration

2.1.1 Feed intake

Experiments using leptin administration can delineate whether or not leptin can affect metabolism and perhaps give clues to how metabolic activity can be altered. Additionally, these studies provide information on the integrated response of a number of tissues. *In vivo* administration demonstrates that leptin can impact a number of metabolic processes resulting in alteration of growth.

As mentioned elsewhere in this review, injection of leptin into the central nervous system of domestic species has been demonstrated to inhibit feeding behavior in swine[9], chickens[10] and fish[11], although no effect in ruminants has been detected.[12,13] Initial experiments with leptin used the route of central administration due to the lack of available recombinant protein and the exorbitant cost for the protein. Several recent studies have demonstrated that peripheral administration of leptin can inhibit feed intake in swine[13,14], chickens[15] and fish.[11] Binding and transport across the blood brain barrier has been demonstrated in sheep[16], swine[17] and rabbits[18]; however this does not exclude the potential for peripheral leptin signals to feedback upon central mechanisms for feed intake regulation, as leptin receptor mRNA has been detected in numerous peripheral tissues of cattle[19], poultry[20,21], sheep[5] and swine.[6]

2.2 Adaptive Metabolism

Numerous adaptive changes occur within metabolically important tissues with the peripheral administration of leptin. Peripheral leptin treatment may alter hormone secretion[14,22,23], metabolite concentrations[13,14], neonatal skeletal growth[24], gut development[25], thermoregulation[26], ovarian function[27,28] and blood flow[29] as described in studies with domestic animal species. These shifts in physiology reflect changes in various metabolic activities, including lipid metabolism, protein metabolism, carbohydrate metabolism, steroid metabolism and heat production. The mechanisms responsible for these metabolic shifts cannot truly be gleaned from *in vivo* studies but require *in vitro* experiments to assess the specific function of leptin in metabolism.

2.2.1 Lipid Metabolism

Peripheral injection of leptin into fasted swine can inhibit the feeding response[14], thereby producing a depression in blood glucose and insulin concentrations with an elevation in plasma free fatty acid and growth hormone (GH) concentrations. The role of the hypoglycemia to produce an increase in serum free fatty acids cannot be excluded. However, Ajuwon et al.[13] clearly demonstrated that serum free fatty acids are elevated in swine following chronic peripheral treatment with a leptin analogue, without a change in blood glucose. Furthermore, Reidy and Weber[30] have reported that peripheral leptin administration increases *in vivo* lipolysis and fatty acid oxidation in rabbits, which indicates that leptin stimulation of lipolysis could contribute to the reported elevation in serum free fatty acids in swine.

Experiments using explant culture have demonstrated that leptin increases lipolytic rates in subcutaneous adipose tissue of swine[13,31]. This appears to be through a specific stimulation in lipolysis and also through suppressing insulin inhibition of lipolysis.[31] Fruhbeck et al.[32] demonstrated that leptin antagonizes the inhibitory action of adenosine on the rat adipocyte, thus suggesting that the mechanism for leptin stimulation of lipolysis is through inhibition of receptor-coupled inhibitory G protein (G_i), which elevating adenylate cyclase activity. Similar experiments using sheep adipose explants could not detect any effect of ovine leptin on lipolysis[33]; however this may have been the consequence of problems with the recombinant ovine leptin as it could not produce any second messenger response.[33]

The peroxisome proliferator activated receptor (PPAR) family of proteins contribute to the regulation of lipid metabolism[34], including lipolysis.[35] Ajuwon et al.[13] examined the *in vivo* and *in vitro* responses of the PPAR family of proteins to leptin treatment. While leptin stimulated lipolysis, no changes in PPARα were detected; the PPAR was associated with changes in lipolytic rate.[35] However, PPARγ was affected by leptin treatment, with an elevation in the *in vitro* expression of PPARγ1. Although no metabolic role has been specifically identified for this PPAR, it may contribute to enhancement of overall insulin sensitivity of the adipocyte.[36] This would imply that leptin may contribute to an enhancement of insulin sensitivity through promoting the expression of PPARγ1. However, leptin inhibits insulin's actions on lipolysis as mentioned above.

Insulin promotes lipid synthesis in porcine adipocytes, but at a more moderate level than in humans or rodents.[37] Leptin was demonstrated to inhibit insulin-stimulated lipid synthesis, thus reducing the rate of lipid synthesis.[38,39] Cohen et al.[40] reported that leptin induces dephosphorylation of IRS-1, thus antagonizing insulin's actions and providing a potential mechanism for leptin's inhibition of lipogenesis. Further studies are necessary to elucidate how leptin binding impacts insulin signaling mechanisms in swine. These studies indicate that the inhibitory effects at the insulin receptor level may preclude the actions of leptin at the level of PPARγ to enhance insulin sensitivity. Even without the use of insulin, leptin can inhibit lipid synthesis within adipose tissue[38,39], reducing endogenous fatty acid synthesis by up to 23% in primary cultures.[38]

The esterification of fatty acids is another mechanism for accretion of lipid within adipocytes. Leptin has been demonstrated to inhibit fatty acid esterification.[38,39] However, it is uncertain if this inhibition of fatty acid incorporation into lipids is the consequence of inhibition of acyl CoA synthetase, diacylglycerol acyltransferase or other enzymes regulating triglyceride synthesis, or whether the inhibition is with glycerol phosphate acyltransferase. The role of leptin in regulating the metabolism of fatty acids through esterification has not been characterized.

The combination of a stimulation of lipolysis and an inhibition of lipogenesis and fatty acid esterification would indicate that leptin promotes the partitioning of energy away from adipose tissue and toward utilization by other tissues, such as the liver, skeletal muscle or the mammary gland. Experiments utilizing muscle cell lines (C_2C_{12}) have demonstrated that porcine leptin can stimulate fatty acid oxidation[41], similar to the effects of murine leptin on skeletal muscle,[42-44] by activating 5´-AMP-activated protein kinase which phosphorylates and inactivates CoA carboxylase.[45] Interestingly, no changes in key oxidative enzymes (citrate synthase, β-hydroxyacyl-CoA dehydrogenase) were detected in mouse skeletal muscle, leading to the suggestion of a potential increase in fatty acid flux through the mitochondrial membrane with carnitine palmitoyltransferase I as responsible for leptin-induced fatty acid oxidation.[46] This still requires specific examination. Steinberg et al.[44] reported that leptin inhibits fatty acid translocase and fatty acid binding protein expression at the plasma membrane, resulting in an overall reduction in fatty acid transport of 45% in red fibers and 80% in white fibers of Sprague-Dawley rats. Therefore, the fatty acids oxidized in muscle may not originate from extracellular sources, through leptin stimulation of the repartitioning of fatty acids from adipose tissue. Rather, de novo lipogenesis may provide the source for the majority of fatty acids that are oxidized in skeletal muscle.[47] This raises the question, where are the elevated plasma NEFA utilized in leptin-treated animals.

A second major site of fatty acid utilization is the mammary gland. Unfortunately no studies have been performed to determine whether uptake, esterification or oxidation of fatty acids is promoted by leptin. However, fatty acid synthesis within the bovine mammary gland is stimulated by leptin, but only in the presence of prolactin which also stimulates expression of the leptin receptor.[48]

2.2.2 Amino Acid Metabolism

Chronic *in vivo* leptin treatment has been demonstrated to reduce feed intake sufficiently to produce negative energy balance, yet the loss of body nitrogen reserves are disproportionately small relative to the loss of adipose mass in rodents.[49-51] Ajuwon et al.[52] reported that exogenous leptin treatment decreases blood urea nitrogen relative to pair fed control swine, suggestive of a protein sparing effect. Acute (3 h) *in vivo* analysis of protein turnover could not detect any effect of a single injection of leptin on protein synthesis or breakdown in the rat[53]; however, that experiment could have been affected by the brevity of the treatment. Protein synthesis was inhibited by leptin in muscles isolated from these rats by approximately 16% during acute (30 minute) *in vitro* experiments, while protein degradation and proteolytic enzymes were unaffected.[53] Incubation of naive rat skeletal muscle with leptin had no effect on protein synthesis, indicating that the effect of *in vivo* leptin treatment may be an indirect action of leptin on rat skeletal muscle. In contrast to the effect on rat skeletal muscle, leptin promotes protein synthesis in embryonic chick muscle cell cultures, while high doses (1000 ng/ml) inhibit protein synthesis in embryonic chick hepatocyte cultures.[54] These contradictory effects on protein synthesis may be a consequence of methodology or species specificity.

Analysis of protein synthesis and breakdown in murine C_2C_{12} myogenic cell cultures demonstrated that leptin does not affect total muscle protein synthesis but can inhibit protein breakdown in C_2C_{12} cells, even under conditions which maximize proteolysis.[41] These data appear to contradict the experiments of Carbó et al.[53]; however leptin treatment of the C_2C_{12} cells was for a much greater period of time. Leptin's inhibitory effect on protein breakdown may contribute to the relative resistance to loss of muscle mass with leptin-induced negative energy balance and body weight loss. Muscle contains multiple proteolytic systems that contribute to protein breakdown, including ubiquitin Ub-ATP-dependent[55], lysosomal[56] and calcium-dependent.[57] Further studies are needed to identify which if any of these proteolytic systems are impacted by leptin.

2.2.3   Carbohydrate Metabolism

As mentioned above, leptin can inhibit endogenous fatty acid synthesis from glucose in porcine adipocyte culture.[38] Leptin can also inhibit glucose oxidation within porcine adipocyte culture.[38] In addition, leptin appears to interfere with insulin stimulation of glucose metabolism by porcine adipose tissue[38,39], as mentioned above. The consequence of these metabolic actions of leptin is to reduce overall metabolism of glucose by adipose tissue, perhaps sparing glucose for utilization by other tissues.

For example, leptin can stimulate glucose oxidation[58] and glycogen synthesis by rodent skeletal muscle *in vitro*[59,60] or *in vivo*[61], although leptin stimulation of glucose transport is debated.[61] No studies of skeletal muscle from domestic species have examined carbohydrate metabolism in response to leptin treatment.

Experiments with porcine hepatocytes have not been able to demonstrate an effect of leptin on gluconeogenesis[62], glycogen synthesis or ketogenesis.[63] Several studies with rodents have demonstrated that leptin can inhibit glycogenolysis or augment insulin inhibition of glycogenolysis[64-66], and inhibit gluconeogensis[62,67,68] in hepatocytes or perfused rodent liver, while stimulating glycogen synthesis.[66] Other studies have demonstrated an elevation in hepatic gluconeogenesis as contributing to the increase in glycogen accumulation.[69] The inability for the hepatic glucose metabolism in the pig to respond to leptin may reflect a species specific variation or may indicate the absence of a functional signaling system for leptin in the pig hepatocyte. While leptin receptor mRNA has been detected[6,62], no studies have been performed to determine whether leptin binding occurs or whether changes in second messenger concentrations occur in response to leptin treatment with the pig hepatocyte.

2.2.4 Energy Expenditure

Leptin is hypothesized to contribute to the maintenance of body mass by altering feed intake and energy expenditure.[70] The effects of leptin on feed intake regulation have already been described in this review. The potential role of leptin in energy expenditure was first suggested following injection of leptin into *ob/ob* mice and a subsequent elevation in body temperature[49,71] and a further study demonstrating an increase in oxygen consumption following leptin injection in *ob/ob* mice[72] and rabbits.[30] However, the role of leptin in energy expenditure and heat production is an area of current contention in human physiology.[73] Resting energy expenditure correlates with serum leptin in many human studies, but serum leptin does not correlate with changes in energy expenditure as the result of manipulating intake[74]. More importantly, increases in serum leptin concentration as a result of leptin injection have not been associated with an increase in energy expenditure in the majority of studies but rather correlated with a depression in feed intake.[73,75] However, the recent study of Rosenbaum et al.[74] reported an increase in total and non-resting energy expenditure with daily injection of leptin at a lower dosage than in previous studies; whether this is the consequence of use of a different formulation of leptin, dosage or differences in experimental design cannot be determined.

If leptin can alter energy expenditure as suggested by the studies of Hwa et al.[76] and Rosenbaum et al.[74], recent studies indicate that a potential source for this energy expenditure is leptin-induced futile cycling within skeletal muscle.[47] Reidy and Weber[30] demonstrated that leptin stimulates an *in vivo* increase in oxygen consumption in rabbits, which is accompanied by elevated triglyceride/fatty acid cycling as a consequence of elevated lipolysis and fatty acid oxidation. Flux through the triglyceride fatty acid and its associated energy cost were 50% higher in leptin-treated rabbits than in control rabbits. Dulloo et al.[77] reported that leptin could stimulate thermogenesis by up to 26% in mouse soleus muscle *in vitro* as measured by indirect microcalorimetry. This thermogenic effect was specific to stimulation of the leptin receptor (long form) as the response could not be detected in muscles derived from *db/db* mice, which lack functional leptin receptors. Solinas et al.[78] extended this research and determined that the increase in thermogenesis is the consequence of substrate cycling between lipogenesis and fatty acid oxidation. Entry of fatty acids into mitochondrial β-oxidation was shown to be necessary for the thermogenic effect of leptin by using the carnitine palmitoyl transferase-1 (CPT-1) inhibitor etomoxir to block the thermogenic response. Addition of 2-deoxyglucose (a nonmetabolizable glucose analogue) to the incubation medium also inhibited the thermogenic response, thereby demonstrating a requirement for glucose metabolism. The final link in demonstrating substrate cycling between lipogensis and fatty acid oxidation was showing that glucose conversion to lipid must occur prior to oxidation, through the use of fatty acid synthase and citrate lyase inhibitors. An estimated loss of 14 ATP is the consequence of the synthesis of one molecule of palmitic acid and its subsequent oxidation in skeletal muscle in response to leptin stimulation of this futile cycle.

Recent studies in fetal and neonatal sheep have suggested that leptin may also function to enhance energy expenditure by stimulation of uncoupling protein activity.[26,79] Uncoupling proteins (UCP) are a group of proteins with similar sequence homology.[80] Uncoupling protein 1 was the first reported UCP and was demonstrated to mediate ATPase independent proton leakage at the inner mitochondrial membrane.[80] UCP1 dissipates the transmembrane electrochemical potential by transporting protons from the intermembrane space back toward the matrix of the mitochondria, promoting a proton leakage and generating energy. The consequence of UCP1 activity is heat production through uncoupling ATP formation from cellular respiration. Additional UCPs (UCP2, 3, 4, 5) were identified subsequently, although their specific role in heat production is unclear.[81,82] Uncoupling protein 1 is almost exclusively found in brown adipose tissue, which is present in fetal and neonatal sheep and cattle[83,84], while UCP2 and UCP3 mRNA can be detected in a variety of tissues including adipose tissue and skeletal muscle in swine.[85,86] Leptin infusion into fetal sheep for 4 days resulted in an increase ($P = 0.06$) in UCP1 expression.[79] During the transition to the early postnatal period, leptin administration was shown to prevent the normal reduction in colonic temperature, followed by accelerating the loss of UCP1 as the brown fat fills with lipid. At seven days of age, colonic temperature was correlated strongly with both mRNA abundance and thermogenic potential of UCP1 in leptin-treated but not control lambs, indicating more effective use of UCP1 for heat production following leptin administration.

Functional analysis has demonstrated that UCP2 and UCP3 can support uncoupling activity.[87-89] However, more recent studies have implicated UCP2 and UCP3 as also functioning as scavengers of mitochondrial free radicals[90,91], with the possibility of functioning in the cycling of fatty acids at the mitochondria.[92] Thus UCP3 can promote fatty acid oxidation by transporting fatty acids out of the skeletal muscle mitochondrial matrix.[93] Therefore, UCPs may contribute to the leptin-induced futile cycling of fatty acids in skeletal muscle as described above.

Uncoupling protein 2 has been detected in the adipose tissues of cattle[94] and sheep[95], although UCP3 has not been monitored, despite sequence identification.[96,97] Uncoupling protein homologues have been reported for chickens[98] that are highly expressed in skeletal muscle. Because of this localized tissue expression pattern and high amino acid sequence homology, it would appear that the uncoupling protein identified in these bird species is most similar to mammalian UCP-3. Injection of recombinant human leptin into chickens did not alter feed intake or UCP expression in skeletal muscle of fed or fasted birds.[99] In swine, leptin increased UCP2 mRNA abundance while suppressing UCP3 mRNA abundance in subcutaneous adipose tissue explants in association with leptin-induced inhibition of lipogenesis.[100] Similarly, Ceddia et al.[101] reported that leptin elevated UCP2 mRNA abundance in rat adipocytes; however, leptin did not affect UCP3 mRNA abundance. *In vivo* studies have demonstrated that the levels of UCP2 mRNA are increased in epididymal fat pads of mice treated with recombinant human leptin[102] and in rats rendered hyperleptinemic by gene therapy[103-105] treatments that produce extensive fat depletion. Ceddia et al.[101] proposed that leptin stimulation produces an increase in UCP2 that may subsequently uncouple mitochondria and thereby increase the capacity of WAT to degrade acetyl CoA and fatty acids and to dissipate energy. However, porcine adipose tissue oxidizes less than 1-2% of the total fatty acids metabolized with >98% esterified.[106] Thus, a role for UCPs in fatty acid oxidation in porcine adipose tissue is probably limited. This does not discount the potential role of leptin in the induction of futile cycling in skeletal muscle through UCP shuttling of fatty acids, however.

2.2.5 Growth

The net result of metabolic activity and positive energy balance is growth through either cell replication or hypertrophy or a combination of both. The potential role of leptin in the growth and development of adipose tissue has already been discussed in this review. However, leptin has been demonstrated to affect the growth of a number of tissues.

2.2.5.1 **Bone and cartilage**

Litten et al.[24] recently reported that four days of peripheral leptin injection in neonatal pigs can increase hind limb length of neonatal meishan pigs and accelerate the growth rate from 0.112 kg/d to 0.184 kg/d. In contrast, Weiler et al.[107] used correlation analysis to demonstrate that serum leptin concentration is highly correlated with bone mass ($R_{adjusted} = 0.72$) and bone area ($R_{adjusted} = 0.57$) in swine. Linear bone growth is the result of proliferation, hypertrophy and calcification of growth plate cartilage while bone mass is the result of bone growth and subsequent modeling and remodeling. These two studies in swine suggest that leptin might have roles in cartilage and bone growth and also in bone remodeling in domestic animals.

Rabbit chondrocytes possess long form leptin receptors as determined by western analysis[108], and rat chondrocytes have recently been reported to express leptin as determined by immunohistochemistry.[109] Nakajima et al.[108] demonstrated that leptin can stimulate ^{3}H-thymidine incorporation into growth plate chondrocytes and increase alkaline phosphatase expression following confluence. Also, mouse chondrocytes derived from the growth centers of mandibular condyle in organ culture proliferate to such an extent that the width of the chondroprogenitor zone can increase by up to 23%, while the length of the condyle is increased by 8%.[110] In addition, leptin treatment promotes chondrocyte differentiation.[110] These studies indicate that leptin may function to promote linear bone growth. The best example for this is the *ob/ob* mouse which has shorter and less dense femurs than wild type mice. Intraperitoneal injection of leptin has been demonstrated to stimulate femoral growth in *ob/ob* mice, despite a leptin-induced reduction in intake.[111] This femoral growth was accompanied by an increase in bone density and mineralization. Peripheral administration is necessary for this growth-promoting response as intracerebroventricular (ICV) administration of leptin inhibits bone growth and promotes a loss in bone density[112], suggesting a level of hypothalamic/neural control and the associated complexity.

Leptin and leptin receptors have also been detected in fetal mouse hypertrophic chondrocytes at the growth plate, in proximity to capillaries[113]. These hypertrophic chondrocytes are specifically involved in bone formation as vascular invasion into hypertrophic cartilage precedes cartilage resorption and subsequent bone formation by osteoblasts, replacing calcified cartilage.[114] Chondrocytes that were not in close proximity to capillaries did not express leptin.[113] This vascular invasion may be the consequence of the angiogenic properties of leptin. Leptin induces both a chemotactic response and structural rearrangements of vascular endothelial cells in culture toward formation of capillary networks.[113] Therefore leptin may contribute to the growth and subsequent resorption of cartilage during the initial steps of bone formation.

Reseland et al.[115] and Kume et al.[113] demonstrated that osteoblasts express leptin. Leptin promotes adult human osteoblast proliferation *in vitro* as measured by ^{3}H-thymidine incorporation[116], a period when leptin expression is low in the osteoblast[115]. Leptin could also chronically induce collagen synthesis in these osteoblasts and could induce mineralization after several weeks.[115,116] Osteoblast differentiation was also induced by leptin in this study, as measured by the expression of marker genes (IGF-1, TGFβ, collagen-Iα, osteocalcin). The mRNA abundance for osteoclast-signaling markers, IL-6 and osteoprotegerin were elevated by leptin and increased with days in culture.[116] These results indicate that leptin promotes bone formation, including mineralization of osteoblasts and may stimulate the production of signals (IL-6 and osteoprotegerin) for the recruitment of osteoclasts for remodeling.

Leptin may modulate bone remodeling as suggested by the *in vitro* study above. *In vivo* experiments have demonstrated that leptin can prevent a decrease in tibia-metaphysis bone mineral density in rats as a result of disuse following tail suspension.[117] In addition, leptin stops the known reduction in bone formation in this model. Leptin treatment of ovariectomized rats reduces the rapid bone loss induced by estrogen deficiency.[118] Lastly, leptin injection into fasted or intake restricted mice prevents the known fall in plasma osteocalcin (an anti-resorptive factor) with these dietary treatments.[119] These data support a role for leptin as a mediator of bone metabolism.

2.2.5.2 Hemopoiesis and Immune Function

Leptin at physiological concentrations has been shown to affect hematopoeis, proinflammatory responses and other immune cell functions in mice, rats and humans *in vivo* or *in vitro*.[120,121,122] The tertiary structural similarity of leptin to the cytokines IL-6, IL-11, 1L-12[123], and a receptor that belongs to the class I cytokine receptor family have suggested a potential role in immune function.[124] Unfortunately there has been no research performed with domestic animals to relate leptin to hemopoiesis.

However, the role of leptin in the proinflammatory response has been examined in domestic animals. This has primarily been through induction of acute endotoxemia with lipopolysaccharide (LPS). The first study to examine this response in swine did not demonstrate a response in leptin mRNA abundance to LPS when animals were fasted.[125] Further studies in swine demonstrated that LPS could reduce leptin mRNA abundance in association with fever, elevated cortisol and TNF-α, while serum glucose, insulin and IGF-1 were reduced.[126] The reduction of leptin mRNA abundance may have been the consequence of the suppressive effect of endotoxemia and fever on feed intake (and shifts in hormones and metabolites to negative energy balance), rather than a direct effect on leptin. Additional research with three genotypes of swine demonstrated a genotype effect in the leptin response to LPS.[127] Two genotypes responded with a decrease in leptin mRNA abundance to LPS while the third genotype demonstrated no change in leptin mRNA abundance, despite similar changes in serum profile as the other breeds. This variation in response may be of significance as efforts are put toward producing leaner breeds of swine, which in some cases have an increased susceptibility to disease.[128] If leptin is involved in the immune response in swine, then an unintentional selection for a depressed leptin secretory response and thus immune response may occur.

In cattle, LPS treatment did not alter serum leptin levels in Holstein cows[129]; this suggests leptin may not have a role in endotoxemia-induced hypophagia in the cow. In addition, injection of recombinant bovine tumor necrosis factor α did not alter serum leptin levels.[129] Waldron et al.[130] confirmed these results, reporting that LPS injection did not alter serum leptin concentration, despite changes in serum cortisol, TNFα and insulin. Similarly, Soliman et al.[131] demonstrated that LPS treatment does not alter serum leptin levels in sheep, which has since been verified by Daniel et al.[132]

Chronic *in vivo* treatment of swine with human recombinant leptin did not affect lymphocyte proliferation or the *in vitro* proliferative response to ConA or hemocyanin.[133] Pigs treated with leptin had lower serum concentrations of antigen-specific IgG1 than the appropriate controls following hemocyanin administration, although the IgG2 response was unaffected. *In vitro* treatment of peripheral blood mononuclear cells (PBMC) with leptin did not alter the proliferation of PBMC or the cytokine response of the PBMC to ConA, which is in disagreement with studies of human or mouse PBMC.[134-136] STAT3 signaling in the porcine PBMC was found to be unresponsive to any treatments, unlike human PBMC[137,138], which may contribute to the lack of an effect of leptin on the porcine PBMC, despite the confirmed presence of leptin receptor mRNA.

In contrast to the pig, leptin treatment of poultry has been shown to stimulate T-lymphocyte proliferation.[139] Chicken leptin induced up to a 400% increase in turkey lymphocyte proliferation *in vitro* following concavalin A treatment. A second experiment demonstrated that *in vivo* leptin treatment of quail by osmotic minipumps produced an increase in web wing thickness, a physiological marker for perivascular accumulation of T-cells, following phytohemagglutinin (PHA) exposure. Once the leptin was no longer secreted by the pumps, web wing thickness response to PHA returned to normal. These data suggest that leptin can modulate the T-cell immune response in birds.

Leptin has been reported to be elevated within wounds during the healing process in swine, although the role for leptin in wound repair and its functions in the immune response within the damaged tissue could not be segregated.[140] A potential role for leptin in the overall healing process has been suggested by the observation that both *ob/ob* (leptin deficient) and *db/db* (leptin resistant) mice are characterized by a reduced ability to repair cutaneous wounds.[141,142] While the metabolic alterations associated with these genetic lines may contribute to the impaired healing, more recent studies have indicated a more direct role for leptin in wound healing.[143-147] In an experiment similar to Marikovsky et al.[140], Murad et al.[147] reported that leptin mRNA abundance within a cutaneous biopsy wound was elevated within six hours of incision and remained elevated for at least five days. Immunohistochemical localization demonstrated that leptin was expressed at elevated levels in keratinocytes in the epidermis, vascular elements and in dermal fibroblasts. Stallmeyer et al.[145] previously demonstrated that keratinocytes express the leptin receptor and proliferate in response to leptin addition. Addition of neutralizing concentrations of anti-leptin antibodies to the wounds for three days reduced reepithelialization by 60% and reduced the thickness of granulation tissue.[147] These data support observations that topical or systemic leptin treatment can promote wound healing in leptin deficient *ob/ob* mice.[144,146] These studies support a potential role for leptin as an endocrine signaling molecule that mediates immune responses in cutaneous wound healing.

2.2.5.3 Angiogenesis

Separating the actions of leptin on angiogenesis from the process of wound healing is difficult as the two processes are critically intertwined during tissue regeneration. For a recent review of this area please see Hausman and Richardson.[148] Bouloumie et al.[149] reported that porcine aortic smooth muscle cells express both the long and short form of the leptin receptor. In addition, these porcine cells proliferate and form capillary-like structures in response to leptin treatment *in vitro*. However, no further studies have been performed with cells from a domestic species.

Additional studies have utilized human umbilical endothelial cells and cell lines to demonstrate that leptin stimulates phosphorylation of the MAP-kinase ERK1/2 and also STAT3.[149,150] The consequences of this tyrosine phosphorylation and subsequent downstream events are to alter endothelial cell proliferation, migration, survival and apoptosis.[149-154] Leptin can also promote the proliferation and migration of smooth muscle cells[155], another critical component of the vascular structure. In addition, leptin can promote the secretion of vascular endothelial cell growth factor (VEGF).[151] Thus leptin may function indirectly through mediating VEGF-mediated angiogenesis.[152]

2.2.5.4 Gastrointestinal tract

Leptin receptor mRNA is detectable by RT-PCR in the brush border throughout the small intestine.[156] Gastric infusion of leptin (10 µg/kg bwt) increases length of the small intestine in milk-formula-fed, neonatal swine.[157] This increase is the result of an increase in length of the jejunum, as length of the ileum was reduced. This growth response is coupled with an increased jejunal and ileal mitotic index, concomitant with a reduction in villi length in the distal half of the jejunum and the ileum. In addition, mucosal thickness is reduced in the jejunum and ileum with leptin treatment of milk-formula-fed swine. Leptin treatment altered the activities of several brush border enzymes within various regions of the jejunum. The major pattern to be discerned from this brush border enzyme data is that leptin reduces the activities of aminopeptidases (A & B) and lactase in the distal half of the jejunum, suggesting a potential maturation of the jejunum relative to control milk-formula-fed pigs. Analysis of marker molecule absorption revealed no effect of leptin on passive transport processes, suggesting the absorptive area of the intestine is not altered by leptin treatment. However, complex molecule absorption (bovine serum albumin) is reduced in leptin supplemented pigs, relative to controls. These data imply that leptin may promote early maturation of the small intestine by leptin treatment, causing a shift from fetal-type enterocytes to adult-type enterocytes. Wolinski et al.[158] also reported that gastric leptin infusion increases motility of the duodenum and reduces motility of the jejunum, suggesting a potential effect on digesta passage.

Systemic administration of leptin to the rat can also produce an increase in total DNA content of the small intestine[159], which supports the gastric infusion data in the pig of Wolinski et al.[157] A 14 day jugular infusion of leptin enhanced mucosal absorptive function as assessed by uptake of ^{14}C-galactose and ^{14}C-glycine. Leptin also increased the mRNA abundance for the sodium/glucose cotransporter and fructose transporter from the intestinal mucosa. These data support the hypothesis that leptin may be a growth promoter for the small intestine. However, Lostao et al.[160] reported that leptin reduced *in vitro* uptake of galactose by intestinal rings through a reduction in apparent Vmax and apparent Km for sugar transport. Comparison of these two studies indicates that leptin may function through intermediary mechanisms, following peripheral infusion, to alter sugar transport *in vivo*.

Besides carbohydrate transport, leptin can promote the absorption of dipeptides following leptin infusion into the lumen of the jejunum.[161] Leptin increases the recruitment of PepT-1 molecules from the intracellular pool to the apical membrane; these transporters can convey dipeptides and tripeptides in association with protons across the brush border.[162]

The source of leptin for promoting intestinal growth and function may be the stomach (for review please see Guilmeau et al.[163]). Leptin can be secreted by chief cells[164] and P cells[165] in the stomach. Gastric leptin secretion has been shown to be regulated by feeding[166], vagal stimulation[167], cholecystokinin[164] and secretin.[168] Gastric leptin secretion occurs rapidly following a meal and is stable in the highly acidic gastric juice.[168] This may permit transfer of leptin to the intestine where it can function following binding to receptors at the brush border as described above, subsequently stimulating CCK release.[169] However, gastric leptin may function at the stomach targeting leptin receptors on vagal afferents[161] and by interacting with cholecystokinin[170] and the CCK intracellular signaling pathway.[171]

2.3.1 Serum Leptin Response to *In Vivo* Metabolic Adjustments

As described by Ingvartsen and Boisclair[76] the leptin level in the bloodstream of domestic animals is the consequence of metabolic state, nutritional status, relative adiposity, secretory characteristics (pulsatility and diurnal rhythms) and the presence of leptin binding proteins. All of these factors may confound our ability to determine what the specific role of leptin may be in these metabolic adjustments. For a definitive review of this research in domestic animals please see Ingvartsen and Boisclair.[76]

At the present time, no evidence has been published to demonstrate that leptin binding proteins contribute to leptin pharmacokinetics in domestic species. Evaluation of leptin disposal in the chicken could not detect the presence of a leptin binding protein.[172] This is not to say that they do not exist, but methods to detect and measure the soluble form of the receptor (Ob-Re) have not been utilized to evaluate the blood from domestic species.

Leptin is secreted in a modest pulsatile manner in swine[173,174]; and sheep.[175,176] Whisnant and Harrell[174] demonstrated that fasting can reduce pulse frequency from 2.7 ± 0.4 per 4 h in full fed pigs to 1.8 ± 0.3 per 4 h in fasted swine without affecting pulse amplitude. The pulse frequency is much less in sheep; the frequency was measured at only 4.8 pulses over 24 hours[176]. The pulsatile secretion in the sheep does not appear to be a regulated phenomenon due to the random nature of the peaks.[175] No diurnal rhythm in leptin secretion has been detected in sheep[175,176] or dairy cattle.[177]

Leptin in the bloodstream may be considered the integrated response of all the peripheral tissues with its primary regulation the overall metabolic status of the animal. This metabolic status is impacted by age, diet, body composition and energy balance, reproductive status, genetics, disease and infection. For a relevant review of the regulation of serum leptin please see Ingvartsen and Boisclair.[76]

3. REGULATION OF LEPTIN GENE EXPRESSION IN ADIPOCYTES

3.1 Leptin gene expression by preadipocytes

Leptin gene expression during porcine preadipocyte differentiation has been examined in primary cultures of adipose tissue stromal- vascular (S-V) cells (for a review see Barb et al.[1]). Leptin gene expression occurs extremely early in culture and may actually precede or coincide with the onset of preadipocyte differentiation. Dexamethasone (Dex) increased leptin mRNA levels and preadipocyte number in a dose dependent manner (for a review see Barb et al.[1]). Furthermore, increases in leptin gene expression and preadipocyte number were positively correlated throughout the culture period. Therefore, these studies indicate that Dex or glucocorticoids may up-regulate leptin expression indirectly by increasing preadipocyte number. Conclusive evidence that the leptin gene is expressed by porcine preadipocytes per se and that preadipocytes express leptin protein was also reviewed by Barb et al.[1]

3.2 Hormonal regulation of leptin gene expression in vitro

Studies in porcine S-V cell cultures showed that leptin expression may be strongly linked to changes in adipocyte size (reviewed by Barb et al.[1]). Leptin gene expression was linked to the degree of adipocyte hypertrophy in vitro, induced regardless of the hormone, growth factor or concentration used. For instance, leptin gene expression and adipocyte size was similar after 1mM and 10 nM insulin treatment while both were markedly lower after 1 nM insulin treatment[1,178]. Furthermore, at similar concentrations, IGF-1 enhanced less leptin gene expression and produced smaller fat cells than did insulin (for a review see Barb et al.[1]). Additionally, TGF-β enhanced leptin expression in S-V cultures was associated with larger lipid droplets in preadipocytes despite a lower proportion of preadipocytes.[1,178]

Several studies indicate that the influence of insulin on leptin expression and lipid accumulation may, in part, be mediated by locally produced IGF-I reviewed by Barb et al.[1] Furthermore, locally produced IGF-1 may mediate TGF-β enhanced leptin expression since TGF β increased levels of IGF-1 (reviewed by Barb et al.[1]). Although growth hormone increases IGF-1 levels and reduces adipocyte size, it does not influence Dex-induced leptin expression in S-V cultures.[1,178]

Studies of adipocytes differentiated in porcine S-V cell cultures suggested that insulin exposure during preadipocyte lipid accretion dictated insulin sensitivity of lipid-filled preadipocytes in regards to expression of leptin mRNA and C/EBPα protein[1]. Furthermore, leptin gene expression and C/EBPα expression were correlated and C/EBPα autoactivation and phosphorylation /dephosphorylation may be involved in maintaining leptin gene expression (reviewed by Barb et al.[1]).

Consideration of short term culture studies of adipose tissue explants from older animals demonstrates similarities between fetal and postnatal hormonal regulation of leptin gene expression. Chronic insulin treatment increased leptin gene expression in adipose tissue explants from young pigs [179] whereas acute exposure to a combination of Dex and insulin increased leptin expression and secretion in explant cultures from market weight pigs[180]. Furthermore, insulin or Dex increased leptin secretion in ovine adipose tissue explant cultures[181] and increased leptin gene expression in bovine explant cultures.[182] Growth hormone alone has either no influence or decreases the influence of insulin or insulin and Dex on leptin expression in explant cultures.[180,182] The results of these adipose tissue explant studies are somewhat limited or confounded since Dex and/or insulin are necessary to maintain explant integrity and viability.[180] Furthermore, as in S-V cell cultures, locally produced IGF-1 in explant cultures may stimulate leptin expression and confound studies of leptin expression. Regardless, it is clear that adipogenic or lipogenic hormones stimulate adipose tissue leptin gene expression in vitro regardless of the age of tissue donor.

Collectively, *in vitro* studies demonstrate that glucocorticoids and insulin are important modulators of adipose tissue leptin gene expression. In this regard, adipose tissue leptin expression is correlated with preadipocyte differentiation and fat cell size or lipogenesis. Furthermore, locally produced IGF-I may confound the effects of hormones on leptin gene expression.

3.2 Insulin regulation of leptin gene expression and CCAAT enhancer binding protein-α (C/EBPα) in porcine S-V cell cultures

C/EBPα is an important transcription factor involved in the mediation of insulin-induced leptin gene expression.[1,183,184] The expression of the leptin gene and C/EBPα protein has been studied in porcine S-V cell cultures.[1,185] During preadipocyte differentiation the expression of leptin and C/EBPα was dependent on insulin and protein synthesis.[185] Exposure to low insulin levels resulted in little leptin expression and low levels of C/EBPα protein.[1,185] Furthermore, when C/EBPα protein was maximally expressed C/EBPα activation was dependent on insulin (reviewed by Ramsay and Richards[180]). Therefore, in vitro studies demonstrate that C/EBPα plays a critical role in mediating insulin driven porcine adipocyte leptin gene expression (reviewed by Ramsay and Richards[180]).

3.3 Regulation of fetal adipose tissue leptin gene expression

Leptin gene expression in adipose tissue is developmentally regulated in fetal sheep and fetal pigs but serum leptin levels are developmentally regulated only in fetal sheep.[186-188] Adipose tissue in fetal sheep develops and matures earlier than in fetal pigs which may account for the capability of fetal sheep adipose tissue to secrete leptin in a developmentally regulated manner.[187,188] Leptin expression is much greater in perirenal adipose tissue than in subcutaneous (s.c.) adipose tissue in fetal sheep which may reflect the much earlier development of the perirenal adipose tissue depot[188]. Fetal adipose tissue leptin gene expression is considerably lower than in maternal sheep or pig adipose tissue.[186,188] Cortisol increases plasma leptin levels in fetal sheep and adrenalectomy abolishes the ontogenic rise in plasma leptin.[189] However, cortisol does not influence leptin expression in fetal sheep adipose tissue[190], whereas indirect evidence indicates that insulin increases fetal sheep adipose tissue leptin expression.[187] In the fetal pig, hypophysectomized (hypox) studies indicated that hydrocortisone or thyroxine (T4) alone slightly increases adipose tissue leptin gene expression, whereas hydrocortisone and T4 together markedly stimulates leptin gene expression with no influence on serum leptin levels.[186] Elevated leptin gene expression by these hormones may be primarily associated with a remarkable increase in apparent fat cell number with hydrocortisone and T4 treatment[191], if leptin expression per adipocyte does not change. The adipogenic hormones, hydrocortisone and T4, indirectly influence leptin gene expression by increasing the number of preadipocytes and/or adipocytes. Similarly, hydrocortisone increases preadipocyte number and increases leptin gene expression in pig cell cultures.[178,192] Earlier maturation of adipose tissue in fetal sheep may indicate relatively less glucocorticoid-driven preadipocyte recruitment and associated increase in leptin gene expression. Therefore, the influence of adipogenic hormones, like the glucocorticoids, on fetal adipose tissue leptin gene expression may simply reflect the particular stage of adipose development. Since the expression of long form leptin receptor mRNA was detected in fetal adipose tissue adipose tissue[186] leptin may act as an autocrine or paracrine factor in the development of fetal adipose tissue.

A new perspective on the regulation of fetal adipose tissue leptin gene expression was provided by studies of fetal sheep infused with leptin, and by related studies.[193,194] A positive relationship was demonstrated between the degree or proportion of unilocular adipocytes or "unilocularity" in fetal adipose tissue, and plasma leptin levels and leptin gene expression.[193,194] Therefore, the increase in adipose tissue leptin gene expression in pig fetuses treated with hydrocortisone and T4 may, in part, be attributable to the greater degree of adipose tissue "unilocularity" in these fetuses compared to untreated controls.[191] However, T4 treatment increased adipose tissue leptin gene expression to the same degree as hydrocortisone treatment[186] despite a much greater degree of "unilocularity" in adipose tissue from T4 treated fetuses.[195,196] Furthermore, serum leptin levels were not influenced by treatment with either T4 or hydrocortisone or the combination of T4 and hydrocortisone.[186] Regardless, fetal adipose tissue leptin gene expression is clearly species dependent and may be associated with the degree of fetal adipose tissue "unilocularity" and the extent of preadipocyte recruitment.

Several studies have examined the influence of maternal nutrition on either circulating leptin levels or adipose tissue leptin expression in fetal sheep. Maternal overnutrition or undernutrition during late gestation had no influence on fetal body weights, plasma leptin levels and adipose tissue leptin gene expression.[188,197,198] However, overfeeding throughout gestation reduced fetal adipose tissue deposition and leptin gene expression despite no influence on fetal weights.[199] These studies indicate that nutrition throughout gestation is more influential on fetal adipose tissue leptin expression than during late gestation. Nutrient availability per se may be important as well since fetal plasma leptin levels and fetal weights were reduced in experimentally induced intrauterine growth-restricted fetal sheep [200]. In this regard, fetal sheep body weights were positively correlated with adipose tissue leptin gene expression.[201] However, two pig studies demonstrated that leptin expression in adipose tissue of 59 day old pigs and plasma leptin levels of 3 and 12 month old pigs were negatively correlated with birth weights.[202,203] Furthermore, moderate overfeeding during the second quarter of gestation in pigs indicated that maternal nutrition during gestation could program postnatal adipose tissue leptin gene expression in females.[202] The influence of birth weight on leptin secretion was also strongest in female pigs.[203] Therefore, estrogen may regulate leptin expression in females as demonstrated in estrogen treated females pigs [204] and estrogen may, therefore, dictate or mediate leptin imprinting in growing animals. However, it is clear that the influence of maternal nutrition on fetal leptin status is species and sex dependent.

4. LEPTIN: A METABOLIC SIGNAL AFFECTING REPRODUCTION

Injection of recombinant leptin reduced feed intake and body weight and restored fertility in the leptin deficient *ob/ob* mouse.[3] Although the hypothalamus appears to be a key site of action[5,6], leptin receptors are also found in other regions within the central nervous system (CNS), pituitary gland[5,6] and ovary.[205] Discovery of leptin has improved our understanding of the relationship between adipose tissue, energy homeostasis and reproductive function.[1,3,206,207] Metabolic perturbations altered endocrine function, delayed onset of puberty and interfered with normal estrous cycles in the gilt[208], heifer[209] and ewe.[210] Thus, leptin may serve as an important link between metabolic status and the neuroendocrine function and subsequent reproductive function.

4.1 Leptin receptor, site of action and leptin secretion

4.1.1 Leptin receptor

The leptin receptor (OB-r) was first identified by expression cloning [211] and has been classified as a member of the class 1 cytokine receptors due to its structural homology to IL-6 receptors and common down-stream signaling pathways.[7] The LR family is comprised of at least 6 receptor isoforms that arise due to alternative splicing. LR isoforms include a long form (OB-rb) and several short forms with varying lengths of the cytoplasmic tail (OB-ra, OB-rc, OB-rd and OB-rf) as well as a soluble form (OB-re), which consists of the extracellular loop and circulates in plasma.[212] Consistent with being a member of the class 1 cytokine receptor family, the long form LR signals via janus-activated kinases (JAK) signal transducers and activators of transcription (STAT) activation.[7]

4.1.2 Site of action

Distribution of OB-rb varies among species, but in general, OB-rb mRNA abundance has been localized in the ventromedial and arcuate nuclei of the hypothalamus and anterior pituitary of the pig[213], ewe[5], rat[214], and mouse.[211] It has been hypothesized that leptin acts directly on GnRH neurons. However, it is more likely that other neuropeptides, such as neuropeptide Y (NPY), proopiomelanocortin (POMC) and gamma-aminobutyric acid (GABA) mediate the action of leptin[215-218,219]. Co-localization of leptin receptor mRNA with NPY gene expression is compelling evidence that hypothalamic NPY is a potential target for leptin.[215,217] In addition, NPY has been implicated in regulation of GnRH/LH secretion in the rodent[220], primate[221], ewe[222], cow[223] and pig.[218,224] Administration of NPY stimulated appetite in the ewe[225] and pig, and this was reversed by central administration of leptin in the pig.[1] Also, other neuronal systems likely mediate the action of leptin, since fertility was partially restored by leptin treatment in the *ob/ob* mouse with a homozygous null mutation for NPY.[226] In support of this idea, leptin treatment did not affect acute release of NPY from mouse[227], rat[228] or pig[218] hypothalamic tissue *in vitro*. However, during periods of nutritional stress, hypothalamic NPY mRNA was elevated.[5] Hence, activation of the NPY system appears to be associated with chronic physiologic changes, such as those occurring during fasting.

Several reports indicate that hypothalamic NPY neurons are not the sole target of leptin.[218,229,230] Neurons expressing the POMC gene, which encodes for beta-endorphin, adrenocorticotropic hormone (ACTH), α-melanocycte-stimulating hormone (α-MSH) and γ-MSH, have direct synaptic contact with GnRH-containing neurons in the ewe[215] and are immunoreactive for OB-rb.[217] Leptin treatment of *ob/ob* mice restored POMC gene expression levels to that of the wild-type animals.[215] The endogenous opioid, beta-endorphin[231,232], as well as the melanocortin system have been implicated in modulating both gonadotropin secretion and feeding behavior,[233,234] Furthermore, a high proportion of the cocaine and amphetamine-regulated transcript (CART), NPY, agouti-related protein (AGRP), orexin, melanin-concentrating hormone (MCH) and galanin hypothalamic neurons express OB-rb, suggesting that these neurons are direct targets of leptin.[217] Thus, potential exists for leptin to influence gonadotropin secretion and subsequent ovarian function via interaction with other neuronal systems (Figure 1).

Leptin in farm animals 283

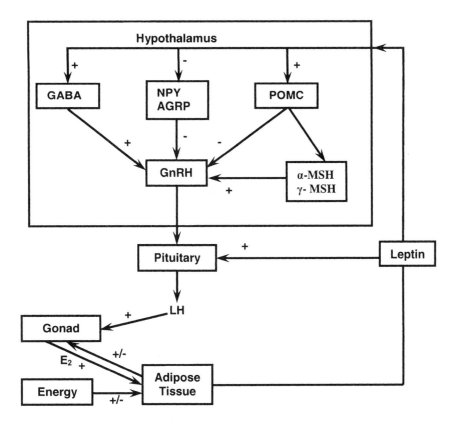

Figure 1. Proposed involvement of leptin in the neuroendocrine regulation of LH secretion and ovarian activity. Leptin secreted from adipose tissue in response to changes in energy balance and/or steroid milieu (E = estrogen) acts through its receptor to: inhibit hypothalamic neuropeptide Y (NPY), stimulate proopiomelanocortin (POMC) activity with α-, γ- melanocyte stimulating hormone (MSH) mediating the effects of leptin, stimulate gamma-aminobutyric acid (GABA)ergic drive to the GnRH neuron, and directly modulate ovarian steroidogenesis.

4.1.3 Leptin secretion

Changes in body weight or nutritional status are characterized by alterations in serum levels of many hormones and growth factors that regulate adipocyte function and development, such as insulin, glucocorticoids, GH and insulin-like growth factor-I (IGF-I).[173,235-237] Administration of glucocorticoids or insulin increased leptin gene expression, demonstrating that other hormonal factors may mediate nutritionally-induced changes in leptin gene expression.[238,239] Acute 48 h fast or chronic feed restriction resulted in a marked decrease in leptin secretion coincident with a reduced LH secretion in the cow[235] and ewe.[240,241] However, acute 28 h fast decreased leptin pulse frequency but not LH secretion in the prepubertal gilt[173], while treatment with a competitive inhibitor of glycolysis suppressed LH secretion without affecting serum leptin concentrations.[173] Furthermore, in the ovariectomized (OVX) prepubertal gilt 7 day feed restriction failed to affect leptin or LH secretion.[242] Conversely, chronic feed restriction for 7 days resulted in a concurrent reduction in serum leptin concentrations and LH secretion in mature OVX gilts.[174] The ability of the pig to maintain euglycemia during acute fast may account for the failure of acute feed deprivation to affect LH secretion in the prepubertal gilt[208], or alternatively, the leptin and LH response to feed restriction in the prepubertal gilt may require energy levels and/or backfat reduction reaching a different putative inhibitory threshold compared to the mature animal. Thus, leptin may serve as a metabolic signal which communicates metabolic status to the brain; the neuroendocrine response to acute energy deprivation may be species dependent and/or age dependent.

The effect of gonadal steroids on leptin secretion and how this relates to LH secretion are poorly understood. Circulating leptin concentrations are lower in males than in females.[243,244] Leptin levels vary during the human menstrual cycle and peak during the luteal phase.[245] In mature heifers and cows, serum leptin concentrations tended to decrease during the late luteal/early follicular phase of the estrous cycle and this was associated with a reduction in adipocyte leptin gene expression.[246] Estrogen treatment induced leptin mRNA expression in adipose tissue in the OVX prepubertal gilt, which occurred at the time of expected puberty in intact contemporaries[204] and was associated with greater LH secretion.[247] In a recent study in ewe lambs[248], pulsatile leptin secretion was independent of LH secretion. Therefore, the physiological relevance of varying levels of circulating leptin during the estrous cycle and pubertal development and its association with LH secretion remains unknown.

4.2 Central effects of leptin on the hypothalamic-pituitary axis

In the pig, leptin treatment stimulated basal LH secretion directly from anterior pituitary cells and GnRH release from hypothalamic-preoptic tissue explants from intact and OVX prepubertal gilts on maintenance rations.[218] Interestingly, intracerebroventricular (ICV) administration of leptin failed to stimulate LH secretion in the intact prepubertal gilt.[218] Obviously, hypothalamic explants are deprived of neuroanatomical connections with other extra-hypothalamic tissues that may convey the heightened negative feedback action of estradiol on the GnRH pulse generator that occurs during pubertal development.

Intracerebroventricular injection of leptin stimulated LH secretion in steroid-implanted castrated male sheep[249], and chronic ICV administration of leptin stimulated LH secretion in the feed-restricted OVX cow[250] and ewe.[251] On the contrary, chronic ICV administration of leptin failed to stimulated LH secretion in well nourished OVX ewes with no steroid replacement[252], and in intact ewe lambs.[241] *In vitro* studies demonstrated that leptin treatment stimulated basal and GnRH-mediated LH secretion from pituitary explants from fasted, but not control-fed cows, while having no effect on GnRH release from hypothalamic explants from either group of cows.[253] Thus, metabolic state appears to be a primary determinant of the hypothalamic-pituitary response to leptin in ruminants.

Thus, in contrast to data obtained from the cow, the effect of leptin on LH secretion in the pig during pubertal development is associated with stage of sexual maturation and subsequent change in the negative feedback action of estradiol on LH secretion.

4.3 Leptin and Onset of Puberty

The endocrine basis for puberty in the gilt, heifer and ewe has been reviewed previously.[247,254,255] Onset of puberty may be linked to attainment of a critical body weight, metabolic mass or a minimum percentage of body fat.[256,257] Initiation of puberty may also be influenced by metabolic factors of peripheral orgin.[208,258,257,259] Identification of such signals has remained elusive. However, the discovery of leptin has improved our understanding of the relationship between adipose tissue and energy homeostasis.[3]

In the rodent, leptin treatment advanced sexual maturation in restricted and *ad lib* fed animals.[260,261] Serum leptin concentrations increased during puberty in the mouse[262], heifer[246] and pig[204], and in the human female, age at first menarche was inversely related to serum leptin concentrations.[263] Thus, leptin may serve as a circulating signal of nutritional status that activates the reproductive axis.

There exists a matter of controversy as to the precise role of leptin in the onset of puberty. Several reports have demonstrated that circulating leptin concentrations remain relatively unchanged during pubertal development in the female mouse or rat[264,265], while leptin administration failed to advance puberty onset in well nourished female mice.[264] Together the above reports suggest that leptin does not serve as a triggering signal but acts mainly as a permissive signal that permits puberty to occur.

Although serum leptin concentrations increased during puberty in the gilt, other factors in addition to leptin may regulate onset of puberty. As indicated above, it is hypothesized that estradiol modulates the hypothalamic-pituitary response to leptin. Moreover, estradiol may regulate the pubertal related changes in leptin gene expression. In the OVX prepubertal gilt, estrogen-induced leptin mRNA expression in adipose tissue occurred at the time of expected puberty but not in younger animals.[204] This was associated with greater LH secretion[247] and an age dependent increase in hypothalamic OB-rb expression.[213]

In the prepubertal heifer and ewe lamb, short term feed restriction reduced adipose leptin gene expression and leptin secretion, but increased hypothalamic OB-rb expression.[5,235] This was associated with decreased serum insulin, IGF-I and LH pulse frequency.[235,241] During pubertal development in heifers, serum leptin concentrations and leptin gene expression increased coincident with increased serum IGF-I concentrations and body weight[246], While short-term fasting failed to reduce pulsatile LH secretion in the mature cow.[250] Thus, there is a heightened sensitivity of the hypothalamic-pituitary axis to variations in energy availability in the heifer compared to the mature cow. With regard to metabolic state, leptin treatment reversed nutrient restriction-induced inhibition of LH secretion in the mature cow[250] ewe[266] and ewe lamb[241] demonstrating a positive association between LH secretion and leptin. However, neither chronic s.c. leptin treatment of normal-fed heifers[267], nor acute i.v. administration of leptin to normal-growth[267] or growth-restricted heifers[268] accelerated the development of a sexually mature pattern of gonadotropin secretion. In support of these observations, developmental constraints prevented the leptin-induced stimulation of LH secretion in the prepubertal gilt,[218] Thus, leptin may act as a metabolic gate for puberty. Accordingly, as circulating leptin concentrations increase during pubertal development, a putative threshold is reached that permits activation of the reproductive axis. In this regard, leptin may serve as a permissive signal for puberty, as apposed to a triggering signal for puberty.

4.4 Seasonal reproduction role of leptin

4.4.1 Temperature

Seasonal and (or) environmental effects have been observed in ruminants. Circulating leptin concentrations were not influenced during winter in OVX cows[246], but blood leptin levels were lower in cows calving in autumn compared to spring.[269] In addition, circulating leptin concentrations increased in early lactating cows exposed to 10 °C compared to animals exposed to 3 °C.[270] Moreover, in the ram, plasma leptin concentrations were lower in animals maintained at 0 °C than in a thermoneutral environment of 20 °C.[271] The authors concluded that lower circulating leptin levels in ruminants exposed to the cold environment could be partly due to the depressed insulin action on leptin secretion, since animals subjected to a euglycemic clamp for 2 h increased circulating leptin concentrations in the thermoneutral, but not the cold, environment.

4.4.2 Day length

In the OVX Lacaune ewe, exposure to long day length (LD) increased leptin mRNA expression in adipose tissue and circulating levels of leptin irrespective of feeding level.[272] Furthermore, leptin mRNA was reduced during short day lengths in the Siberian hamster.[273] Circulating leptin concentrations increased in mature OVX estradiol-implanted cows from January to the summer solstice[246], which was similar to observations reported in mares.[274] In Soay rams fed ad libitum, LD increased plasma leptin concentrations compared to short day length (SD).[275] Furthermore, appetite response to central administration of leptin was sex and seasonal dependent in mature gonadectomized Rommey Marsh sheep; leptin had a profound inhibitory effect on feeding behavior in females during the spring compared to males.[276] The physiological significance of photoperiod regulation of leptin expression in adipose tissue and secretion may be related to seasonal changes in reproductive activity. Day length has been reported to affect the age at which puberty occurs in beef and dairy heifers.[277,278] Spring-born heifers exposed to 18 h of daylight reached puberty earlier than those raised under natural photoperiod.[279] Hence, mechanisms through which seasonal changes in day-length affect puberty appear to involve photo-regulated factors that may include not only leptin but also melatonin. In the rat, melatonin administered to mimic SD decreased plasma leptin and insulin concentrations and intra-abdominal fat.[280] In contrast, melatonin treatment for 3 months to mimic SD in sheep did not change plasma leptin concentrations but did increase LH and prolactin secretion.[236] Thus, mechanisms through which seasonal changes in day length affect reproductive activity may involve melatonin, but the role of leptin is unclear.

Seasonal anestrous mares exhibited low leptin levels.[281] Similarly, in Siberian hamsters, serum leptin levels were significantly reduced in SD when compared to LD. Leptin secretion increased from anestrus to follicular and luteal phases subsequent to the first ovulation in mares.[282] Thus it appears that the transition from ovarian activity to anestrus is preceded by a decrease in plasma leptin concentrations. Conversely, resumption of ovarian activity may require increasing leptin concentrations during this transition period.

4.5 Leptin and Ovarian Function

Leptin receptors have been observed in both the granulosa and theca cells of the human[283,284], bovine[205,285] and porcine.[286] Circulating concentrations of leptin are generally below 10 ng/ml[173,287,288], and both physiological and supra-physiological leptin concentrations have been reported to affect steroid synthesis *in vitro* and *in vivo*. *In vitro* studies demonstrated that treatment with supra-physiological concentrations of leptin inhibited steroidogenesis in bovine granulosa[205,289] and theca cells.[285] Similar results have been reported for the human[290,291], rodent[292,293], sheep[294] and pig.[295] In contrast, physiological doses of leptin have been reported to stimulate steroidogenesis in granulosa in the pig[295] in the presence or absence of IGF-I. Taken together, the above reports support the idea that leptin has a direct role in modulating follicular development. A critical blood level of leptin may be necessary to initiate follicular development, stimulatory threshold, and elevated circulating leptin concentrations may reach a putative inhibitory threshold.

Kendall et al.[296] reported that passive immunization against leptin during the follicular phase of the estrous cycle in the ewe increased ovarian estradiol secretion but had no effect on gonadotropin secretion, ovulation or subsequent luteal function. In contrast, direct ovarian arterial infusion of high dose (20 µg/h) or low dose (2 µg/h) of leptin had no effect on estradiol production but increased the progesterone production from the subsequent corpus luteum. This paradox may in part be explained by activation of alternate pathways which stimulate ovarian function. Such pathways would include: the GnRH-LH axis[218,297], GH/IGF axis[216,298] and altered ovarian blood flow[299,300] via the angiotensin II system.[301] Lastly, supra-physiological doses of leptin may have down-regulated OB-rb expression.[302,303]

The fact that exposure of the somatic cells of the preovulatory follicle to leptin enhanced the steroidogenic capacity of the luteal cells suggests a role for leptin in corpus luteum development. In support of this idea, increased progesterone production from porcine granulasa cells due to leptin treatment was associated with enhanced expression of steroidogenic acute regulatory protein (StAR), which may be a key regulatory event in the action of leptin on steroidogenesis.[295] Moreover, leptin receptor mRNA abundance increased during *in vitro* luteinization and was greatest in luteal tissue collected during the mid luteal phase in the pig.[286] This, evidence demonstrates that leptin plays a role in both follicular development and subsequent luteal function.

4.6 Lactation

4.6.1 Lactating sow

During lactation, feed intake of sows is often inadequate to meet nutrient requirements for maintenance and lactation. There is increasing evidence that nutrition, reduction in backfat, changes in metabolic state, and associated changes in metabolite and metabolic hormones such as insulin, IGF-I, GH, and leptin, influence the reproductive axis in the sow.[304]

In the primaparous and multiparous lactating sow, serum and milk leptin concentrations were positively correlated with backfat thickness and level of dietary energy fed during gestation, as well as feed consumption.[305,306] A positive correlation was observed among plasma insulin, leptin and LH concentrations in lactating sows fed ad libitum compared to feed-restricted sows. Moreover, the weaning to estrus interval was greater in the feed-restricted sows compared to controls.[307] These findings provide evidence that circulating leptin, LH concentrations and feed consumption during lactation are influenced by dietary energy intake during pregnancy or lactation in the sow. Thus, the role of leptin in modulating feed intake during lactation and post-weaning reproductive function remains to be determined.

4.6.2 Lactating ruminants

Generally, energy balance and adiposity is positively correlated to postpartum reproductive function in ruminants.[308,309] Postpartum reproductive performance in cows was associated with greater IGF-I[310] and increasing leptin concentrations during the postpartum period.[311] Cows with decreased leptin level exhibited delayed onset of reproductive function during the post-partum period.[311,312] In addition, peripartum plasma leptin concentrations were associated with parity and body condition score (BCS) at calving.[309] Circulating leptin concentrations during lactation were also associated with BCS. Cows and heifers with BCS greater than 3 had greater blood leptin and IGF-I levels, and the peripartum decrease in leptin was more pronounced in heifers and occurred later in fat animals. Leptin levels greater than 5 ng/ml in lean heifers, multiparous cows and fat heifers resulted in resumption of ovarian follicular development earlier than animals with lower circulating leptin concentrations.[309] Theses observations support the hypothesis that leptin may play a permissive role in activation of the reproductive axis in the postpartum animal as previously reported.[218,308,313]

5. CONCLUSION

Evidence has been presented demonstrating that leptin may act beyond its role as a satiety signal. Leptin serves as a metabolic signal interacting with neuropeptides that link energy status with the neuroendocrine axis. Furthermore, leptin may play a direct role in modulating ovarian activity. Leptin may act as a metabolic gate during the onset of puberty and during the resumption of postpartum reproductive function. We suggest a putative stimulatory threshold is reached which permits activation of the hypothalamic-pituitary-gonadal axis and subsequent reproductive function.

REFERENCES

1. C.R. Barb, G.J. Hausman, and K.L. Houseknecht, Biology of leptin in the pig. *Domest Anim Endocrinol,* **21**:297-317 (2001).
2. C.R. Barb and R.R. Kraeling, Role of leptin in the regulation of gonadotropin secretion in farm animals. *Anim Reprod Sci,* **82-83**:155-167 (2004).
3. L.A. Campfield, F.J. Smith, Y. Guisez, R. Devos, and P. Burn, Recombinant mouse ob protein: Evidence for a peripheral signal linking adiposity and the central neural networks. *Science,* **269**:546-549 (1995).
4. Y. Zhang, R. Proenca, M. Maffel, M. Barone, L. Leopold, and J.M. Friedman, Positional clonong of the mouse obese gene and its human homologue. *Nature,* **372**:425-432 (1994).
5. C.J. Dyer, J.M. Simmons, R.L. Matteri, and D.H. Keisler, Leptin receptor mRNA is expressed in ewe anterior pituitary and adipose tissue and is differentially expressed in hypothalamic regions of well-fed and feed-restricted ewes. *Domest Anim Endocrinol,* **14**:119-128 (1997).
6. J. Lin, C.R. Barb, R.L. Matteri, R.R. Kraeling, X. Chen, R.J. Meinersmann, and G.B. Rampacek, Long form leptin receptor mRNA expression in the brain, pituitary, and other tissues in the pig. *Domest Animl Endocrinol,* **19**:53-61 (2000).
7. K.L. Houseknecht and C.P. Portocarrero, Leptin and its receptors: regulators of whole-body energy homeostasis. *Domest Anim Endocrinol,* **15**:457-475 (1998).
8. G.C. Kennedy, The role of depot fat in the hypothalamic control of food intake in the rat. *Proc Roy Soc,* **140**:578-592 (1953).
9. C.R. Barb, X. Yan, M.J. Azain, R.R. Kraeling, G.B. Rampacek, and T.G. Ramsay, Recombinant porcine leptin reduces feed intake and stimulates growth hormone secretion in swine. *Domest Anim Endocrino,* **15**:77-86 (1998).
10. D.M. Denbow, S. Meade, A. Robertson, J.P. McMurtry, M. Richards, and C. Ashwell, Leptin-induced decrease in food intake in chickens. *Physiol Behav,* **69**:359-362 (2000).
11. H. Volkoff and R.E. Peter, Characterization of two forms of cocaine- and amphetamine-regulated transcript (CART) peptide precursors in goldfish: molecular cloning and distribution, modulation of expression by nutritional status, and interactions with leptin. *Endocrinology,* **142**:5076-5088 (2001).
12. C.D. Morrison, R. Wood, E.L. McFadin, N.C. Whitley, and D.H. Keisler, Effect of intravenous infusion of recombinant ovine leptin on feed intake and serum concentrations of GH, LH, insulin, IGF-1, cortisol, and thyroxine in growing prepubertal ewe lambs. *Domest Anim Endocrinol,* **22**:103-112 (2002).
13. K.M. Ajuwon, J.L. Kuske, D.B. Anderson, D.L. Hancock, K.L. Houseknecht, O. Adeola, and M.E. Spurlock, Chronic leptin administration increases serum NEFA in the pig and differentially regulates PPAR expression in adipose tissue. *J Nutr Biochem,* **14**:576-583 (2003).
14. T.G. Ramsay, J.A. Bush, J.P. McMurtry, M.C. Thivierge, and T.A. Davis, Peripheral leptin administration alters hormone and metabolite levels in the young pig. *Comp Biochem Physiol A Mol Integr Physiol,* **138**:17-25 (2004).
15. S. Dridi, N. Raver, E.E. Gussakovsky, M. Derouet, M. Picard, A. Gertler, and M. Taouis, Biological activities of recombinant chicken leptin C4S analog compared with unmodified leptins. *Am J Physiol Endocrinol Metab,* **279**:E116-E123 (2000).
16. S.A. Thomas, J.E. Preston, M.R. Wilson, C.L. Farrell, and M.B. Segal, Leptin transport at the blood--cerebrospinal fluid barrier using the perfused sheep choroid plexus model. *Brain Res,* **895**:283-290 (2001).

17. C. Peiser, G.P. McGregor, and R.E. Lang, Binding and internalization of leptin by porcine choroid plexus cells in culture. *Neurosci Lett,* **283**:209-212 (2000).
18. S.L. Karonen, H.A. Koistinen, P. Nikkinen, and V.A. Koivisto, Is brain uptake of leptin in vivo saturable and reduced by fasting? *Eur J Nucl Med,* **25**:607-612 (1998).
19. P.K. Chelikani, D.R. Glimm, and J.J. Kennelly, Short communication: Tissue distribution of leptin and leptin receptor mRNA in the bovine. *J Dairy Sci,* **86**:2369-2372 (2003).
20. T. Ohkubo, M. Tanaka, and K. Nakashima, Structure and tissue distribution of chicken leptin receptor (cOb-R) mRNA. *Biochim Biophys Acta,* **1491**:303-308 (2000).
21. M.P. Richards and S.M. Poch, Molecular cloning and expression of the turkey leptin receptor gene. *Comp Biochem Physiol B Biochem Mol Biol,* **136**:833-847 (2003).
22. S. Nagatani, Y. Zeng, D.H. Keisler, D.L. Foster, and C.A. Jaffe, Leptin regulates pulsatile luteinizing hormone and growth hormone secretion in the sheep. *Endocrinology,* **141**:3965-3975 (2000).
23. D.A. Zieba, M. Amstalden, M.N. Maciel, D.H. Keisler, N. Raver, A. Gertler, and G.L. Williams, Divergent effects of leptin on luteinizing hormone and insulin secretion are dose dependent. *Exp Biol Med (Maywood),* **228**:325-330 (2003).
24. J.C. Litten, A. Mostyn, K.S. Perkins, A.M. Corson, M.E. Symonds, and L. Clarke, Effect of administration of recombinant human leptin during the neonatal period on the plasma concentration and gene expression of leptin in the piglet. *Biol Neonate,* **87**:1-7 (2005).
25. J. Wolinski, M. Biernat, P. Guilloteau, B.R. Westrom, and R. Zabielski, Exogenous leptin controls the development of the small intestine in neonatal piglets. *J Endocrinol,* **177**:215-222 (2003).
26. A. Mostyn, J. Bispham, S. Pearce, Y. Evens, N. Raver, D.H. Keisler, R. Webb, T. Stephenson, and M.E. Symonds, Differential effects of leptin on thermoregulation and uncoupling protein abundance in the neonatal lamb. *FASEB J,* **16**:1438-1440 (2002).
27. H.E. Paczoska-Eliasiewicz, A. Gertler, M. Proszkowiec, J. Proudman, A. Hrabia, A. Sechman, M. Mika, T. Jacek, S. Cassy, N. Raver, and J. Rzasa, Attenuation by leptin of the effects of fasting on ovarian function in hens (Gallus domesticus). *Reproduction,* **126**:739-751 (2003).
28. N.R. Kendall, C.G. Gutierrez, R.J. Scaramuzzi, D.T. Baird, R. Webb, and B.K. Campbell, Direct in vivo effects of leptin on ovarian steroidogenesis in sheep. *Reproduction,* **128**:757-765 (2004).
29. S.H. Schirmer, I.R. Buschmann, M.M. Jost, I.E. Hoefer, S. Grundmann, J.P. Andert, S. Ulusans, C. Bode, J.J. Piek, and N. van Royen, Differential effects of MCP-1 and leptin on collateral flow and arteriogenesis. *Cardiovasc Res,* **64**:356-364 (2004).
30. S.P. Reidy and J.M. Weber, Accelerated substrate cycling: a new energy-wasting role for leptin in vivo. *Am J Physiol Endocrinol Metab,* **282**:E312-E317 (2002).
31. T.G. Ramsay, Porcine leptin alters insulin inhibition of lipolysis in porcine adipocytes in vitro. *J Anim Sci,* **79**:653-657 (2001).
32. G. Frühbeck, M. Aguado, and J.A. Martínez, *In vitro* lipolytic effect of leptin on mouse adipocytes: Evidence for a possible autocrine/paracrine role of leptin. *Biocheml Biophys Res Commun,* **240**:590-594 (1997).
33. D. Newby, A. Gertler, and R.G. Vernon, Effects of recombinant ovine leptin on in vitro lipolysis and lipogenesis in subcutaneous adipose tissue from lactating and nonlactating sheep. *J Anim Sci,* **79**:445-452 (2001).

34. R.M. Evans, G.D. Barish, and Y.X. Wang, PPARs and the complex journey to obesity. *Nat Med,* **10**:355-361 (2004).
35. M.Y. Wang, Y. Lee, and R.H. Unger, Novel form of lipolysis induced by leptin. *J Biol Chem,* **274**:17541-17544 (1999).
36. M.A. Lazar, PPAR gamma, 10 years later. *Biochimie,* **87**:9-13 (2005).
37. H.J. Mersmann, The effect of insulin on porcine adipose tissue lipogenesis. *Comp Biochem Physiol B,* **94**:709-713 (1989).
38. T.G. Ramsay, Porcine leptin inhibits lipogenesis in porcine adipocytes. *J Anim Sci,* **81**:3008-3017 (2003).
39. T.G. Ramsay, Porcine leptin alters isolated adipocyte glucose and fatty acid metabolism. *Domest Anim Endocrinol,* **26**:11-21 (2004).
40. B. Cohen, D. Novick, and M. Rubinstein, Modulation of insulin activities by leptin. *Science,* **274**:1185-1188 (1996).
41. T.G. Ramsay, Porcine leptin inhibits protein breakdown and stimulates fatty acid oxidation in C2C12 myotubes. *J Anim Sci,* **81**:3046-3051 (2003).
42. D.M. Muoio, G.L. Dohm, F.T. Fiedorek, Jr., E.B. Tapscott, and R.A. Coleman, Leptin directly alters lipid partitioning in skeletal muscle. *Diabetes,* **46**:1360-1363 (1997).
43. R. Lau, W.D. Blinn, A. Bonen, and D.J. Dyck, Stimulatory effects of leptin and muscle contraction on fatty acid metabolism are not additive. *Am J Physiol Endocrinol Metab,* **281**:E122-E129 (2001).
44. G.R. Steinberg, D.J. Dyck, J. Calles-Escandon, N.N. Tandon, J.J. Luiken, J.F. Glatz, and A. Bonen, Chronic leptin administration decreases fatty acid uptake and fatty acid transporters in rat skeletal muscle. *J Biol Chem,* **277**:8854-8860 (2002).
45. Y. Minokoshi, Y.B. Kim, O.D. Peroni, L.G. Fryer, C. Muller, D. Carling, and B.B. Kahn, Leptin stimulates fatty-acid oxidation by activating AMP-activated protein kinase. *Nature,* **415**:268-269 (2002).
46. G.R. Steinberg, A. Bonen, and D.J. Dyck, Fatty acid oxidation and triacylglycerol hydrolysis are enhanced after chronic leptin treatment in rats. *Am J Physiol Endocrinol Metab,* **282**:E593-E600 (2002).
47. A.G. Dulloo, M. Gubler, J.P. Montani, J. Seydoux, and G. Solinas, Substrate cycling between de novo lipogenesis and lipid oxidation: a thermogenic mechanism against skeletal muscle lipotoxicity and glucolipotoxicity. *Int J Obes Relat Metab Disord,* **28 Suppl 4**:S29-37.:S29-S37 (2004).
48. Y. Feuermann, S.J. Mabjeesh, and A. Shamay, Leptin affects prolactin action on milk protein and fat synthesis in the bovine mammary gland. *J Dairy Sci,* **87**:2941-2946 (2004).
49. M.A. Pellymounter, J.J. Cullen, M.B. Baker, R. Hecht, D. Winters, T. Boone, and F. Collins, Effects of the obese gene product on body weight regulation in *ob/ob* mice. *Science,* **269**:540-546 (1995).
50. N. Levin, C. Nelson, A. Gurney, R. Vandlen, and F. de Sauvage, Decreased food intake does not completely account for adiposity reduction after ob protein infusion. *Proc Natl Acad Sci U S A,* %20;**93**:1726-1730 (1996).
51. I.S. Farooqi, S.A. Jebb, G. Langmack, E. Lawrence, C.H. Cheetham, A.M. Prentice, I.A. Hughes, M.A. McCamish, and S. O'Rahilly, Effects of recombinant leptin therapy in a child with congenital leptin deficiency. *N Engl J Med,* **341**:879-884 (1999).
52. K.M. Ajuwon, J.L. Kuske, D. Ragland, O. Adeola, D.L. Hancock, D.B. Anderson, and M.E. Spurlock, The regulation of IGF-1 by leptin in the pig is tissue specific and independent of changes in growth hormone. *J Nutr Biochem,* **14**:522-530 (2003).

53. N. Carbo, V. Ribas, S. Busquets, B. Alvarez, F.J. Lopez-Soriano, and J.M. Argiles, Short-term effects of leptin on skeletal muscle protein metabolism in the rat. *J Nutr Biochem,* **11**:431-435 (2000).
54. D. Lamosova and M. Zeman, Effect of leptin and insulin on chick embryonic muscle cells and hepatocytes. *Physiol Res,* **50**:183-189 (2001).
55. J.M. Fagan, L. Waxman, and A.L. Goldberg, Skeletal muscle and liver contain a soluble ATP + ubiquitin-dependent proteolytic system. *Biochem J,* **243**:335-343 (1987).
56. J.W. Bird, J.H. Carter, R.E. Triemer, R.M. Brooks, and A.M. Spanier, Proteinases in cardiac and skeletal muscle. *Fed Proc,* **39**:20-25 (1980).
57. W.R. Dayton, D.E. Goll, M.G. Zeece, R.M. Robson, and W.J. Reville, A Ca2+-activated protease possibly involved in myofibrillar protein turnover. Purification from porcine muscle. *Biochemistry,* **15**:2150-2158 (1976).
58. R.B. Ceddia, W.N. William, Jr., and R. Curi, Comparing effects of leptin and insulin on glucose metabolism in skeletal muscle: evidence for an effect of leptin on glucose uptake and decarboxylation. *Int J Obes Relat Metab Disord,* **23**:75-82 (1999).
59. L. Berti, M. Kellerer, E. Capp, and H.U. Haring, Leptin stimulates glucose transport and glycogen synthesis in C2C12 myotubes: evidence for a P13-kinase mediated effect. *Diabetologia,* **40**:606-609 (1997).
60. R.B. Ceddia, W.N. William, Jr., and R. Curi, Leptin increases glucose transport and utilization in skeletal muscle in vitro. *Gen Pharmacol,* **31**:799-801 (1998).
61. R.B. Harris, Acute and chronic effects of leptin on glucose utilization in lean mice. *Biochem Biophys Res Commun,* **245**:502-509 (1998).
62. P. Raman, S.S. Donkin, and M.E. Spurlock, Regulation of hepatic glucose metabolism by leptin in pig and rat primary hepatocyte cultures. *Am J Physiol Regul Integr Comp Physiol,* **286**:R206-R216 (2004).
63. I. Fernandez-Figares, A.E. Shannon, D. Wray-Cahen, and T.J. Caperna, The role of insulin, glucagon, dexamethasone, and leptin in the regulation of ketogenesis and glycogen storage in primary cultures of porcine hepatocytes prepared from 60 kg pigs. *Domest Anim Endocrinol,* **27**:125-140 (2004).
64. L. Rossetti, D. Massillon, N. Barzilai, P. Vuguin, W. Chen, M. Hawkins, J. Wu, and J. Wang, Short term effects of leptin on hepatic gluconeogenesis and in vivo insulin action. *J Biol Chem,* **272**:27758-27763 (1997).
65. R.B. Ceddia, G. Lopes, H.M. Souza, G.R. Borba-Murad, W.N. William, Jr., R.B. Bazotte, and R. Curi, Acute effects of leptin on glucose metabolism of in situ rat perfused livers and isolated hepatocytes. *Int J Obes Relat Metab Disord,* **23**:1207-1212 (1999).
66. R.M. O'Doherty, P.R. Anderson, A.Z. Zhao, K.E. Bornfeldt, and C.B. Newgard, Sparing effect of leptin on liver glycogen stores in rats during the fed-to-fasted transition. *Am J Physiol,* **277**:E544-E550 (1999).
67. M. Nemecz, K. Preininger, R. Englisch, C. Furnsinn, B. Schneider, W. Waldhausl, and M. Roden, Acute effect of leptin on hepatic glycogenolysis and gluconeogenesis in perfused rat liver. *Hepatology,* **29**:166-172 (1999).
68. G.R. Borba-Murad, M. Vardanega-Peicher, S.B. Galende, R. Curi, H.M. Souza, E.G. Mario, B.K. Bassoli, and R.B. Bazotte, Central role of cAMP in the inhibition of glycogen breakdown and gluconeogenesis promoted by leptin and insulin in perfused rat liver. *Pol J Pharmacol,* **56**:223-231 (2004).
69. S.M. Cohen, J.G. Werrmann, and M.R. Tota, 13C NMR study of the effects of leptin treatment on kinetics of hepatic intermediary metabolism. *Proc Natl Acad Sci U S A,* **95**:7385-7390 (1998).
70. J.S. Flier, Leptin expression and action: new experimental paradigms. *Proc Natl Acad Sci ,USA,* **94**:4242-4245 (1999).

71. J.L. Halaas, K.S. Gajiwala, M. Maffei, S.L. Cohen, B.T. Chait, D. Rabinowitz, R.L. Lallone, S.K. Burley, and J.M. Friedman, Weight-reducing effects of the plasma protein encoded by the obese gene. *Science*, **269**:543-546 (1995).
72. J.J. Hwa, A.B. Fawzi, M.P. Graziano, L. Ghibaudi, P. Williams, M. Van Heek, H. Davis, M. Rudinski, E. Sybertz, and C.D. Strader, Leptin increases energy expenditure and selectively promotes fat metabolism in *ob/ob* mice. *Am J Physiol*, **272**:R1204-R1209 (1997).
73. C.J. Hukshorn and W.H. Saris, Leptin and energy expenditure. *Curr Opin Clin Nutr Metab Care*, **7**:629-633 (2004).
74. M. Rosenbaum, K. Vandenborne, R. Goldsmith, J.A. Simoneau, S. Heymsfield, D.R. Joanisse, J. Hirsch, E. Murphy, D. Matthews, H.R. Segal, and Leibel, Effects of experimental weight perturbation on skeletal muscle work efficiency in human subjects. *Am J Physiol Regul Integr Comp Physiol*, **285**:R183-R192 (2003).
75. R.M. Mackintosh and J. Hirsch, The effects of leptin administration in non-obese human subjects. *Obes Res*, **9**:462-469 (2001).
76. K.L. Ingvartsen and Y.R. Boisclair, Leptin and the regulation of food intake, energy homeostasis and immunity with special focus on periparturient ruminants. *Domest Anim Endocrinol*, **21**:215-250 (2001).
77. A.G. Dulloo, M.J. Stock, G. Solinas, O. Boss, J.P. Montani, and J. Seydoux, Leptin directly stimulates thermogenesis in skeletal muscle. *FEBS Lett*, **515**:109-113 (2002).
78. G. Solinas, S. Summermatter, D. Mainieri, M. Gubler, L. Pirola, M.P. Wymann, S. Rusconi, J.P. Montani, J. Seydoux, and A.G. Dulloo, The direct effect of leptin on skeletal muscle thermogenesis is mediated by substrate cycling between de novo lipogenesis and lipid oxidation. *FEBS Lett*, %19;**577**:539-544 (2004).
79. B.S. Yuen, P.C. Owens, B.S. Muhlhausler, C.T. Roberts, M.E. Symonds, D.H. Keisler, J.R. McFarlane, K.G. Kauter, Y. Evens, and I.C. McMillen, Leptin alters the structural and functional characteristics of adipose tissue before birth. *FASEB J*, **17**:1102-1104 (2003).
80. D. Ricquier and F. Bouillaud, Mitochondrial uncoupling proteins: from mitochondria to the regulation of energy balance. *J Physiol*, **529 Pt 1:3-10.**:3-10 (2000).
81. P. Jezek, Possible physiological roles of mitochondrial uncoupling proteins--UCPn. *Int J Biochem Cell Biol*, **34**:1190-1206 (2002).
82. C. Erlanson-Albertsson, The role of uncoupling proteins in the regulation of metabolism. *Acta Physiol Scand*, **178**:405-412 (2003).
83. L. Casteilla, C. Forest, J. Robelin, D. Ricquier, A. Lombet, and G. Ailhaud, Characterization of mitochondrial-uncoupling protein in bovine fetus and newborn calf. *Am J Physiol*, **252**:E627-E636 (1987).
84. G.S. Martin, G.E. Carstens, M.D. King, A.G. Eli, H.J. Mersmann, and S.B. Smith, Metabolism and morphology of brown adipose tissue from Brahman and Angus newborn calves. *J Anim Sci*, **77**:388-399 (1999).
85. M. Damon, A. Vincent, A. Lombardi, and P. Herpin, First evidence of uncoupling protein-2 (UCP-2) and -3 (UCP-3) gene expression in piglet skeletal muscle and adipose tissue. *Gene*, **246**:133-141 (2000).
86. A. Mostyn, J.C. Litten, K.S. Perkins, M.C. Alves-Guerra, C. Pecqueur, B. Miroux, M.E. Symonds, and L. Clarke, Influence of genotype on the differential ontogeny of uncoupling protein 2 and 3 in subcutaneous adipose tissue and muscle in neonatal pigs. *J Endocrinol*, **183**:121-131 (2004).
87. D.W. Gong, Y. He, M. Karas, and M. Reitman, Uncoupling protein-3 is a mediator of thermogenesis regulated by thyroid hormone, beta3-adrenergic agonists, and leptin. *J Biol Chem*, **272**:24129-24132 (1997).

88. M.A. Paulik, R.G. Buckholz, M.E. Lancaster, W.S. Dallas, E.A. Hull-Ryde, J.E. Weiel, and J.M. Lenhard, Development of infrared imaging to measure thermogenesis in cell culture: thermogenic effects of uncoupling protein-2, troglitazone, and beta-adrenoceptor agonists. *Pharm Res,* **15**:944-949 (1998).
89. M. Jaburek, M. Varecha, R.E. Gimeno, M. Dembski, P. Jezek, M. Zhang, P. Burn, L.A. Tartaglia, and K.D. Garlid, Transport function and regulation of mitochondrial uncoupling proteins 2 and 3. *J Biol Chem,* **274**:26003-26007 (1999).
90. L.X. Li, F. Skorpen, K. Egeberg, I.H. Jorgensen, and V. Grill, Uncoupling protein-2 participates in cellular defense against oxidative stress in clonal beta-cells. *Biochem Biophys Res Commun,* **282**:273-277 (2001).
91. K.S. Echtay, D. Roussel, J. St Pierre, M.B. Jekabsons, S. Cadenas, J.A. Stuart, J.A. Harper, S.J. Roebuck, A. Morrison, S. Pickering, J.C. Clapham, and M.D. Brand, Superoxide activates mitochondrial uncoupling proteins. *Nature,* **415**:96-99 (2002).
92. K.D. Garlid, M. Jaburek, P. Jezek, and M. Varecha, How do uncoupling proteins uncouple? *Biochim Biophys Acta,* **1459**:383-389 (2000).
93. A.G. Dulloo and S. Samec, Uncoupling proteins: their roles in adaptive thermogenesis and substrate metabolism reconsidered. *Br J Nutr,* **86**:123-139 (2001).
94. S.H. Lee, T.E. Engle, and K.L. Hossner, Effects of dietary copper on the expression of lipogenic genes and metabolic hormones in steers. *J Anim Sci,* **80**:1999-2005 (2002).
95. S.H. Lee and K.L. Hossner, Coordinate regulation of ovine adipose tissue gene expression by propionate. *J Anim Sci,* **80**:2840-2849 (2002).
96. R.T. Stone, C.E. Rexroad, III, and T.P. Smith, Bovine UCP2 and UCP3 map to BTA15. *Anim Genet,* **30**:378-381 (1999).
97. Sadiq, F., Karamanlidis, G., Hazlerigg, D. G., and Lomax, M. A. Ovis aries uncoupling protein 3 (UCP3) mRNA, partial cds. Genbank Accession # AY371069 (2005).
98. S. Raimbault, S. Dridi, F. Denjean, J. Lachuer, E. Couplan, F. Bouillaud, A. Bordas, C. Duchamp, M. Taouis, and D. Ricquier, An uncoupling protein homologue putatively involved in facultative muscle thermogenesis in birds. *Biochem J,* **353**:441-444 (2001).
99. C.M. Evock-Clover, S.M. Poch, M.P. Richards, C.M. Ashwell, and J.P. McMurtry, Expression of an uncoupling protein gene homolog in chickens. *Comp Biochem Physiol A Mol Integr Physiol,* **133**:345-358 (2002).
100. T.G. Ramsay and R.W. Rosebrough, Regulation of uncoupling proteins 2 and 3 in porcine adipose tissue. *Domest Anim Endocrinol,* **28**:351-366 (2005).
101. R.B. Ceddia, W.N. William, Jr., F.B. Lima, P. Flandin, R. Curi, and J.P. Giacobino, Leptin stimulates uncoupling protein-2 mRNA expression and Krebs cycle activity and inhibits lipid synthesis in isolated rat white adipocytes. *Eur J Biochem,* **267**:5952-5958 (2000).
102. U. Sarmiento, B. Benson, S. Kaufman, L. Ross, M. Qi, S. Scully, and C. DiPalma, Morphologic and molecular changes induced by recombinant human leptin in the white and brown adipose tissues of C57BL/6 mice. *Lab Invest,* **77**:243-256 (1997).
103. G. Chen, K. Koyama, X. Yuan, Y. Lee, Y.T. Zhou, R. O'Doherty, C.B. Newgard, and R.H. Unger, Disappearance of body fat in normal rats induced by adenovirus-mediated leptin gene therapy. *Proc Natl Acad Sci U S A,* **93**:14795-14799 (1996).
104. Y.T. Zhou, M. Shimabukuro, K. Koyama, Y. Lee, M.Y. Wang, F. Trieu, C.B. Newgard, and R.H. Unger, Induction by leptin of uncoupling protein-2 and enzymes of fatty acid oxidation. *Proc Natl Acad Sci U S A,* **94**:6386-6390 (1997).

105. Y.T. Zhou, Z.W. Wang, M. Higa, C.B. Newgard, and R.H. Unger, Reversing adipocyte differentiation: implications for treatment of obesity. *Proc Natl Acad Sci U S A,* **96**:2391-2395 (1999).
106. K.C. Lee, M.J. Azain, D.B. Hausman, and T.G. Ramsay, Somatotropin and adipose tissue metabolism: substrate and temporal effects. *J Anim Sci,* **78**:1236-1246 (2000).
107. H.A. Weiler, H. Kovacs, C. Murdock, J. Adolphe, and S. Fitzpatrick-Wong, Leptin predicts bone and fat mass after accounting for the effects of diet and glucocorticoid treatment in piglets. *Exp Biol Med (Maywood),* **227**:639-644 (2002).
108. R. Nakajima, H. Inada, T. Koike, and T. Yamano, Effects of leptin to cultured growth plate chondrocytes. *Horm Res,* **60**:91-98 (2003).
109. M. Morroni, R. De Matteis, C. Palumbo, M. Ferretti, I. Villa, A. Rubinacci, S. Cinti, and G. Marotti, In vivo leptin expression in cartilage and bone cells of growing rats and adult humans. *J Anat,* **205**:291-296 (2004).
110. G. Maor, M. Rochwerger, Y. Segev, and M. Phillip, Leptin acts as a growth factor on the chondrocytes of skeletal growth centers. *J Bone Miner Res,* **17**:1034-1043 (2002).
111. C.M. Steppan, D.T. Crawford, K.L. Chidsey-Frink, H. Ke, and A.G. Swick, Leptin is a potent stimulator of bone growth in *ob/ob* mice. *Regul Pept,* **92**:73-78 (2000).
112. P. Ducy, M. Amling, S. Takeda, M. Priemel, A.F. Schilling, F.T. Beil, J. Shen, C. Vinson, J.M. Rueger, and G. Karsenty, Leptin inhibits bone formation through a hypothalamic relay: a central control of bone mass. *Cell,* **100**:197-207 (2000).
113. K. Kume, K. Satomura, S. Nishisho, E. Kitaoka, K. Yamanouchi, S. Tobiume, and M. Nagayama, Potential role of leptin in endochondral ossification. *J Histochem Cytochem,* **50**:159-169 (2002).
114. G.A. Wallis, Bone growth: coordinating chondrocyte differentiation. *Curr Biol,* **6**:1577-1580 (1996).
115. J.E. Reseland, U. Syversen, I. Bakke, G. Qvigstad, L.G. Eide, O. Hjertner, J.O. Gordeladze, and C.A. Drevon, Leptin is expressed in and secreted from primary cultures of human osteoblasts and promotes bone mineralization. *J Bone Miner Res,* **16**:1426-1433 (2001).
116. J.O. Gordeladze, C.A. Drevon, U. Syversen, and J.E. Reseland, Leptin stimulates human osteoblastic cell proliferation, de novo collagen synthesis, and mineralization: Impact on differentiation markers, apoptosis, and osteoclastic signaling. *J Cell Biochem,* **85**:825-836 (2002).
117. A. Martin, R. de Vittoris, V. David, R. Moraes, M. Begeot, M.H. Lafage-Proust, C. Alexandre, L. Vico, and T. Thomas, Leptin modulates both resorption and formation while preventing disuse-induced bone loss in tail-suspended female rats. *Endocrinology,* **146**:3652-3659 (2005).
118. B. Burguera, L.C. Hofbauer, T. Thomas, F. Gori, G.L. Evans, S. Khosla, B.L. Riggs, and R.T. Turner, Leptin reduces ovariectomy-induced bone loss in rats. *Endocrinology,* **142**:3546-3553 (2001).
119. A.P. Goldstone, J.K. Howard, G.M. Lord, M.A. Ghatei, J.V. Gardiner, Z.L. Wang, R.M. Wang, S.I. Girgis, C.A. Baile, and S.R. Bloom, Leptin prevents the fall in plasma osteocalcin during starvation in male mice. *Biochem Biophys Res Commun,* **295**:475-481 (2002).
120. T. Gainsford and W.S. Alexander, A role for leptin in hemopoieses? *Mol Biotechnol,* **11**:149-158 (1999).
121. G. Fantuzzi and R. Faggioni, Leptin in the regulation of immunity, inflammation, and hematopoiesis. *J Leukoc Biol,* **68**:437-446 (2000).
122. G. Matarese, S. Moschos, and C.S. Mantzoros, Leptin in immunology. *J Immunol,* **174**:3137-3142 (2005).

123. F. Zhang, M.B. Basinski, J.M. Beals, S.L. Briggs, L.M. Churgay, D.K. Clawson, R.D. DiMarchi, T.C. Furman, J.E. Hale, H.M. Hsiung, B.E. Schoner, D.P. Smith, X.Y. Zhang, J.P. Wery, and R.W. Schevitz, Crystal structure of the obese protein leptin-E100. *Nature (London),* **387**:206-209 (1997).
124. H. Baumann, K.K. Morella, D.W. White, M. Dembski, P.S. Bailon, H. Kim, C.F. Lai, and L.A. Tartaglia, The full-length leptin receptor has signaling capabilities of interleukin 6-type cytokine receptors. *Proc Natl Acad Sci U S A,* **93**:8374-8378 (1996).
125. M.E. Spurlock, M.A. Ranalletta, S.G. Cornelius, G.R. Frank, G.M. Willis, S. Ji, A.L. Grant, and C.A. Bidwell, Leptin expression in porcine adipose tissue is not increased by endotoxin but is reduced by growth hormone. *J Interfer Cytok Res,* **18**:1051-1058 (1998).
126. M.T. Leininger, C.P. Portocarrero, C.A. Bidwell, M.E. Spurlock, and K.L. Houseknecht, Leptin expression is reduced with acute endotoxemia in the pig: correlation with glucose, insulin, and insulin-like growth factor-1 (IGF-1). *J Interfer Cytok Res,* **20**:99-106 (2000).
127. M.T. Leininger, C.P. Portocarrero, A.P. Schinckel, M.E. Spurlock, C.A. Bidwell, J.N. Nielsen, and K.L. Houseknecht, Physiological response to acute endotoxemia in swine: effect of genotype on energy metabolites and leptin. *Domest Anim Endocrinol,* **18**:71-82 (2000).
128. Kendall, D. C., Rihert, B. T., and Schinckel, A. P. Evaluation of Genotype, therapeutic antibiotic and health management effects and interactions on lean growth rate. Research Investment Report, National Pork Producers Council (2000).
129. M. Soliman, K. Ishioka, K. Kimura, S. Kushibiki, and M. Saito, Plasma leptin responses to lipopolysaccharide and tumor necrosis factor alpha in cows. *Jpn J Vet Res,* **50**:107-114 (2002).
130. M.R. Waldron, T. Nishida, B.J. Nonnecke, and T.R. Overton, Effect of lipopolysaccharide on indices of peripheral and hepatic metabolism in lactating cows. *J Dairy Sci,* **86**:3447-3459 (2003).
131. M. Soliman, S. Abdelhady, I. Fattouh, K. Ishioka, H. Kitamura, K. Kimura, and M. Saito, No alteration in serum leptin levels during acute endotoxemia in sheep. *J Vet Med Sci,* **63**:1143-1145 (2001).
132. J.A. Daniel, T.H. Elsasser, C.D. Morrison, D.H. Keisler, B.K. Whitlock, B. Steele, D. Pugh, and J.L. Sartin, Leptin, tumor necrosis factor-alpha (TNF), and CD14 in ovine adipose tissue and changes in circulating TNF in lean and fat sheep. *J Anim Sci,* **81**:2590-2599 (2003).
133. T.E. Weber and M.E. Spurlock, Leptin alters antibody isotype in the pig in vivo, but does not regulate cytokine expression or stimulate STAT3 signaling in peripheral blood monocytes in vitro. *J Anim Sci,* **82**:1630-1640 (2004).
134. G.M. Lord, G. Matarese, J.K. Howard, R.J. Baker, S.R. Bloom, and R.I. Lechler, Leptin modulates the T-cell immune response and reverses starvation-induced immunosuppression. *Nature,* **394**:897-901 (1998).
135. H. Zarkesh-Esfahani, G. Pockley, R.A. Metcalfe, M. Bidlingmaier, Z. Wu, A. Ajami, A.P. Weetman, C.J. Strasburger, and R.J. Ross, High-dose leptin activates human leukocytes via receptor expression on monocytes. *J Immunol,* **167**:4593-4599 (2001).
136. G.M. Lord, G. Matarese, J.K. Howard, S.R. Bloom, and R.I. Lechler, Leptin inhibits the anti-CD3-driven proliferation of peripheral blood T cells but enhances the production of proinflammatory cytokines. *J Leukoc Biol,* **72**:330-338 (2002).
137. V. Sanchez-Margalet and C. Martin-Romero, Human leptin signaling in human peripheral blood mononuclear cells: activation of the JAK-STAT pathway. *Cell Immunol,* **211**:30-36 (2001).

138. M. Maccarrone, M. Di Rienzo, A. Finazzi-Agro, and A. Rossi, Leptin activates the anandamide hydrolase promoter in human T lymphocytes through STAT3. *J Biol Chem*, **278**:13318-13324 (2003).
139. M. Lohmus, M. Olin, L.F. Sundstrom, M.H. Troedsson, T.W. Molitor, and M. El Halawani, Leptin increases T-cell immune response in birds. *Gen Comp Endocrinol*, **139**:245-250 (2004).
140. M. Marikovsky, C.I. Rosenblum, Z. Faltin, and M. Friedman-Einat, Appearance of leptin in wound fluid as a response to injury. *Wound Repair Regen*, **10**:302-307 (2002).
141. W.H. Goodson, III and T.K. Hunt, Wound collagen accumulation in obese hyperglycemic mice. *Diabetes*, **35**:491-495 (1986).
142. R. Tsuboi, C.M. Shi, D.B. Rifkin, and H. Ogawa, A wound healing model using healing-impaired diabetic mice. *J Dermatol*, **19**:673-675 (1992).
143. S. Frank, B. Stallmeyer, H. Kampfer, N. Kolb, and J. Pfeilschifter, Leptin enhances wound re-epithelialization and constitutes a direct function of leptin in skin repair. *J Clin Invest*, **106**:501-509 (2000).
144. B.D. Ring, S. Scully, C.R. Davis, M.B. Baker, M.J. Cullen, M.A. Pelleymounter, and D.M. Danilenko, Systemically and topically administered leptin both accelerate wound healing in diabetic *ob/ob* mice. *Endocrinology*, **141**:446-449 (2000).
145. B. Stallmeyer, H. Kampfer, M. Podda, R. Kaufmann, J. Pfeilschifter, and S. Frank, A novel keratinocyte mitogen: regulation of leptin and its functional receptor in skin repair. *J Invest Dermatol*, **117**:98-105 (2001).
146. I. Goren, H. Kampfer, M. Podda, J. Pfeilschifter, and S. Frank, Leptin and wound inflammation in diabetic *ob/ob* mice: differential regulation of neutrophil and macrophage influx and a potential role for the scab as a sink for inflammatory cells and mediators. *Diabetes*, **52**:2821-2832 (2003).
147. A. Murad, A.K. Nath, S.T. Cha, E. Demir, J. Flores-Riveros, and M.R. Sierra-Honigmann, Leptin is an autocrine/paracrine regulator of wound healing. *FASEB J*, **17**:1895-1897 (2003).
148. G.J. Hausman and R.L. Richardson, Adipose tissue angiogenesis. *J Anim Sci*, **82**:925-934 (2004).
149. A. Bouloumie, H.C. Drexler, M. Lafontan, and R. Busse, Leptin, the product of Ob gene, promotes angiogenesis. *Circ Res*, **83**:1059-1066 (1998).
150. M.R. Sierra-Honigmann, A.K. Nath, C. Murakami, G. Garcia-Cardena, A. Papapetropoulos, W.C. Sessa, L.A. Madge, J.S. Schechner, M.B. Schwabb, P.J. Polverini, and J.R. Flores-Riveros, Biological action of leptin as an angiogenic factor. *Science*, **281**:1683-1686 (1998).
151. H.Y. Park, H.M. Kwon, H.J. Lim, B.K. Hong, J.Y. Lee, B.E. Park, Y. Jang, S.Y. Cho, and H.S. Kim, Potential role of leptin in angiogenesis: leptin induces endothelial cell proliferation and expression of matrix metalloproteinases in vivo and in vitro. *Exp Mol Med*, **33**:95-102 (2001).
152. R. Cao, E. Brakenhielm, C. Wahlestedt, J. Thyberg, and Y. Cao, Leptin induces vascular permeability and synergistically stimulates angiogenesis with FGF-2 and VEGF. *Proc Natl Acad Sci U S A*, **98**:6390-6395 (2001).
153. M. Artwohl, M. Roden, T. Holzenbein, A. Freudenthaler, W. Waldhausl, and S.M. Baumgartner-Parzer, Modulation by leptin of proliferation and apoptosis in vascular endothelial cells. *Int J Obes Relat Metab Disord*, **26**:577-580 (2002).
154. S. Goetze, A. Bungenstock, C. Czupalla, F. Eilers, P. Stawowy, U. Kintscher, C. Spencer-Hansch, K. Graf, B. Nurnberg, R.E. Law, E. Fleck, and M. Grafe, Leptin induces endothelial cell migration through Akt, which is inhibited by PPARgamma-ligands. *Hypertension*, **40**:748-754 (2002).
155. A. Oda, T. Taniguchi, and M. Yokoyama, Leptin stimulates rat aortic smooth muscle cell proliferation and migration. *Kobe J Med Sci*, **47**:141-150 (2001).

156. N.M. Morton, V. Emilsson, Y.L. Liu, and M.A. Cawthorne, Leptin action in intestinal cells. *J Biol Chem*, **273**:26194-26201 (1998).
157. J. Wolinski, M. Biernat, P. Guilloteau, B.R. Westrom, and R. Zabielski, Exogenous leptin controls the development of the small intestine in neonatal piglets. *J Endocrinol*, **177**:215-222 (2003).
158. J. Wolinski, V. Seniewska, M. Biernat, M. Babelewska, W. Korczynski, and R. Zabielski, Exogenous leptin influences gastrointestinal growth and in vitro small intestinal motility in neonatal piglets-preliminary results. *J Anim Feed Sci*, **10**(Suppl 2):249-254 (2001).
159. K. Alavi, M.Z. Schwartz, R. Prasad, D. O'connor, and V. Funanage, Leptin: a new growth factor for the small intestine. *J Pediatr Surg*, **37**:327-330 (2002).
160. M.P. Lostao, E. Urdaneta, E. Martinez-Anso, A. Barber, and J.A. Martinez, Presence of leptin receptors in rat small intestine and leptin effect on sugar absorption. *FEBS Lett*, **423**:302-306 (1998).
161. M. Buyse, F. Berlioz, S. Guilmeau, A. Tsocas, T. Voisin, G. Peranzi, D. Merlin, M. Laburthe, M.J. Lewin, C. Roze, and A. Bado, PepT1-mediated epithelial transport of dipeptides and cephalexin is enhanced by luminal leptin in the small intestine. *J Clin Invest*, **108**:1483-1494 (2001).
162. Y.J. Fei, Y. Kanai, S. Nussberger, V. Ganapathy, F.H. Leibach, M.F. Romero, S.K. Singh, W.F. Boron, and M.A. Hediger, Expression cloning of a mammalian proton-coupled oligopeptide transporter. *Nature*, **368**:563-566 (1994).
163. S. Guilmeau, M. Buyse, and A. Bado, Gastric leptin: a new manager of gastrointestinal function. *Curr Opin Pharmacol*, **4**:561-566 (2004).
164. A. Bado, S. Levasseur, S. Attoub, S. Kermorgant, J.P. Laigneau, M.N. Bortoluzzi, L. Moizo, T. Lehy, M. Guerre-Millo, Y. Marchand-Brustel, and M.J. Lewin, The stomach is a source of leptin. *Nature*, **394**:790-793 (1998).
165. S. Cinti, R.D. Matteis, C. Pico, E. Ceresi, A. Obrador, C. Maffeis, J. Oliver, and A. Palou, Secretory granules of endocrine and chief cells of human stomach mucosa contain leptin. *Int J Obes Relat Metab Disord*, **24**:789-793 (2000).
166. S. Attoub, S. Levasseur, M. Buyse, H. Goiot, J.P. Laigneau, L. Moizo, F. Hervatin, Y. Marchand-Brustel, J.M. Lewin, and A. Bado, Physiological role of cholecystokinin B/gastrin receptor in leptin secretion. *Endocrinology*, **140**:4406-4410 (1999).
167. I. Sobhani, M. Buyse, H. Goiot, N. Weber, J.P. Laigneau, D. Henin, J.C. Soul, and A. Bado, Vagal stimulation rapidly increases leptin secretion in human stomach. *Gastroenterology*, **122**:259-263 (2002).
168. I. Sobhani, A. Bado, C. Vissuzaine, M. Buyse, S. Kermorgant, J.P. Laigneau, S. Attoub, T. Lehy, D. Henin, M. Mignon, and M.J. Lewin, Leptin secretion and leptin receptor in the human stomach. *Gut*, **47**:178-183 (2000).
169. S. Guilmeau, M. Buyse, A. Tsocas, J.P. Laigneau, and A. Bado, Duodenal leptin stimulates cholecystokinin secretion: evidence of a positive leptin-cholecystokinin feedback loop. *Diabetes*, **52**:1664-1672 (2003).
170. M.D. Barrachina, V. Martinez, L. Wang, J.Y. Wei, and Y. Tache, Synergistic interaction between leptin and cholecystokinin to reduce short-term food intake in lean mice. *Proc Natl Acad Sci U S A*, **94**:10455-10460 (1997).
171. Y.H. Wang, Y. Tache, A.B. Sheibel, V.L. Go, and J.Y. Wei, Two types of leptin-responsive gastric vagal afferent terminals: an in vitro single-unit study in rats. *Am J Physiol*, **273**:R833-R837 (1997).
172. J.P. McMurtry, C.M. Ashwell, D.M. Brocht, and T.J. Caperna, Plasma clearance and tissue distribution of radiolabeled leptin in the chicken. *Comp Biochem Physiol A Mol Integr Physiol*, **138**:27-32 (2004).
173. C.R. Barb, J.B. Barrett, R.R. Kraeling, and G.B. Rampacek, Serum leptin concentrations, luteinizing hormone and growth hormone secretion during feed and

metabolic fuel restriction in the prepuberal gilt. *Dom Anim Endocrinol,* **20**:47-63 (2001).

174. C.S. Whisnant and R.J. Harrell, Effect of short-term feed restriction and refeeding on serum concentrations of leptin, luteinizing hormone and insulin in ovariectomized gilts. *Domest Anim Endocrinol,* **22**:73-80 (2002).

175. D. Blache, R.L. Tellam, L.M. Chagas, M.A. Blackberry, P.E. Vercoe, and G.B. Martin, Level of nutrition affects leptin concentrations in plasma and cerebrospinal fluid in sheep. *J Endocrinol,* **165**:625-637 (2000).

176. T. Tokuda, T. Matsui, and H. Yano, Effects of light, and food on plasma leptin concentrations in ewes. *J Anim Sci,* **71**:235-242 (2000).

177. S.S. Block, W.R. Butler, R.A. Ehrhardt, A.W. Bell, M.E. Van Amburgh, and Y.R. Boisclair, Decreased concentration of plasma leptin in periparturient dairy cows is caused by negative energy balance. *J Endocrinol,* **171**:339-348 (2001).

178. X.L. Chen, D.B. Hausman, R.G. Dean, and G.J. Hausman, Hormonal regulation of leptin mRNA expression and preadipocyte recruitment and differentiation in porcine primary cultures of S-V cells. *Obes Res,* **6**:164-172 (1998).

179. T.G. Ramsay and M.E. White, Insulin regulation of leptin expression in streptozotocin diabetic pigs. *J Anim Sci,* **78**:1497-1503 (2000).

180. T.G. Ramsay and M.P. Richards, Hormonal regulation of leptin and leptin receptor expression in porcine subcutaneous adipose tissue. *J Anim Sci,* **82**:3486-3492 (2004).

181. Y. Faulconnier, C. Delavaud, and Y. Chilliard, Insulin and (or) dexamethasone effects on leptin production and metabolic activities of ovine adipose tissue explants. *Reprod Nutr Dev,* **43**:237-250 (2003).

182. K.L. Houseknecht, C.P. Portocarrero, R.P. Lemenager, and M.E. Spurlock, Growth hormone regulates leptin gene expression in bovine adipose tissue: correlation with adipose IGF-I expression. *J Endocrinol,* **164**:51-57 (2000).

183. C.S. Hwang, S. Mandrup, O.A. MacDougald, D.E. Geiman, and M.D. Lane, Transcriptional activation of the mouse obese (ob) gene by CCAAT/enhancer binding protein alpha. *Proc Natl Acad Sci USA,* **93**:873-877 (1996).

184. S.G. Miller, P. De Vos, M. Guerre-Millo, K. Wong, T. Hermann, B. Staels, M.R. Briggs, and J. Auwerx, The adipocyte specific transcription factor C/EBPalpha modulates human ob gene expression. *Proc Natl Acad Sci USA,* **93**:5507-5511 (1996).

185. X.L. Chen, R.G. Dean, and G.J. Hausman, Expression of leptin mRNA and CCAAT-enhancer binding proteins in response to insulin deprivation during preadipocyte differentiation in primary cultures of porcine stromal-vascular cells. *Domest Anim Endocrinol,* **17**:389-401 (1999).

186. X. Chen, J. Lin, D.B. Hausman, R.J. Martin, R.G. Dean, and G.J. Hausman, Alterations in fetal adipose tissue leptin expression correlate with the development of adipose tissue. *Biol Neonate,* **78**:41-47 (2000).

187. S.U. Devaskar, R. Anthony, and W. Hay, Jr., Ontogeny and insulin regulation of fetal ovine white adipose tissue leptin expression. *Am J Physiol Regul Integr Comp Physiol,* **282**:R431-R438 (2002).

188. R.A. Ehrhardt, A.W. Bell, and Y.R. Boisclair, Spatial and developmental regulation of leptin in fetal sheep. *Am J Physiol Regul Integr Comp Physiol,* **282**:R1628-R1635 (2002).

189. A.J. Forhead, L. Thomas, J. Crabtree, N. Hoggard, D.S. Gardner, D.A. Giussani, and A.L. Fowden, Plasma leptin concentration in fetal sheep during late gestation: ontogeny and effect of glucocorticoids. *Endocrinology,* **143**:1166-1173 (2002).

190. A. Mostyn, S. Pearce, H. Budge, M. Elmes, A.J. Forhead, A.L. Fowden, T. Stephenson, and M.E. Symonds, Influence of cortisol on adipose tissue

development in the fetal sheep during late gestation. *J Endocrinol,* **176**:23-30 (2003).
191. G.J. Hausman, The interaction of hydrocortisone and thyroxine during fetal adipose tissue differentiation: CCAAT enhancing binding protein expression and capillary cytodifferentiation. *J Anim Sci,* **77**:2088-2097 (1999).
192. X. Chen, D.B. Hausman, R.G. Dean, and G.J. Hausman, Differentiation-dependent expression of obese (ob) gene by preadipocytes and adipocytes in primary cultures of porcine stromal-vascular cells. *Biochim Biophys Acta,* **1359**:136-142 (1997).
193. B.S. Yuen, P.C. Owens, B.S. Muhlhausler, C.T. Roberts, M.E. Symonds, D.H. Keisler, J.R. McFarlane, K.G. Kauter, Y. Evens, and I.C. McMillen, Leptin alters the structural and functional characteristics of adipose tissue before birth. *FASEB J,* **17**:1102-1104 (2003).
194. I.C. McMillen, B.S. Muhlhausler, J.A. Duffield, and B.S. Yuen, Prenatal programming of postnatal obesity: fetal nutrition and the regulation of leptin synthesis and secretion before birth. *Proc Nutr Soc,* **63**:405-412 (2004).
195. G.J. Hausman, The influence of thyroxine on the differentiation of adipose tissue and skin during fetal development. *Pediatr Res,* **32**:204-211 (1992).

196. J.T. Wright and G.J. Hausman, Flow cytometric analysis of porcine preadipocyte replication. *J Anim Sci,* **72**:1712-1718 (1994).
197. B.S. Muhlhausler, C.T. Roberts, J.R. McFarlane, K.G. Kauter, and I.C. McMillen, Fetal leptin is a signal of fat mass independent of maternal nutrition in ewes fed at or above maintenance energy requirements. *Biol Reprod,* **67**:493-499 (2002).
198. B.S. Yuen, P.C. Owens, J.R. McFarlane, M.E. Symonds, L.J. Edwards, K.G. Kauter, and I.C. McMillen, Circulating leptin concentrations are positively related to leptin messenger RNA expression in the adipose tissue of fetal sheep in the pregnant ewe fed at or below maintenance energy requirements during late gestation. *Biol Reprod,* **67**:911-916 (2002).
199. J. Bispham, G.S. Gopalakrishnan, J. Dandrea, V. Wilson, H. Budge, D.H. Keisler, P.F. Broughton, T. Stephenson, and M.E. Symonds, Maternal endocrine adaptation throughout pregnancy to nutritional manipulation: consequences for maternal plasma leptin and cortisol and the programming of fetal adipose tissue development. *Endocrinology,* **144**:3575-3585 (2003).
200. A. Buchbinder, U. Lang, R.S. Baker, J.C. Khoury, J. Mershon, and K.E. Clark, Leptin in the ovine fetus correlates with fetal and placental size. *Am J Obstet Gynecol,* **185**:786-791 (2001).
201. B.S. Yuen, I.C. McMillen, M.E. Symonds, and P.C. Owens, Abundance of leptin mRNA in fetal adipose tissue is related to fetal body weight. *J Endocrinol,* **163**:R11-R14 (1999).
202. J.E. Eckert, K.L. Gatford, B.G. Luxford, R.G. Campbell, and P.C. Owens, Leptin expression in offspring is programmed by nutrition in pregnancy. *J Endocrinol,* **165**:R1-R6 (2000).
203. K.R. Poore and A.L. Fowden, The effects of birth weight and postnatal growth patterns on fat depth and plasma leptin concentrations in juvenile and adult pigs. *J Physiol,* **558**:295-304 (2004).
204. H. Qian, C.R. Barb, M.M. Compton, G.J. Hausman, M.J. Azain, R.R. Kraeling, and C.A. Baile, Leptin mRNA expression and serum leptin concentrations as influenced by age, weight and estradiol in pigs. *Domest Anim Endocrinol,* **16**:135-143 (1999).
205. L.J. Spicer and C.C. Francisco, The adipose obese gene product, leptin: evidence of a direct inhibitory role in ovarian function. *Endocrinology,* **138**:3374-3379 (1997).
206. M. Macajova, D. Lamosova, and M. Zeman, Role of leptin in farm animals: a review. *J Vet Med,* **A 51**:157-166 (2004).

207. D.A. Zieba, M. Amstalden, and G.L. Williams, Regulatory roles of leptin in reproduction and metabolism: a comparative review. *Domest Anim Endocrinol*, **29**:166-185 (2005).
208. C.R. Barb, R.R. Kraeling, G.B. Rampacek, and C.R. Dove, Metabolic changes during the transition from the fed to the acute feed-deprived state in prepuberal and mature gilts. *J Anim Sci*, **75**:781-789 (1997).
209. K.L. Houseknecht, D.L. Boggs, D.R. Campion, J.L. Sartin, T.E. Kiser, G.B. Rampacek, and H.E. Amos, Effect of dietary energy source and level on serum gorwth hormone, insulin-like growth factor-I, growth and body composition in beef heifers. *J Anim Sci*, **66**:2916-2923 (1988).
210. M.J. Estienne, K.K. Schillo, S.M. Hileman, M.A. Green, S.H. Hayes, and J.A. Boling, Effects of free fatty acids on luteinizing hormone and growth hormone secretion in ovariectomized lambs. *Endocrinology*, **126**:1934-1940 (1990).
211. L.A. Tartaglia, M. Dembski, X. Weng, N. Deng, J. Culpepper, R. Deros, G.J. Richards, L.A. Camfield, F.T. Clark, J. Deeds, C. Muri, S. Sanker, A. Moriarty, K.J. Moore, J.S. Smutko, G.G. Mays, E.A. Woolf, C.A. Monore, and R.I. Tepper, Identification and expression cloning of leptin receptor, OB-R. *Cell*, **83**:1263-1271 (1995).
212. L.A. Tartaglia, The leptin receptor. *J Biol Chem*, **272**:6093-6096 (1997).
213. J. Lin, C.R. Barb, R.R. Kraeling, and G.B. Rampacek, Developmental changes in the long form leptin receptor and related neuropeptide gene expression in the pig brain. *Biol Reprod*, **64**:1614-1618 (2001).
214. P.L. Zamorano, V.B. Mahesh, L.M. De Sevilla, L.P. Chorich, G.K. Bhat, and D.W. Brann, Expression and localization of the leptin receptor in endocrine and neuroendocrine tissues of the rat. *Neuroendocrinology*, **65**:223-228 (1997).
215. M.J. Cunningham, D.K. Clifton, and R.A. Steiner, Leptin's action on the reproductive axis: perspectives and mechanisms. *Biol Reprod*, **60**:216-222 (1999).
216. G.L. Williams, M. Amstalden, M.R. Garcia, R.L. Stanko, S.E. Nizielski, C.D. Morrison, and D.H. Keisler, Leptin and its role in the central regulation of reproduction in cattle. *Domest Anim Endocrinol*, **23**:339-349 (2002).
217. J. Iqbal, S. Pompolo, T. Murakami, E. Grouzmann, T. Sakurai, B. Meister, and I.J. Clarke, Immunohistochemical characterization of localization of long-form leptin receptor (OB-Rb) in neurochemically defined cells in the ovine hypothalamus. *Brain Res*, **920**:55-64 (2001).
218. C.R. Barb, J.B. Barrett, and R.R. Kraeling, Role of leptin in modulating the hypothalamic-pituitary axis in the pig. *Domest Anim Endocrinol*, **26**:201-214 (2004).
219. S.D. Sullivan and S.M. Moenter, ã-Aminobutyric acid neurons intergrate and repidly transmit permissive and inhibitory metabolic cues to gonadotropin-releasing hormone neurons. *Endocrinology*, **145**:1194-1202 (2004).
220. S.P. Kalra, Mandatory neuropeptide-steroid signaling for the preovulatory luteinizing hormone-releasing hormone discharge. *Endocr Rev*, **14**:507-538 (1993).
221. A.H. Kaynard, K.-Y.F. Pau, D.L. Hess, and H.G. Spies, Third-ventricular infusion of neuropeptide Y suppresses luteinizing hormone secretion in ovariectomized rhesus macaques. *Endocrinology*, **127**:2437-2444 (1990).
222. C.D. Morrison, J.A. Daniel, J.H. Hampton, P.R. Buff, T.M. McShane, M.G. Thomas, and D.H. Keisler, Luteinizing hormone and growth hormone secretion in ewes infused intracerebroventricularly with neuropeptide Y. *Domest Anim Endocrinol*, **24**:69-80 (2003).
223. M.G. Thomas, O.S. Gazal, G.L. Williams, R.L. Stanko, and D.H. Keisler, Injection of neuropeptide Y into the third cerebroventricle differentially influences pituitary secretion of luteinizing hormone and growth hormone in ovariectomized cows. *Domest Anim Endocrinol*, **16**:159-169 (1999).

224. C.R. Barb and J.B. Barrett, Neuropeptide Y modulstes growth hormone secretion but not luteinizing hormone secretion from porcine pituitary cells in culture derived from the prepuberal gilt. *Domest Anim Endocrinol,* **29**:548-555 (2005).
225. J.L. Miner, Recent advances in the central control of intake in ruminants. *J Anim Sci,* **70**:1283-1289 (1992).
226. J.C. Erickson, G. Hollopeter, and R.D. Palmiter, Attenuation of the obesity syndrome of *ob/ob* mice by the loss of neuropeptide Y. *Science,* **274**:1704-1707 (1996).
227. M. Jang, A. Mistry, A.G. Swick, and D.R. Romsos, Leptin rapidly inhibits hypothalamic neuropeptide Y secretion and stimulates corticotropin-releasing hormone secretion in adrenalectomized mice. *J Nutr,* **130**:2813-2820 (2000).
228. P.J. King, P.S. Widdowson, H. Doods, and G. Williams, Regulation of neuropeptide Y release from hypothalamic slices by melanocortin-4 agonists and leptin. *Peptides,* **21**:45-48 (2000).
229. A. Sahu, Evidence suggesting that galanin (GAL), melanin-concentrating hormone (MCH), neurotensin (NT), proopiomelanocortin (POMC) and neuropetide Y (NPY) are targets fo leptin signaling in the hypothalamus. *Endocrinology,* **139**:795-798 (1998).
230. R.L. Matteri, Overview of central targets for appetite regulation. *J Anim Sci,* **79**:E148-E158 (2001).
231. P.V. Malven, Inhibition of pituitary LH release resulting from endogenous opioid peptides. *Domest Anim Endocrinol,* **3 (3)**:135-144 (1986).
232. C.R. Barb, R.R. Kraeling, and G.B. Rampacek, Opioid modulation of gonadotropin and prolactin secretion in domestic farm animals. *Domes Anim Endocrinol,* **8**:15-27 (1991).
233. K.S. Kim, N. Larsen, T. Short, G. Plastow, and M.F. Rothschild, A missence variant of the porcine melanocortin-4 receptor (MC4R) gene is associated with fatness, growth, and feed intake traits. *Mamm Genome,* **11**:131-135 (2000).
234. C.R. Barb, A.S. Robertson, J.B. Barrett, R.R. Kraeling, and K.L. Houseknecht, The role of melanocortin-3 and -4 receptor in regulating appetite, energy homeostasis and neuroendocrine function in the pig. *J Endocrinol,* **181**:39-52 (2004).
235. M. Amstalden, M.R. Garcia, S.W. Williams, R.L. Stanko, S.E. Nizielski, C.D. Morrison, D.H. Keisler, and G.L. Williams, Leptin gene expression, circulating leptin, and luteinizing hormone pulsatility are acutely responsive to short-term fasting in prepubertal heifers: relationships to circulating insulin and insulin-like growth factor I. *Biol Reprod,* **63**:127-133 (2000).
236. Y. Chilliard, M. Bonnet, C. Delavaud, Y. Faulconnier, C. Leroux, J. Djiane, and F. Bocquier, Leptin in ruminants. Gene expression in adipose tissue and mammary gland, and regulation of plasma concentration. *Domest Anim Endocrinol,* **21**:271-295 (2001).
237. Y. Chilliard, C. Delavaud, and M. Bonnet, Leptin expression in ruminants: nutritional and physiological regulations in relation with energy metabolism. *Domest Anim Endocrinol,* **29**:3-22 (2(•)5).
238. P. De Vos, R. Saladin, J. Auwerx, and B. Staels, Induction of ob gene expression by corticosteroids is accompanied by body weight loss and reduced food intake. *J Biol Chem,* **270**:15958-15961 (1995).
239. R. Saladin, P. De Vos, M. Guerre Millo, A. Leturque, J. Girard, B. Staels, and J. Auwerx, Transient increase in obese gene expression after food intake or insulin administration. *Nature,* **377**:527-529 (1995).
240. B.A. Henry, J.W. Goding, A.J. Tilbrook, F.R. Dunshea, and I.J. Clarke, Intracerebroventricular infusion of leptin elevates the secretion of luteinising hormone without affecting food intake in long-term food-restricted sheep, but

increases growth hormone irrespective of bodyweight. *J Endocrinol,* **168**:67-77 (2001).
241. C.D. Morrison, J.A. Daniel, B.J. Holmberg, J. Djiane, N. Raver, A. Gertler, and D.H. Keisler, Central infusion of leptin into well-fed and undernourished ewe lambs: effects on feed intake and serum concentrations of growth hormone and luteinizing hormone. *J Endocrinol,* **168**:317-324 (2001).
242. H.A. Hart, M.J. Azain, G.J. Hausman, Reeves.D.E., and C.R. Barb, Failure of short term feed restriction to effect leptin secretion and subcutaneous adipose tissue expression of leptin or long form leptin receptor (Ob-rb) in the prepuberal gilt. *J Anim Sci,* **83**:40 (2005).
243. H. Shimizu, Y. Shimomura, Y. Nakanishi, aT. Futawatari, K. Ohtani, N. Sato, and M. Mori, Estrogen increases in vivo leptin production in rats and human subjects. *J Endocrinol,* **154**:285-292 (1997).
244. W.F. Blum, Leptin: The voice of the adipose tissue. *Horm Res,* **48**:2-8 (1997).
245. M. Ludwig, H.H. Klein, K. Diedrich, and O. Ortmann, Serum leptin concentrations throughout the menstrual cycle. *Arch Gynecol Obstet,* **263**:99-101 (2000).
246. M.R. Garcia, M. Amstalden, S.W. Williams, R.L. Stanko, C.D. Morrison, D.H. Keisler, S.E. Nizielski, and G.L. Williams, Serum leptin and its adipose gene expression during pubertal development, the estrous cycle, and different seasons in cattle. *J Anim Sci,* **80**:2158-2167 (2002).
247. C.R. Barb, R.R. Kraeling, G.B. Rampacek, and M.J. Estienne, Current concepts of the onset of puberty in the gilt. *Reprod Domest Anim Suppl,* **6**:82-89 (2000).
248. S.E. Recabarren, A. Lobos, C. Vilches, P. Munoz, and T. Sir-Petermann, Pulsatile leptin secretion is independent of luteinizing hormone secretion in prepubertal sheep. *Endocrine,* **17**:175-184 (2002).
249. D.W. Miller, P.A. Findlay, M.A. Morrison, N. Raver, and C.L. Adam, Seasonal and dose-dependent effects of intracerebroventricular leptin on LH secretion and appetite in sheep. *J Endocrinol,* **175**:395-404 (2002).
250. M. Amstalden, M.R. Garcia, R.L. Stanko, S.E. Nizielski, C.D. Morrison, D.H. Keisler, and G.L. Williams, Central infusion of recombinant ovine leptin normalizes plasma insulin and stimulates a novel hypersecretion of luteinizing hormone after short-term fasting in mature beef cows. *Biol Reprod,* **66**:1555-1561 (2002).
251. B.A. Henry, J.W. Goding, A.J. Tilbrook, F.R. Dunshea, and I.J. Clarke, Intracerebroventricular infusion of leptin elevates the secretion of luteinising hormone without affecting food intake in long-term food-restricted sheep, but increases growth hormone irrespective of bodyweight. *J Endocrinol,* **168**:67-77 (2001).
252. B.A. Henry, J.W. Goding, W.S. Alexander, A.J. Tilbrook, B.J. Canny, F. Dunshea, A. Rao, A. Mansell, and I.J. Clarke, Central administration of leptin to ovariectomized ewes inhibits food intake without affecting the secretion of hormones from the pituitary gland: evidence for a dissociation of effects on appetite and neuroendocrine function. *Endocrinology,* **140**:1175-1182 (1999).
253. M. Amstalden, D.A. Zieba, J.F. Edwards, P.G. Harms, T.H. Welsh Jr, R.L. Stanko, and G.L. Williams, Leptin Acts at the Bovine Adenohypophysis to Enhance Basal and Gonadotropin Releasing Hormone-Mediated Release of Luteinizing Hormone: Differential Effects Are Dependent upon Nutritional History. *Biol Reprod,* **69**:1539-1544 (2003).
254. J.E. Kinder, M.L. Day, and R.J. Kittok, Endocrine regulation of puberty in cows and ewes. *J Reprod Fertil Suppl,* **34**:167-186 (1987).
255. J.D. Armstrong, R.L. Stanko, W.S. Cohick, R.B. Simpson, R.W. Harvey, B.G. Huff, D.R. Clemmons, M.D. Whitacre, R.M. Campbell, and E.P. Heimer, Endocrine events prior to puberty in heifers: role of somatotropin, insulin-like

growth factor-I and insulin-like growth factor binding proteins. *J Physiol Pharmacol*, **43**:179-193 (1992).
256. R.E. Frisch, Body fat, puberty and fertility. *Biol Rev*, **59**:161-188 (1984).
257. J.E. Schneider, Energy balance and reproduction. *Physiol Behav*, **81**:289-317 (2004).
258. J.L. Cameron, D.J. Koerker, and R.A. Steiner, Metabolic changes during maturation of male monkeys: possible sign for onset of puberty. *Am J of Physiol*, **249**:E385-E391 (1985).
259. C.R. Barb, G.J. Hausman, and K. Czaja, Leptin: A metabolic signal affecting central regulation of reproduction in the pig. *Domest Anim Endocrinol*, **29**:186-192 (2005).
260. I.A. Barash, C.C. Cheung, D.S. Weigle, H.P. Ren, E.B. Kabigting, J.L. Kuijper, D.K. Clifton, and R.A. Steiner, Leptin is a metabolic signal to the reproductive system. *Endocrinology*, **137**:3144-3147 (1996).
261. R.S. Ahima, J. Dushay, S.N. Flier, D. Prabakaran, and J.S. Flier, Leptin accelerates the onset of puberty in normal mice. *J Clin Invest*, **99**:391-395 (1997).
262. F. Chehab, K. Mounzih, R. Lu, and M. Lim, Early onset of reproductive function in normal female mice treated with leptin. *Science*, **275**:88-90 (1997).
263. V. Matkovic, J.Z. Ilich, M. Skugor, N.E. Badenhop, P. Goel, A. Clairmont, D. Klisovic, R.W. Nahhas, and J.D. Landoll, Leptin is inversely related to age at menarche in human females. *J Clin Endocrinol Metab*, **82**:3239-3245 (1997).
264. C.C. Cheung, J.E. Thornton, S.D. Nurani, D.K. Clifton, and R.A. Steiner, A reassessment of leptin's role in triggering the onset of puberty in the rat and mouse. *Neuroendocrinology*, **74**:12-21 (2001).
265. F.H. Bronson, Puberty in female mice is not associated with increases in either body fat or leptin. *Endocrinology*, **142**:4758-4761 (2001).
266. B.A. Henry, J.W. Goding, A.J. Tilbrook, F.R. Dunshea, and I.J. Clarke, Intracerebroventricular infusion of leptin elevates the secretion of luteinizing hormone without affecting food intake in long-term food-restricted sheep, but increases growth hormone irrespective of bodyweight. *J Endocrinol*, **168**:67-77 (2001).
267. M.N. Maciel, D.A. Zieba, M. Amstalden, D.H. Keisler, J.P. Neves, and G.L. Williams, Chronic administration of recombinant ovine leptin in growing beef heifers: effects on secretion of LH, metabolic hormones, and timing of puberty. *J Anim Sci*, **82**:2930-2936 (2004).
268. D.A. Zieba, M. Amstalden, S. Morton, M.N. Maciel, D.H. Keisler, and G.L. Williams, Regulatory roles of leptin at the hypothalamic-hypophyseal axis before and after sexual maturation in cattle. *Biol Reprod*, **71**:804-812 (2004).
269. M. Reist, D. Erdin, D. von Euw, K. Tschuemperlin, H. Leuenberger, C. Delavaud, Y. Chilliard, H.M. Hammon, N. Kuenzi, and J.W. Blum, Concentrate feeding strategy in lactating dairy cows: metabolic and endocrine changes with emphasis on leptin. *J Dairy Sci*, **86**:1690-1706 (2003).
270. T. Kokkonen, J. Taponen, S. Alasuuatari, M. Nousiainen, T. Anttila, L. Syrjala-Qvist, .Plasma leptin in transition dairy cows. Effects of body fatness, ambient temperature and dietary factors. *Proceedings of the British Society of Animal Science*,92 (2002).
271. S. Asakuma, H. Morishita, T. Sugino, Y. Kurose, S. Kobayashi, and Y. Terashima, Circulating leptin response to feeding and exogenous infusion of insulin in sheep exposed to thermoneutral and cold environments. *Comp Biochem Physiol A Mol Integr Physiol*, **134**:329-335 (2003).
272. F. Bocquier, M. Bonnet, Y. Faulconnier, M. Guerre-Millo, P. Martin, and Y. Chilliard, Effects of photoperiod and feeding level on perirenal adipose tissue

metabolic activity and leptin synthesis in the ovariectomized ewe. *Reprod Nutr Dev,* **38**:489-498 (1998).

273. Z.F. Atcha, F.R.A. Cagampang, J.A. Stirland, I.D. Morris, A.N. Brooks, F.J.P. Ebling, M. Klingenspor, and A.S.I. Loudon, Leptin acts on metabolism in a photoperiod-dependent manner, but has no effect on reproductive function in the seasonally breeding Siberian hamster (Phodopus sungorus). *Endocrinology,* **141**:4128-4135 (2000).

274. B.P. Fitzgerald and C.J. McManus, Photoperiodic versus metabolic signals as determinants of seasonal anestrus in the mare. *Biol Reprod,* **63**:335-340 (2000).

275. M. Marie, P.A. Findlay, L. Thomas, and C.L. Adam, Daily patterns of plasma leptin in sheep: effects of photoperiod and food intake. *J Endocrinol,* **170**:277-286 (2001).

276. I.J. Clarke, A.J. Tilbrook, A.I. Turner, B.W. Doughton, and J.W. Goding, Sex, fat and the tilt of the earth: effects of sex and season on the feeding response to centrally administered leptin in sheep. *Endocrinology,* **142**:2725-2728 (2001).

277. K.K. Schillo, P.J. Hansen, L.A. Kamwanja, D.J. Dierschke, and E.R. Hauser, Influence of season on sexual development in heifers: age at puberty as related to growth and serum concentrations of gonadotropins, prolactin, thyroxine and progesterone. *Biol Reprod,* **28**:329-341 (1983).

278. D. Petitclerc, L.T. Chapin, R.S. Emery, and H.A. Tucker, Body growth, growth hormone, prolactin and puberty response to photoperiod and plane of nutrition in Holstein heifers. *J Anim Sci,* **57**:892-898 (1983).

279. P.J. Hansen, L.A. Kamwanja, and E.R. Hauser, Photoperiod influenced age at puberty in heifers. *J Anim Sci,* **57**:985-992 (1983).

280. T. Wolden-Hanson, D.R. Mitton, R.L. McCants, S.M. Yellon, C.W. Wilkinson, A.M. Matsumoto, and D.D. Rasmussen, Daily melatonin administration to middle-aged male rats suppresses body weight, intraabdominal adiposity, and plasma leptin and insulin independent of food intake and total body fat. *Endocrinology,* **141**:487-497 (2000).

281. L.R. Gentry, D.L. Thompson, Jr., G.T. Gentry, Jr., K.A. Davis, R.A. Godke, and J.A. Cartmill, The relationship between body condition, leptin, and reproductive and hormonal characteristics of mares during the seasonal anovulatory period. *J Anim Sci,* **80**:2695-2703 (2002).

282. G. Ferreira-Dias, F. Claudino, H. Carvalho, R. Agricola, J. Alpoim-Moreira, and S.J. Robalo, Seasonal reproduction in the mare: possible role of plasma leptin, body weight and immune status. *Domest Anim Endocrinol,* **29**:203-213 (2005).

283. J.A. Cioffi, J. Van Blerkom, M. Antczak, A. Shafer, S. Wittmer, and H.R. Snodgrass, The expression of leptin and its receptors in pre-ovulatory human follicles. *Mol Hum Reprod,* **3**:467-472 (1997).

284. C. Karlsson, K. Lindell, E. Svensson, C. Bergh, P. Lind, H. Billig, L.M.S. Carlsson, and B. Carlsson, Expression of functional leptin receptors in the human ovary. *J Clin Endocrinol Metab,* **82**:4144-4148 (1997).

285. L.J. Spicer and C.C. Francisco, Adipose obese gene product, leptin, inhibits bovine ovarian thecal cell steroidogenesis. *Biol Reprod,* **58**:207-212 (1998).

286. Z.T. Ruiz-Cortes, T. Men, M.F. Palin, B.R. Downey, D.A. Lacroix, and B.D. Murphy, Porcine leptin receptor: molecular structure and expression in the ovary. *Mol Reprod Dev,* **56**:465-474 (2000).

287. C. Delavaud, F. Bocquier, Y. Chilliard, D.H. Keisler, A. Gertler, and G. Kann, Plasma leptin determination in ruminants: effect of nutritional status and body fatness on plasma leptin concentration assessed by a specific RIA in sheep. *J Endocrinol,* **165**:519-526 (2000).

288. H.V. Leon, J. Hernandez-Ceron, D.H. Keislert, and C.G. Gutierrez, Plasma concentrations of leptin, insulin-like growth factor-I, and insulin in relation to changes in body condition score in heifers. *J Anim Sci,* **82**:445-451 (2004).
289. L.J. Spicer, C.S. Chamberlain, and C.C. Francisco, Ovarian action of leptin: effects on insulin-like growth factor-I-stimulated function of granulosa and thecal cells. *Endocrine,* **12**:53-59 (2000).
290. S.K. Agarwal, K. Vogel, S.R. Weitsman, and D.A. Magoffin, Leptin antagonizes the insulin-like growth factor-I augmentation of steroidogenesis in granulosa and theca cells of the human ovary. *J Clin Endocrinol Metab,* **84**:1072-1076 (1999).
291. J.D. Brannian, Y. Zhao, and M. McElroy, Leptin inhibits gonadotrophin-stimulated granulosa cell progesterone production by antagonizing insulin action. *Hum Reprod,* **14**:1445-1448 (1999).
292. R.J. Zachow and D.A. Magoffin, Direct intraovarian effects of leptin: impairment of the synergistic action of insulin-like growth factor-I on the follicle-stimulating hormone-dependent estradiol-17B production by rat ovarian granulosa cells. *Endocrinology,* **138**:847-850 (1997).
293. R.J. Zachow, S.R. Weitsman, and D.A. Magoffin, Leptin impairs the synergistic stimulation by transforming growth factor-beta of follicle-stimulating hormone-dependent aromatase activity and messenger ribonucleic acid expression in rat ovarian granulosa cells. *Biol Reprod,* **61**:1104-1109 (1999).
294. B.K. Campbell, C.G. Guitierrez, D.G. Armstrong, R. Webb, and D.T. Baird, Leptin: *in vitro* and *in vivo* evidence for direct effects on the ovary in monovulatory ruminants. *Human Reprod,* **14**:15-16 (2000).
295. Z.T. Ruiz-Cortes, Y. Martel-Kennes, N.Y. Gevry, B.R. Downey, M.F. Palin, and B.D. Murphy, Biphasic effects of leptin in porcine granulosa cells. *Biol Reprod,* **68**:789-796 (2003).
296. N.R. Kendall, C.G. Gutierrez, R.J. Scaramuzzi, D.T. Baird, R. Webb, and B.K. Campbell, Direct in vivo effects of leptin on ovarian steroidogenesis in sheep. *Reproduction,* **128**:757-765 (2004).
297. M. Kimura, M. Irahara, T. Yasui, S. Saito, M. Tezuka, S. Yamano, M. Kamada, and T. Aono, The obesity in bilateral ovariectomized rats is related to a decrease in the expression of leptin receptors in the brain. *Biochem Biophys Res Commun,* **290**:1349-1353 (2002).
298. K.L. Houseknecht, M.K. McGuire, C.P. Portocarrero, M.A. McGuire, and K. Beerman, Leptin is present in human milk and is related to maternal plasma leptin concentration and adiposity. *Biochem Biophys Res Commun,* **240**:742-747 (1997).
299. B. Berisha, D. Schams, and A. Miyamoto, The expression of angiotensin and endothelin system members in bovine corpus luteum during estrous cycle and pregnancy. *Endocrine,* **19**:305-312 (2002).
300. D. Schams, B. Berisha, T. Neuvians, W. Amselgruber, and W.D. Kraetzl, Real-time changes of the local vasoactive peptide systems (angiotensin, endothelin) in the bovine corpus luteum after induced luteal regression. *Mol Reprod Dev,* **65**:57-66 (2003).
301. A. Fortuno, A. Rodriguez, J. Gomez-Ambrosi, P. Muniz, J. Salvador, J. Diez, and G. Fruhbeck, Leptin inhibits angiotensin II-induced intracellular calcium increase and vasoconstriction in the rat aorta. *Endocrinology,* **143**:3555-3560 (2002).
302. R.L. Martin, E. Perez, Y.J. He, R. Dawson, and W.J. Millard, Leptin resistance is associated with hypothalamic leptin receptor mRNA and protein downregulation. *Metabolism,* **49**:1478-1484 (2000).
303. A. Sahu, Resistance to the satiety action of leptin following chronic central leptin infusion is associated with the development of leptin resistance in neuropeptide Y neurones. *J Neuroendocrinol,* **14**:796-804 (2002).

304. A. Prunier and H. Quesnel, Nutritional influences on the hormonal control of reproduction in female pigs. *Livest Prod Sci,* **63**:1-16 (2000).
305. M.J. Estienne, A.F. Harper, D.M. Kozink, and J.W. Knight, Serum and milk concentrations of leptin in gilts fed a high- or low-energy diet during gestation. *Anim Reprod Sci,* **75**:95-105 (2003).
306. M.J. Estienne, A.F. Harper, C.R. Barb, and M.J. Azain, Concentrations of leptin in serum and milk collected from lactating sows differing in body condition [In Process Citation]. *Domest Anim Endocrinol,* **19**:275-280 (2000).
307. J. Mao, L.J. Zak, J.R. Cosgrove, S. Shostak, and G.R. Foxcroft, Reproductive, metabolic, and endocrine responses to feed restriction and GnRH treatment in primiparous, lactating sows. *J Anim Sci,* **77**:724-735 (1999).
308. N.C. Friggens, Body lipid reserves and the reproductive cycle: towards a better understanding. *Livest Prod Sci,* **83**:219-236 (2003).
309. A. Meikle, M. Kulcsar, Y. Chilliard, H. Febel, C. Delavaud, D. Cavestany, and P. Chilibroste, Effects of parity and body condition at parturition on endocrine and reproductive parameters of the cow. *Reproduction,* **127**:727-737 (2004).
310. W.R. Butler, Nutritional interactions with reproductive performance in dairy cattle. *Anim Reprod Sci,* **60-61**:449-457 (2000).
311. H. Kadokawa, J.R. Briegel, M.A. Blackberry, D. Blache, G.B. Martin, and N.R. Adams, Relationships between plasma concentrations of leptin and other metabolic hormones in GH-transgenic sheep infused with glucose. *Domest Anim Endocrinol,* **24**:219-229 (2003).
312. S.C. Liefers, R.F. Veerkamp, M.F. te Pas, C. Delavaud, Y. Chilliard, and L.T. van der, Leptin concentrations in relation to energy balance, milk yield, intake, live weight, and estrus in dairy cows. *J Dairy Sci,* **86**:799-807 (2003).
313. I.J. Clarke and B.A. Henry, Leptin and reproduction. *Rev Reprod,* **4**:48-55 (1999).

Chapter 15

GENETIC DISORDERS INVOLVING LEPTIN AND THE LEPTIN RECEPTOR

I. S. Farooqi
University Department of Clinical Biochemistry, Cambridge Institute for Medical Research, Addenbrooke's Hospital, Cambridge, CB2 2XY, United Kingdom

Abstract: There has been a major increase in the scale of scientific activity devoted to the study of energy balance and obesity in the last 10 years. This explosion of interest has to a large extent been driven by the identification of genes responsible for murine obesity syndromes and the novel physiological pathways that have been delineated by these genetic discoveries. Several single gene defects causing severe human obesity have been identified. Many of these defects have been in molecules identical or similar to those identified as a cause of obesity in rodents. In this chapter, I will review two of the human monogenic obesity syndromes that have been characterized to date and discuss how far such observations support the physiological role of leptin in the regulation of human body weight and neuroendocrine function

Key words: obesity, genetics, leptin, leptin receptor

1. INTRODUCTION

The concept that mammalian body fat mass is likely to be regulated has its underpinning in experimental science going back over 50 yrs. Thus, the adipostatic theory of Kennedy, which emerged in the 1950s, was based on his own observations of the responses of rodents to perturbations of food intake[1]. The hypothalamic lesioning studies of Hetherington[2] and Anand[3] and the parabiosis experiments of Hervey[4] established that the hypothalamus was central to energy homeostasis. The subsequent emergence of several murine genetic models of obesity[5], and their study in parabiosis experiments by Coleman[6] led to the consolidation of the concept that a circulating factor might be involved in the mediation of energy homeostasis. However, it was not until the 1990s when the precise molecular basis for the *agouti, ob/ob, db/db and fat/fat* mouse models emerged, that the molecular components of an energy balance regulatory network began to be pieced together[7]. The use of gene targeting technology has gone on to demonstrate the critical roles of certain other key molecules such as the melanocortin 4 receptor (MC4R)[8] and melanin concentrating hormone (MCH)[9-10] in that network.

A critical question raised by these discoveries is the extent to which these regulatory pathways are operating in the control of human body weight. Over the past few years a number of novel monogenic disorders causing human obesity have emerged[11]. In many cases the mutations are found in components of the regulatory pathways identified in rodents. The importance of these human studies is several fold. Firstly, they have established for the first time that humans can become obese due to a simple inherited defect. Secondly, it has been notable that in all cases the principle effect of the genetic mutation has been to disrupt mechanisms regulating food intake. Thirdly, some defects, although rare, are amenable to rational therapy. Fourthly, although the physiological consequences of mutations in the same gene in humans and mice are frequently very similar, there are certain key inter-species differences in phenotype. These studies have been particularly informative in dissecting complex human phenotypes.

2. CONGENITAL LEPTIN DEFICIENCY

In 1997, we reported two severely obese cousins from a highly consanguineous family of Pakistani origin[12]. Serum leptin levels were undetectable in these children and direct nucleotide sequencing of the *ob* gene revealed the children to be homozygous for deletion of a single guanine nucleotide in codon 133 of the open reading frame which resulted in a truncated protein that was not secreted[12-13]. The deletion was present in the heterozygous state in both parents. We have since identified three further affected individuals from two other families[14] (and unpublished observations) who are also homozygous for the same mutation in the leptin gene. All the families are of Pakistani origin but not known to be related over five generations. A large Turkish family who carry a homozygous missense mutation have also been described[15]. All subjects in these families are characterised by severe early onset obesity and intense hyperphagia[14,16,17]. Hyperinsulinaemia and an advanced bone-age are also common features[14,16]. Some of the Turkish subjects are adults with hypogonadotropic hypogonadism[17]. Although normal pubertal development did not occur there was some evidence of a delayed but spontaneous pubertal development in one person[17].

We demonstrated that children with leptin deficiency had profound abnormalities of T cell number and function[14], consistent with high rates of childhood infection and a high reported rate of childhood mortality from infection in obese Turkish subjects[17]. Most of these phenotypes closely parallel those seen in murine leptin deficiency (Table 1). However, there are some phenotypes where the parallels between human and mouse are not as clear-cut. Thus, while *ob/ob* mice are stunted[18], it appears that growth retardation is not a feature of human leptin deficiency [14,16], although abnormalities of dynamic growth hormone secretion have been reported in one human subject[17]. *Ob/ob* mice have marked activation of the hypothalamic pituitary adrenal axis with very elevated corticosterone levels[19]. In humans, abnormalities of cortisol secretion are not seen[14]. The contribution of reduced energy expenditure to the obesity of the *ob/ob* mouse is reasonably well established[20]. In leptin deficient humans we found no detectable changes in resting or free-living energy expenditure[14], although it was not possible to examine how such systems adapted to stressors such as cold. Ozata et al reported abnormalities of sympathetic nerve function in leptin deficient humans consistent with defects in the efferent sympathetic limb of thermogenesis[17]. It may be that any deficits in energy expenditure in humans are difficult to measure in the basal state and may only be revealed with dynamic perturbations of energy balance.

3. PHYSIOLOGICAL CONSEQUENCES OF LEPTIN THERAPY

Recently we reported the dramatic and beneficial effects of daily subcutaneous injections of leptin reducing body weight and fat mass in three congenitally leptin deficient children[14]. We have recently commenced therapy in the other two children and seen comparably beneficial results (personal observations). All children showed a response to initial leptin doses (that were) designed to produce plasma leptin levels at only 10% of those predicted by height and weight (i.e. approximately 0.01mg/kg of lean body mass)[14]. The most dramatic example of leptin's effects was with a 3 year old boy, severely disabled by gross obesity (wt 42kg), who now weighs 32kg (75th centile for weight) after 48 months of leptin therapy (Figure 1).

The major effect of leptin was on appetite with normalisation of hyperphagia. Leptin therapy reduced energy intake during an 18MJ adlibitum test meal by up to 84% (5MJ ingested pre-treatment vs 0.8MJ post-treatment in the child with the greatest response)[14.] We were unable to demonstrate a major effect of leptin on basal metabolic rate or free-living energy expenditure[14], but, as weight loss by other means is associated with a decrease in (BMR) basal metabolic rate[21], the fact that energy expenditure did not fall in our leptin deficient subjects is notable.

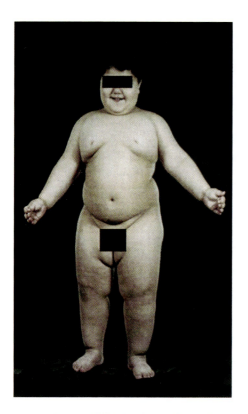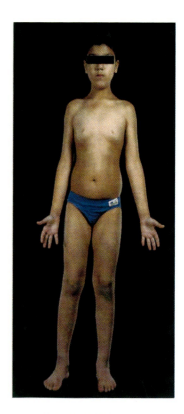

Figure 1. Effects of recombinant human leptin treatment in leptin deficiency

The administration of leptin permitted progression of appropriately timed pubertal development in the single child of appropriate age and did not cause the early onset of puberty in the younger children[14]. Free thyroxine and TSH levels, although in the normal range before treatment, had consistently increased at the earliest post-treatment time point and subsequently stabilized at this elevated level[14]. In a recently reported leptin deficient patient, we observed subclinical hypothyroidism for which thyroxine therapy had been started[22]. Her thyroid function completely normalized once leptin therapy was established, allowing withdrawal of thyroxine. Thus it appears that leptin deficiency is a cause of reversible subclinical hypothyroidism. Evidence from rodents suggests that leptin is necessary for the normal biosynthesis and secretion of TRH and that complete leptin deficiency is associated with a moderate degree of central hypothyroidism[23-25]. Prior to this report, thyroid biochemistry has been reported in seven subjects with congenital leptin deficiency, three children and four adults. In all cases, plasma free thyroxine concentrations have been within the normal range, but four children had significantly elevated TSH levels. The pulsatility of TSH secretion was studied in a single subject with congenital leptin deficiency and demonstrated to have a markedly disorganized secretory pattern[26]. Mantzoros et al. recently examined the ability of leptin to influence the responses of the hypothalamic-pituitary-thyroidal axis to three days starvation[27]. They showed that while leptin abrogated the effects of starvation on integrated TSH levels and on TSH pulsatility, the fasting induced drop in plasma free T3 was not altered by leptin. By contrast Rosenbaum et al. showed that low dose leptin replacement therapy prevented the drop in free T4 and free T3 resulting from a more chronic but lesser degree of caloric restriction[21]. The latter study was conducted over a longer interval, which may explain the observed differences in the reported effects of leptin on the thyroid axis in these groups of patients subjected to caloric restriction.

If leptin is having a significant effect in circulating thyroid hormone concentrations, at what level is this effect operating? On the basis of the high expression of leptin receptors in the arcuate nucleus, the known projection of the arcuate to the paraventricular nucleus where the cell bodies are located, and the demonstrated effects of leptin on TRH biosynthesis and release, a central role of leptin seems most likely. There is no evidence to date for leptin having a direct role on the pituitary thyrotroph. Thus, the bulk of evidence favors a role for leptin in the hypothalamic control of TRH release as the major mediator of its effects on thyroidal function[25].

Throughout the trial of leptin administration, weight loss continued in all subjects, albeit with refractory periods which were overcome by increases in leptin dose[14]. The families in the UK harbour a mutation which leads to a prematurely truncated form of leptin and thus wild-type leptin is a novel antigen to them. Thus, all subjects developed anti-leptin antibodies after ~6 weeks of leptin therapy, which interfered with interpretation of serum leptin levels and in some cases were capable of neutralising leptin in a bioassay[14]. These antibodies are the likely cause of refractory periods occurring during therapy. The fluctuating nature of the antibodies probably reflects the complicating factor that leptin deficiency is itself an immuno-deficient state[28] and administration of leptin leads to a change from the secretion of predominantly Th2 to Th1 cytokines, which may directly influence antibody production. Thus far, we have been able to regain control of weight loss by increasing the dose of leptin.

Table 1. Phenotypes associated with leptin deficiency in rodents (*ob/ob*) and humans

PHENOTYPE	MOUSE	HUMAN
Total Body Weight	3 x normal	mean BMI sds = 6.2
Fat mass	over 50%	mean 57% of body weight
Lean mass	decreased	normal for age
Bone mineral content	increased	normal for age
Food intake	inc meal size	inc meal size and frequency
Basal metabolic rate	decreased	appropriate for body composition
Physical activity	reduced	reduced
SNS activation	decreased	reduced in response to cold
Diabetes	yes	normoglycaemia
Hyperinsulinaemia	severe	appropriate for degree of obesity
Immunity	dec CD4 cells	dec CD4 cells
Reproductive	hypogonadism	hypogonadism
Thyroid	hypothyroid	hypothalamic hypothyroidism
Growth	stunted	normal linear growth and IGF-1
Adrenal	corticosterone excess	normal cortisol and ACTH levels

4. IS HAPLO-INSUFFICIENCY BENEFICIAL?

The major question with respect to the potential therapeutic use of leptin in more common forms of obesity relates to the shape of the leptin dose response curve. We have clearly shown that at the lower end of plasma leptin levels, raising leptin levels from undetectable to detectable has profound effects on appetite and weight[14]. Heymsfield et al administered supraphysiological doses (0.1–0.3 mg/kg body weight) of leptin to obese subjects for 28 weeks[29]. On average, subjects lost significant weight, but the extent of weight loss and the variability between subjects has led many to conclude that the leptin resistance of common obesity cannot be usefully overcome by leptin supplementation, at least when administered peripherally. However, on scientific rather than pragmatic grounds, it is of interest that there was a significant effect on weight, suggesting that plasma leptin can continue to have a dose/response effect on energy homeostasis across a wide plasma concentration range. To test this hypothesis, we studied the heterozygous relatives of our leptin deficient subjects. Serum leptin levels in the heterozygous subjects were found to be significantly lower than expected for % body fat and they had a higher prevalence of obesity than seen in a control population of similar age, sex and ethnicity[30]. Additionally, % body fat was higher than predicted from their height and weight in the heterozygous subjects compared to control subjects of the same ethnicity[30]. These findings closely parallel those in heterozygous ob- and db/- mice [31,32]. These data provide further support for the possibility that leptin can produce a graded response in terms of body composition across a broad range of plasma concentrations.

All heterozygous subjects had normal thyroid function and appropriate gonadotropins, normal development of secondary sexual characteristics, normal menstrual cycles and fertility suggesting that low leptin levels are sufficient to preserve these functions. This is consistent with the data of Ioffe and colleagues who demonstrated that several of the neuroendocrine features associated with leptin deficiency were abolished in low level leptin transgenic mice, which were fertile with normal corticosterone levels[33]. However, these low level leptin transgenic mice still exhibited an abnormal thermoregulation in response to cold exposure and had mildly elevated plasma insulin concentrations, suggesting that there are different thresholds for the various biological responses elicited by changes in serum leptin concentration and that these could be reversed by leptin administration.

Our findings in the heterozygous individuals have some potential implications for the treatment of common forms of obesity. Whilst serum leptin concentrations correlate positively with fat mass, there is considerable inter-individual variation at any particular fat mass. Leptin is inappropriately low in some obese individuals and the relative hypoleptinemia in these subjects may be actively contributing to their obesity and may be responsive to leptin therapy[34]. Heymsfield et al, found no relationship between baseline plasma leptin levels and therapeutic response[29], however, study subjects were not preselected for relative hypoleptinemia. A therapeutic trial in a subgroup of subjects selected for disproportionately low circulating leptin levels would be of great interest.

5. LEPTIN RECEPTOR DEFICIENCY

A mutation in the leptin receptor has been reported in one consanguineous family with three affected subjects[35]. Affected individuals were found to be homozygous for a mutation that truncates the receptor before the transmembrane domain. The mutant receptor ectodomain is shed from cells and circulates bound to leptin. The phenotype has similarities to that of leptin deficiency. Leptin receptor deficient subjects were also of normal birthweight but exhibited rapid weight gain in the first few months of life, with severe hyperphagia and aggressive behaviour when food was denied[35]. Basal temperature and resting metabolic rate were normal, cortisol levels were in the normal range and all individuals were normoglycaemic with mildly elevated plasma insulins similar to leptin-deficient subjects. Leptin receptor deficiency subjects had some unique neuroendocrine features not seen with leptin deficiency. Evidence of mild growth retardation in early childhood, with impaired basal and stimulated growth hormone secretion and decreased IGF-1 and IGF-BP3 levels alongside features of hypothalamic hypothyroidism in these subjects, suggest that loss of the leptin receptor results in a more severe neuroendocrine phenotype than loss of leptin itself.

6. SUMMARY

Several monogenic forms of human obesity have now been identified by searching for mutations homologous to those causing obesity in mice. Although such monogenic obesity syndromes are rare, the successful use of murine models to study human obesity indicates that substantial homology exists across mammalian species in the functional organisation of the weight regulatory system. More importantly, the identification of molecules that control food intake has generated new targets for drug development in the treatment of obesity and related disorders. These considerations indicate that an expanded ability to diagnose the pathophysiological basis of human obesity will have direct applications to its treatment. A more detailed understanding of the molecular pathogenesis of human obesity may ultimately guide treatment of affected individuals.

REFERENCES

1. Kennedy GC 1953 The role of depot fat in the hypothalamic control of food intake in the rat. *Proc R Soc London* **140**:578-96
2. Hetherington AW, Ranson SW 1940 Hypothalamic lesions and adiposity in the rat. *Anat Rec* **78**:149-172
3. Anand BK, Brobeck JR 1951 Hypothalamic control of food intake in rats and cats. *Yale J Biol Med* **24**:123-146
4. Hervey GR 1959 The effects of lesions in the hypothalamus in parabiotic rats. *J Physiol London* **145**:336
5. Bray GA, York DA 1971 Genetically transmitted obesity in rodents. *Physiol.Rev.* **51**:598-646
6. Coleman DL 1973 Effects of parabiosis of obese with diabetes and normal mice. *Diabetologia* **9**:294-8
7. Leibel RL, Chung WK, Chua SC, Jr. 1997 The molecular genetics of rodent single gene obesities. *J Biol Chem* **272**:31937-40.
8. Huszar D, Lynch CA, Fairchild-Huntress V, et al. 1997 Targeted disruption of the melanocortin-4 receptor results in obesity in mice. *Cell* **88**:131-41
9. Shimada M, Tritos NA, Lowell BB, Flier JS, Maratos-Flier E 1998 Mice lacking melanin-concentrating hormone are hypophagic and lean. *Nature* **396**:670-4
10. Chen Y, Hu C, Hsu CK, et al. 2002 Targeted disruption of the melanin-concentrating hormone receptor-1 results in hyperphagia and resistance to diet-induced obesity. *Endocrinology* **143**:2469-77
11. Barsh GS, Farooqi IS, O'Rahilly S 2000 Genetics of body-weight regulation. *Nature* **404**:644-51.
12. Montague CT, Farooqi IS, Whitehead JP, et al. 1997 Congenital leptin deficiency is associated with severe early-onset obesity in humans. *Nature* **387**:903-8
13. Rau H, Reaves BJ, O'Rahilly S, Whitehead JP 1999 Truncated human leptin (delta133) associated with extreme obesity undergoes proteasomal degradation after defective intracellular transport. *Endocrinology* **140**:1718-23
14. Farooqi IS, Matarese G, Lord GM, et al. 2002 Beneficial effects of leptin on obesity, T cell hyporesponsiveness, and neuroendocrine/metabolic dysfunction of human congenital leptin deficiency. *J Clin Invest* **110**:1093-103
15. Strobel A, Issad T, Camoin L, Ozata M, Strosberg AD 1998 A leptin missense mutation associated with hypogonadism and morbid obesity. *Nat Genet* **18**:213-5.
16. Farooqi IS, Jebb SA, Langmack G, et al. 1999 Effects of recombinant leptin therapy in a child with congenital leptin deficiency. *N Engl J Med* **341**:879-84.
17. Ozata M, Ozdemir IC, Licinio J 1999 Human leptin deficiency caused by a missense mutation: multiple endocrine defects, decreased sympathetic tone, and immune system dysfunction indicate new targets for leptin action, greater central than peripheral resistance to the effects of leptin, and spontaneous correction of leptin-mediated defects. *J Clin Endocrinol Metab* **84**:3686-95.
18. Dubuc PU, Carlisle HJ 1988 Food restriction normalizes somatic growth and diabetes in adrenalectomized *ob/ob* mice. *Am J Physiol* **255**:R787-93
19. Dubuc PU 1977 Basal corticosterone levels of young og/ob mice. *Horm Metab Res* **9**:95-7
20. Trayhurn P, Thurlby PL, James WPT 1977 Thermogenic defect in pre-obese *ob/ob* mice. *Nature* **266**:60-62

21. Rosenbaum M, Murphy EM, Heymsfield SB, Matthews DE, Leibel RL 2002 Low dose leptin administration reverses effects of sustained weight-reduction on energy expenditure and circulating concentrations of thyroid hormones. *J Clin Endocrinol Metab* **87**:2391.
22. Gibson WT, Farooqi IS, Moreau M, DePaoli AM, Lawrence E, O'Rahilly S, Trussell RA. 2004 Congenital leptin deficiency due to homozygosity for the Delta133G mutation: report of another case and evaluation of response to four years of leptin therapy. *J Clin Endocrinol Metab* **89**:4821-6.
23. Legradi G, Emerson CH, Ahima RS, Flier JS, Lechan RM 1997 Leptin prevents fasting-induced suppression of prothyrotropin-releasing hormone messenger ribonucleic acid in neurons of the hypothalamic paraventricular nucleus. *Endocrinology* **138**:2569-76
24. Nillni EA, Vaslet C, Harris M, Hollenberg A, Bjorbak C, Flier JS 2000 Leptin regulates prothyrotropin-releasing hormone biosynthesis. Evidence for direct and indirect pathways. *J Biol Chem 275*:36124-33.
25. Harris M, Aschkenasi C, Elias CF, et al. 2001 Transcriptional regulation of the thyrotropin-releasing hormone gene by leptin and melanocortin signaling. *J Clin Invest* **107**:111-20.
26. Mantzoros CS, Ozata M, Negrao AB, et al. 2001 Synchronicity of frequently sampled thyrotropin (TSH) and leptin concentrations in healthy adults and leptin-deficient subjects: evidence for possible partial TSH regulation by leptin in humans. *J Clin Endocrinol Metab* **86**:3284-91.
27. Chan JL, Heist K, DePaoli AM, Veldhuis JD, Mantzoros CS 2003 The role of falling leptin levels in the neuroendocrine and metabolic adaptation to short-term starvation in healthy men. *J Clin Invest* **111**:1409-21
28. Lord GM, Matarese G, Howard JK, Baker RJ, Bloom SR, Lechler RI 1998 Leptin modulates the T-cell immune response and reverses starvation-induced immunosuppression. *Nature* **394**:897-901
29. Heymsfield SB, Greenberg AS, Fujioka K, et al. 1999 Recombinant leptin for weight loss in obese and lean adults: a randomized, controlled, dose-escalation trial. *JAMA* **282**:1568-75.
30. Farooqi IS, Keogh JM, Kamath S, et al. 2001 Partial leptin deficiency and human adiposity. *Nature* **414**:34-5
31. Coleman DL 1979 Obesity genes: beneficial effects in heterozygous mice. *Science* **203**:663-5
32. Chung WK, Belfi K, Chua M, et al. 1998 Heterozygosity for Lep(ob) or Lepr(db) affects body composition and leptin homeostasis in adult mice. *Am J Physiol* **274**:R985-90.
33. Ioffe E, Moon B, Connolly E, Friedman JM 1998 Abnormal regulation of the leptin gene in the pathogenesis of obesity. *Proc Natl Acad Sci U S A* **95**:11852-7
34. Ravussin E, Pratley RE, Maffei M, et al. 1997 Relatively low plasma leptin concentrations precede weight gain in Pima Indians. *Nat Med* **3**:238-40
35. Clement K, Vaisse C, Lahlou N, et al. 1998 A mutation in the human leptin receptor gene causes obesity and pituitary dysfunction. *Nature* **392**:398-401

Chapter 16

IMMUNOASSAYS FOR LEPTIN AND LEPTIN RECEPTORS

Jehangir Mistry
Department of Research and Development, Linco Research, Inc., St. Charles, MO

Abstract: Availability of methods for accurate and reproducible quantification of leptin in various biological fluids in humans and in animals has greatly facilitated research leading to the understanding of its role in various physiological and pathophysiological conditions. Immunoassay techniques provide a simple and robust tool for measurement of biomolecules. In this chapter, I describe the principles behind various types of immunoassay methods, features of several commercially available leptin and leptin receptor immunoassays, and factors that influence leptin measurement using immunoassays.

Key words: Immunoassays, RIA, ELISA, antibodies, immunofunctional

1. INTRODUCTION

To gain understanding of the biological functions of any molecule, it is critical to develop simple, accurate and reproducible tools that enable the measurement of the molecule in various biological fluids. Following its discovery, methods for measuring circulating concentrations of leptin in the human and other animal species were developed rapidly. The first assays were based on the immunoprecipitation/Western blotting techniques and were not only semi-quantitative but also tedious[1]. Therefore, there was an immediate need for precise and quantitative methods. The first commercial assay was introduced by Linco Research, Inc. as described by Ma et al.[2]. This simple and robust assay has been used in majority of the published literature on the measurement of circulating levels of leptin in human serum, plasma or tissue culture media. Leptin circulates in the blood as "free" hormone as well as bound to the extra cellular domain of its soluble receptor. The objective of this chapter is to familiarize the reader with (a) various immunoassay methods and formats available for human leptin and soluble leptin receptor measurement in biological fluids, (b) parameters such as calibration, analyte stability, interference from endogenous molecules, assay characteristics and lot-to-lot variability may influence leptin measurement in various biological matrices, and (c) the availability of various animal leptin assays.

2. COMPETITIVE IMMUNOASSAYS FOR LEPTIN

The competitive immunoassays utilize either radioactive (usually ^{125}I-labeled) or non-radioactive leptin (usually enzyme-labeled or biotin labeled) as the tracer and only one antibody (called primary antibody) raised against the full-length or a peptide fragment of leptin. The method involves competition between the labeled and unlabeled leptin to bind to a fixed number of binding sites[3]. The amount of labeled leptin bound to the antibody is inversely proportional to the concentration of unlabeled leptin present. The separation of the free and bound leptin is achieved by using a double antibody system. The advantage of competitive immunoassays is that they do not require purified antibodies (e.g., antigen affinity purification or other chromatographic steps) and therefore, they are relatively easy to develop for the measurement of large peptides or proteins. The first commercial assay introduced by Linco utilizes ^{125}I-labeled human recombinant leptin, human recombinant calibrators and antiserum raised by immunizing rabbits with highly purified recombinant leptin. This radioimmunoassay (RIA) has been used extensively to determine leptin concentrations in serum, plasma or tissue culture media[4, 5]. In addition, Linco has developed a sensitive leptin RIA suitable for measurement of very low leptin concentrations in biological matrices such as cerebrospinal fluid[6].

3. "TWO-SITE" SANDWICH IMMUNOASSAYS FOR LEPTIN

The sandwich immunoassays are non-competitive assays in which the analyte (e.g., leptin) to be measured is "sandwiched" between two antibodies[7]. The first antibody is immobilized to a solid support (e.g., inside walls of plastic tubes or microtiter wells) and the other antibody is labeled (e.g. ^{125}I label or enzyme or fluorescence tag) for detection of the analyte. The analyte present in the standards or unknown samples is bound by both antibodies to form a "sandwich" complex. Unbound reagents are removed by washing the tubes or microtiter wells or the solid support. Examples of sandwich immunoassays include Immunoradiometric Assay (IRMA) or Enzyme-Linked Immunosorbent Assay (ELISA). Several leptin immunoassays kits are now available in the ELISA format. Table 1 shows compilation of a list of commercially available human leptin immunoassays from various manufacturers and suppliers, with their essential characteristics.

Table 1. Comparison of Human Leptin Assays from Various Commercial Sources*

Company	Assay Format	Dynamic Range	Sample Volume	Incubation Time	Sensitivity	Sample Treatment
ALPCO Diagnostics/ BioVendor	ELISA	1-50 ng/ml	33 µl	2.5 hr.	0.5 ng/ml	Dilution
Assay Designs	ELISA	195-12,500 pg/ml	100 µl	2 hr.	25.5 pg/ml	None
B-Bridge	ELISA	1-50 ng/ml	100l µl	2.5 hr.	Not Described	Dilution
DSL	IRMA	0.25-120 ng/ml	100 µl	Overnight	0.1 ng/ml	None
DSL	ELISA	0.5-50 ng/ml	25 µl	3.5 hr.	0.05 ng/ml	None
LINCO Research	RIA	0.5-100 ng/ml	≤100 µl	Overnight	0.1 ng/ml	None
LINCO Research	RIA	0.05-10 ng/ml	≤100 µl	Two-day	0.01 ng/ml	None
LINCO Research	ELISA	0.125-20 ng/ml	50 µl	3.5 hr.	0.05 ng/ml	None
		0.5-100 ng/ml	25 µl	3.5 hr.	0.2 ng/ml	None
LINCO Research	Luminex Multiplex	6.2-4,500 pM	25 µl	Overnight	8.7 pM	None
R&D Systems	ELISA	30-2,000 pg/ml	100 µl	5 hr.	Not Described	Dilution

*Information was obtained from various manufacturers' kit inserts.

4. MEASUREMENT OF FREE FORM OF LEPTIN IN HUMAN SERUM

Circulating leptin in humans is bound to high-molecular-weight components, as demonstrated by traditional methods using ^{125}I-labeled recombinant leptin and size exclusion chromatography[8-10]. Furthermore, a spun-column assay was used to determine leptin-binding activity in human serum[11]. Horn and Lewandowski[12,13] used an innovative approach to measure selectively only the free leptin by developing an RIA with antibodies raised against a C-terminal leptin fragment (leptin$_{126-140}$). Lewandowskin et al. also raised antibodies against an N-terminal fragment of leptin (leptin$_{26-39}$) which was shown to recognize only the soluble receptor bound leptin. Free and bound forms of leptin have also been quantified by HPLC separation of serum samples followed by measurement of leptin with Linco's RIA[14].

5. SOLUBLE LEPTIN RECEPTOR ASSAYS

At least two commercial immunoassays, one from Diagnostic Systems Laboratories, Inc. (Webster, Texas) and the other from BioVendor (Czech Republic), are currently available to measure the soluble form of leptin receptor. Both assays utilize the sandwich ELISA format in which the "capture" and "detection" antibodies are raised against the soluble receptor protein. Wu et al.[15] developed a Ligand-Mediated Immunofunctional Assays (LIFA) for measurement of (a) circulating endogenous leptin/soluble leptin receptor complexes and (b) total soluble leptin receptor. The soluble leptin receptor is captured by a monoclonal antibody which binds to an epitope on the soluble receptor away from the ligand-receptor binding site and equally recognizes both free leptin receptor and leptin/leptin receptor complexes. Addition of anti-leptin monoclonal antibody alone detects pre-existing endogenous leptin/soluble leptin receptor complexes only, whereas addition of the anti-leptin monoclonal antibody together with an excess of recombinant leptin allows for the measurement of total soluble receptor[15].

6. ANIMAL LEPTIN IMMUNOASSAYS

The study of leptin physiology in animals such as mice, rats, non-human primates and pigs has been greatly facilitated due to the availability of simple, robust RIAs for the measurement of this hormone. Linco Research,

Inc has also developed a multi-species RIA; the antibody used in this kit was raised against human leptin but displays broad cross-reactivity to leptin molecules of many, but not all, species. Richards et al.[16] developed a rabbit polyclonal antiserum to an epitope containing a specific eight amino acid sequence (GLDFIPGL) found in the AB loop portion of most leptin proteins, such as pig, chicken, human, rat, mouse, bovine, sheep and dog. The antiserum apparently recognizes the full-length protein, regardless of the species of origin using Western blot, Slot blot or Immuno-histochemistry techniques. This is typical of many antisera which are raised against a small peptide where they can only detect the intact molecule in a denatured form but not in its native form in solution. The rodent leptin assays are now commercially available in the ELISA format as well. Antibodies raised against human, mouse and rat leptin do not appear to show any significant cross-reactivity to canine leptin. There is only one report in the literature where Kimura et al.[17] developed a sandwich ELISA for canine leptin. Table 2 shows compilation of a list of commercially available animal leptin immunoassays from various manufacturers and suppliers, with their essential characteristics.

Table 2. Comparison of Animal Leptin Assays From Various Commercial Sources*

Company	Species	Assay Format	Dynamic Range	Sample Volume	Incubation Time	Sensitivity	Sample Treatment
ALPCO Diagnostics	Mouse/Rat	ELISA	25-1,600 pg/ml	25 µl	4 hr.	10 pg/ml	Dilution
Assay Design	Mouse	ELISA	12.5-800 pg/ml	100 µl	2 hr.	1.74 pg/ml	None
Assay Design	Rat	ELISA	56-3,600 pg/ml	100 µl	2 hr.	46.7 pg/ml	None
B-Bridge	Mouse/Rat	ELISA	62.5-4,000 pg/ml	100 µl	2.5 hr.	Not described	Dilution
BioVendor	Mouse/Rat	ELISA	62.5-4,000 pg/ml	100 µl	2.5 hr.	Not described	Dilution
DSL	Murine	ELISA	0.5-50 ng/ml	25 µl	4.5 hr.	0.04 ng/ml	None
DSL	Porcine	ELISA	0.5-50 ng/ml	50 µl	2.5 hr.	Not described	None
LINCO Research	Mouse	RIA	0.2-20 ng/ml	≤100 µl	Two-day	0.05 ng/ml	None
LINCO Research	Rat	RIA	0.5-50 ng/ml	≤100 µl	Two-day	0.1 ng/ml	None
LINCO Research	Mouse	ELISA	0.2-30 ng/ml	10 µl	4 hr.	0.1 ng/ml	None
LINCO Research	Rat	ELISA	0.2-30 ng/ml	10 µl	4 hr.	0.1 ng/ml	None
LINCO Research	Mouse/Rat	Luminex Multiplex	6.2-4,500 pM	10 µl	Overnight	6.2 pM	None
LINCO Research	Primate	RIA	0.5-100 ng/ml	≤100 µl	Overnight	0.1 ng/ml	None
LINCO Research	Multi-species	RIA	1-50 ng/ml	≤100 µl	Two-day	0.5 ng/ml	None
R&D Systems	Mouse/Rat	ELISA	31.25-2,000 pg/ml	50 µl	5 hr.	22 pg/ml	Dilution

*Information was obtained from various manufacturers' kit inserts.

7. FACTORS INFULENCING LEPTIN MEASUREMENT

For accurate and reproducible measurement of leptin, it is important to select an immunoassay that is analytically robust in terms of its performance characteristics such as precision, cross-reactivity, linearity of dilution of the biological sample, recovery of exogenously added leptin to the sample and, shows minimum batch-to-batch variability. The long-term batch-to-batch variability, specifically for different lots of standard preparation, should be monitored by using aliquots of quality control serum samples stored at ≤-20 ^{0}C containing a range of leptin concentrations, obtained by pooling samples from volunteers of variable body mass index. Similarly, serum pools for animal leptin assays are also needed to monitor lot-to-lot consistency.

The assay format (e.g., competitive vs. sandwich) and the antibodies used in various assays have significant influence in the measurement of various molecular forms of leptin (e.g., free vs. receptor-bound leptin, truncated form(s) of leptin). In the author's own experience, the RIA format can generally recognize multiple molecular forms of leptin but the sandwich format may measure only selected molecular forms of leptin. For example, in an RIA format, a rabbit polyclonal antibody was able to recognize leptin in monkey serum/plasma samples but the same antibody used in the sandwich format, was unable to recognize monkey leptin.

Human leptin, as measured by RIAs in serum, plasma or cerebrospinal fluid has been found to be stable at -20 ^{0}C for over two years, at 4 0C for at least two months, and over at least five freeze/thaw cycles[2, 12, 18]. However, this needs to be confirmed in all new assays.

It has been documented that leptin secretion is pulsatile. The peak leptin concentration occurs between 00:00 and 4:00 hr and is approximately 30-40% higher than the nadir occurring between 8:00 and 12:00 h[19, 20]. It is therefore important to standardize the timing of sample collection. Modest intra-individual differences may also exist in leptin concentration over a prolonged period. For example, Ma et al.[2] have reported approximately 30% variability in two subjects in whom leptin was measured on eight consecutive mornings. Non-fasting samples are acceptable and normal feeding does not significantly affect circulating leptin concentrations. However, sudden and extreme alterations in feeding patterns should be avoided. Within 24 hr of fasting, leptin concentrations decline to about 30% of initial basal values whereas massive overfeeding over a 12-hr period increases leptin concentrations by about 50% of basal values[21].

There is little evidence of interferences in leptin immunoassays. Leptin appears to be a unique molecule with no known circulating interfering immunoassay cross-reactants. Although there is evidence that a proportion of leptin in the circulation is bound to binding proteins, majority of immunoassays have been shown to measure total leptin most likely because the affinity of antibodies for leptin exceeds that of endogenous binding components. Commercial sandwich immunoassays that use monoclonal antibodies for capture and detection of human leptin may be prone to falsely elevated leptin values because of heterophilic interference occurring due to the presence of human anti-mouse antibodies or rheumatoid factors present in some human serum samples. The heterophilic interference can be eliminated or minimized by using normal mouse IgG in the assay.

8. CONCLUSIONS

Despite the widespread availability of other bioanalytical techniques such as HPLC, mass spectrometry and gel electrophoresis for the measurement of proteins, immunoassays remain of critical importance for protein quantitation in biological fluids due to their simplicity and ability to rapidly & reproducibly measure the concentration of proteins in multiple numbers of samples at one time. Due to the availability of robust immunoassays for leptin measurement, an incredible amount of research has been conducted since its discovery about a decade ago resulting in the emergence of a much wider physiological role of leptin in the last few years.

REFERENCES

1. M. Maffei, J. Halaas, A. Ravussin, Leptin levels in human and rodent: measurement of plasma leptin and *ob* RNA in obese and weight-reduced subjects. *Nat Med* 1995; **1**: 1151-61
2. Z.M. Ma, R.L. Gingerich, J.V. Santiago, S. Klein, C.H. Smith, M. Landt, Radioimmunoassay of leptin in human plasma. *Clin Chem* 1996; **42**: 942-6
3. R. Yalow, S. Barou, Introduction and general considerations. In: Odel, WD, Daughady WH (eds): Principles of competitive protein binding assays. *J.B. Lippincott Co., Philadelphia* 1971; pp 1-19
4. L.B. Williams, R.L. Fawcett, A.S. Waechter, P. Zhang, B.E. Kogon, R. Jones, M. Inman, J. Huse, R.V. Considine, Leptin production in adipocytes from morbidly obese subjects: stimulation by dexamethasone, inhibition with troglitazone, and influence of gender. *J Clin Endocrinol Metab* 2000; Vol. 85, No. 8 2678-2684
5. F. Parhami, Y. Tintut, A. Ballard, A.M. Fogelman, L.L. Demer, Leptin enhances the calcification of vascular cells. *Circulation Research* 2001; **88**: 954

6. J.F. Caro, J.W. Kolacznski, M.R. Nyce, J.P. Ohannesian, I. Opentanova, W.H. Goldman, et al. Decreased cerebrospinal-fluid/serum leptin ratio in obesity: a possible mechanism for leptin resistance. *Lancet* 1996; **348**: 159-61
7. L.E.M. Miles, D.A. Lipschitz, C.P. Bieber, J.D. Cook, Measurement of serum ferritin by a 2-site immunoradiometric assay. *Analyt. Biochem* 1974; **61**: 209-22
8. F.B. Diamond, D.C. Eichler, G. Duckett, E.V. Jorgensen, D. Shulman, A.W. Root, Demonstration of a leptin binding factor in human serum. *Biochem Biophys Res Commun* 1997; **233**: 818-822
9. K.L. Houseknecht, C.S. Mantzoros, R. Kuliawat, E. Hadro, J.S. Flier, B.B. Kahn, Evidence for leptin binding to proteins in serum of rodents and humans: modulation with obesity. *Diabetes* 1996; **45**: 1638-1643
10. M.K. Sinha, I. Opentanova, J.P. Ohannesian, J.W. Kolaczynski, M.L. Heiman, J. Hale, G.W. Becker, R.R. Bowsher, T.W. Stephens, J.F. Caro, Evidence of free and bound leptin in human circulation. Studies in lean and obese subjects and during short-term fasting. *J Clin Invest* 1996; **98**: 1277-1282
11. D.C. Eichler, A.W. Root, G. Duckett, K.L. Moore,F. B. Diamond, A spun-column assay for determination of leptin binding in serum. *Anal Biochem* 1999; **267**: 100-103
12. R. Horn, R. Geldszus, E. Potter, A.B. von Zur Muhlen, G. Rabat, Radioimmunoassay for the detection of leptin in human serum. *Exp Clin Endocrinol Diabetes* 1996; **104:** 454-8
13. K. Lewandoqski, R. Horn, C.J. O'Callaghan, D. Dunlop, G.F. Medley, P. O'Hare, et al. Free leptin, bound leptin, and soluble leptin receptor in normal and diabetic pregnancies. *J Clin Endocrinol Metab* 1999; **84**: 300-6
14. M. Landt, Leptin binding and binding capacity in serum. *Clin Chem* 2000; **46**: 379-384
15. Z. Wu, M. Bidlingmaier, C. Liu, E.B. DeSouza, M. Tschop, K. M. Morrison, C.J. Strasburger, Quantification of the soluble leptin receptor in human blood by ligand-mediated immunofunctional assay. *J Clin Endocrinol Metab* 2002; Vol. 87, No. 6 2931-2939
16. M.P. Richards, T.J. Caperna, T.H. Elsasser, C.M. Ashwell, J.P. McMurtry, Design and application of a polyclonal peptide antiserum for the universal detection of leptin protein. *J Biochem Biophys Methods* 2000; **45**: 147-156
17. M. Iwase, K. Kimura, R. Komagome, N. Sasaki, K. Ishioka, T. Honjoh, M. Saito, Sandwich enzyme-linked immunosorbent assay of canine leptin. *J Vet Med Sci.* Feb. 2000; **62** (2): 207-9
18. A.M. Wallace, Measurement of leptin and leptin binding in the human circulation. *Ann Clin Biochem* 2000: **37**: 244-252
19. M.K. Sinha, J. Sturis, J. Ohannesian, S. Magosin, T. Stephens, M. Heiman, et al. Nocturnal rise and pulsatile secretion of leptin in humans. *Diabetes* 1996; **45**: 386
20. J. Licinio, A.B. Negrao, C. Mantzoros, V. Kaklamani, M.L. Wong, P.B. Bongiorno, et al. Sex differences in circulating human leptin pulse amplitude: clinical implications. *J Clin Endocrinol Metab* 1998; **83**: 4140-7
21. M.K. Sinha, J.F. Caro, Clinical aspects of leptin. *Vitam Horm* 1998; **54**: 1-30

Chapter 17

CLINICAL APPLICATIONS OF LEPTIN

Elif Arioglu Oral [1] and Alex M. DePaoli [2]
[1] Division of Metabolism, Endocrinology and Diabetes, Department of Internal Medicine, University of Michigan, Ann Arbor, MI [2] Amgen Inc., Thousand Oaks, CA

Abstract: The discovery of the adipocyte hormone leptin has had a profound impact on our understanding of obesity and the role of the adipose tissue as an endocrine organ. Due primarily to the weight reducing effect of leptin in the *ob/ob* mouse, the initial enthusiasm for leptin clinical investigation was in human obesity. This review will trace the clinical studies from states of leptin deficiency ('*Ob/Ob*', lipodystrophy, hypothalamic amenorrhea), a physiological replacement paradigm, to the pharmacological applications in obesity (a purported state of leptin insensitivity). This chapter reviews the clinical applications of two leptin analogs for which there is relevant clinical data available (A-200, a long acting analog, will not be discussed, as there is little available data). Both animal and clinical data in multiple disease states provide strong support for a leptin analogue as a potent physiological replacement therapy in states of 'leptin deficiency'. The pharmacological applications in obesity will require further work to identify populations that might respond to leptin alone or in combination with agents impacting other pathways. The available clinical studies provide invaluable insights into furthering our understanding of the relevance of this hormone in health and disease states. Future studies are needed to explore the many potential applications of this remarkable cytokine hormone.

Key words: obesity; lipodystrophy; insulin resistance; dyslipidemia; adipocytokines; reproductive endocrinology; hypothalamic amenorrhea, neuroendocrine; therapeutics

INTRODUCTION

The discovery of leptin and other adipocyte-derived hormones has completely changed our view of the adipocyte as a cell with an important role in the regulation of metabolism. We now know that the fat cells have an endocrine function and can secrete a variety of proteins including leptin, adinopectin[1], resistin[2], TNFα[3], and IL-6 [4,5]. This list has grown to include other secreted factors such as adiponutrin, visfatin[6,7], omentin[8], etc. Leptin, by virtue of its rapid development for therapeutic applications and its projected therapeutic potential in obesity, has received the most attention. In addition to its regulatory effect in energy homeostasis and metabolism, there is a growing body of evidence that suggests involvement of leptin in the regulation of the immune system [9], reproduction [10], coagulation, sympathetic nervous system [11,12], blood pressure[12], growth [13], steroid hormone production, fetal development [14], hematopoiesis [15], angiogenesis [4,5,14,16-19] and wound repair [20,21]. When the effects of a cytokine hormone are so diverse, finding its clinical utility becomes challenging. A logical approach toward developing clinical uses of the pathway begins with the lessons from the knockout ob/ob mouse. Since the most obvious effect observed in the ob/ob mouse was dramatic weight loss, the drug was quickly embraced as the potential "magic bullet" for the rising epidemic of obesity in the Western World.

Since the story originates from the ob/ob mouse and begins with the discovery of leptin, it is useful to briefly review the physiology of leptin. Leptin is a protein structurally similar to cytokines [22,23]. It is the protein product of the ob gene in mice and humans [24] [25]. The main site of leptin synthesis is adipose tissue (white more than brown) and blood levels of leptin correlate with total body fat; the circulating leptin level is elevated in obese rodents and humans[26,27] [28] and lower in lean subjects. Its main function is thought to be as an energy sensor via informing the brain of the energy storage level of the body [16,29,30]. In response to this signal, the brain makes appropriate adjustments to change food intake and energy expenditure to reestablish the energy homeostasis [16,29-34]. The ob/ob mouse, which has complete deficiency of leptin, are hyperphagic, hypothermic and morbidly obese, marked by increased energy intake with reduced energy expenditure [16,35] [36,37]. Treatment of ob/ob mice with leptin causes a decrease in appetite and promotes weight loss, the majority of which is the body fat [35-37]. These mice also have a marked hepatic steatosis coupled with hepatic insulin resistance and hyperglycemia. In addition, the ob/ob mice are infertile and have a number of other hypothalamic pituitary axes abnormalities such as central hypothyroidism, hypercorticisterosenemia due to central CRF neuron activation, and linear growth impairment. More recently, immunological

abnormalities such as decreased CD4 counts, impaired activation of peripheral blood mononuclear cells and a protective effect against permissive autoimmunity have been observed in the murine ob/ob model. Replacement of leptin in the ob/ob mouse significantly reverses or corrects all of these abnormalities. Leptin is now viewed, not as a simple signal that mediates eating behavior, but rather an integrative control switch, signaling status of energy stores to the brain that in turn controls adaptive response to a state of low energy availability. In this paradigm, a low leptin level or the fall in circulating leptin levels will manifest a robust signal that mediates a coordinated set of responses. Although the animal model can be quite informative, there are differences in metabolic and hormonal effects in leptin-deficient humans and rodents.

1. THERAPEUTIC EFFECTS OF LEPTIN IN CONGENITAL LEPTIN DEFICIENCY

Ob gene and leptin receptor mutations are rare in humans [5,38-41]. In humans, ob gene mutations resulting in leptin deficiency, are associated with morbid obesity, hyperphagia, and hypothalamic hypogonadism [39,40,42]. Unlike ob/ob mice, hypothermia, and decreased basal energy expenditure, are not observed in humans. Hyperinsulinemia consistent with the overweight state is evident, but hyperglycemia is only observed in older patients[40 39]. Leptin-deficient ob/ob mice have elevated serum glucocorticoid insulin resistance and impaired linear growth, whereas leptin-deficient human subjects with mutations in the ob gene- have normal plasma glucocorticoid levels [39-41,43,44] and do not show evidence of growth impairment [45].

Farooqi et al. described a homozygous frame-shift mutation involving the deletion of a single guanine nucleotide in codon 133 of the leptin gene in three children [39,45,46]. These children had very low plasma leptin levels, marked hyperphagia, excessive weight gain in early life, and severe obesity [39]. Leptin treatment, in the form of r-metHuLeptin (recombinant methionyl Human Leptin) in these children (Figure 1) resulted in a marked reduction in food intake, accompanied by a significant loss of body weight[45]. Ninety-five percent of the weight loss was body fat. Energy intake at a test meal after the initiation of treatment decreased by 42 percent, to 930 kcal, and the rate of food consumption decreased markedly. The reduction in food intake was sustained throughout the study, with mean energy consumption during therapy of 1000 kcal. Bone mineral mass increased by 0.15 kg.

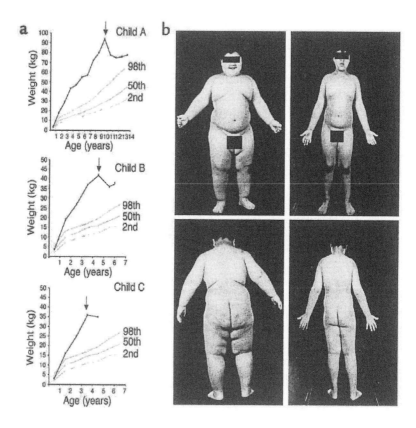

Figure 1: (a) The weight loss effect of r-metHuleptin in three children with congenital leptin mutations as a function of time on therapy as taken from their lifetime weight charts. (b) Remarkable weight loss is demonstrated with pictures of Child B before and after therapy. Reproduced with permission [46].

In addition to marked weight loss due to significant decrease in energy consumption, there was a gradual decline in fasting insulin (baseline hyperinsulinemia), total cholesterol, LDL and triglyceride levels, and a gradual incline in HDL. It is of note that, the patients had episodes of weight gain which were overcome and reversed by increments in leptin dose. Approximately 98% of the weight loss was due to a reduction in fat mass in these growing children. The weight loss was apparently accounted for through suppressive effects on food intake, since there was no identified change in basal metabolic rate and total energy expenditure[45].

Another form of congenital leptin deficiency due to a non-conservative mis-sense leptin gene mutation (Cys-to-Thr in codon 105) was demonstrated

Clinical applications of leptin

in a highly consanguineous Turkish family [47,48]. Four homozygous and 19 heterozygous subjects were identified [49]. Three morbidly obese and hypogonadal homozygous leptin-deficient adult patients (two female and one male) were treated with r-metHuLeptin at low, physiological replacement doses for 18 months[50]. Weight loss was noticeable as early as one week after the initiation of the treatment in association with a 49% decrease in daily food intake in two weeks. The mean BMI dropped from 51 to 26.9 at the end of the study period. It should be noted that the dose of r-metHuLeptin was reduced accordingly as the patients dropped their weights (Figure 2).

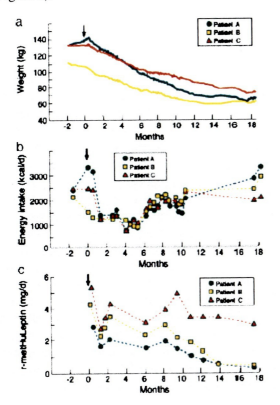

Figure 2: Body weight (a), energy intake (b) and daily r-metHuLeptin dose (c) in 3 adult Turkish leptin deficient patients. Reproduced with permission [50].

The striking finding in this study is that leptin replacement is effective after morbid obesity is established for several decades[49]. Although one patient had type 2 diabetes, the other two subjects had normal baseline fasting glucose and insulin concentrations, and a normal oral glucose tolerance test [50]. The fasting insulin and C-peptide levels in these 2 subjects showed a decrease to less than half of their original values at the end of 18 months. Interestingly, all three congenitally leptin-deficient children reported by Farooqi had baseline hyperinsulinemia [46]. Whether the differences in pretreatment insulin levels is due to differences in the nature of genetic abnormalities between two groups of patients or to a difference in age (children versus adults) remains to be elucidated.

The data on the effect of r-metHuLeptin replacement on other adipokines and potential circulating factors controlling appetite are limited. The available data does not suggest that the effects of leptin are mediated by effects on other adipocytokines such as adiponectin.

Neuroendocrine effects of r-metHuLeptin therapy in leptin deficient humans

As indicated above, ob mice display profound abnormalities in their neuroendocrine regulation that manifest with impaired linear growth, infertility, abnormal thyroid hormone status and hypercorticosteronemia. Replacement with leptin improves all of these abnormalities (see above). The effects of leptin therapy on the various endocrine axes controlled via the neuroendocrine system were evaluated in a limited fashion in the patients with congenital leptin deficiency. In the two prepubertal children reported by Farooqi[46], basal FSH and LH concentrations and sex steroid concentrations remained in the prepubertal range after a maximum of 36 months of r-metHuLeptin therapy. In contrast, there was a gradual increase in gonadotropins and estradiol in the first patient after 24 months of r-metHuLeptin therapy at age 11 years. She had multiple synchronous nocturnal pulses of LH and FSH and subsequently progressed through the clinical stages of pubertal development. This was associated with a growth spurt, behavioral changes associated with pubertal development, enlargement of the ovaries on ultrasound with observation of follicles, and an increase in uterine size. She had her menarche at 12.1 years and reportedly continues to have regular menstrual cycles. The changes in the LH and FSH pulsatility in this girl and two other prepubertal children are shown in Figure 3.

In the report of Licínio and colleagues, there was rescue of gonadal/reproductive function in all three adult patients after r-metHuLeptin therapy[50]. In this small group, there were two female patients who had baseline regular menstrual periods characterized by a luteal phase defect with low midluteal phase progesterone levels. After leptin replacement both patients had regular menstrual periods that were associated with serial midluteal phase progesterone measurements >10 ng/ml, which are indicative of ovulation. The male patient had evidence for hypogonadotropic hypogonadism that was corrected after 6 months of therapy with r-

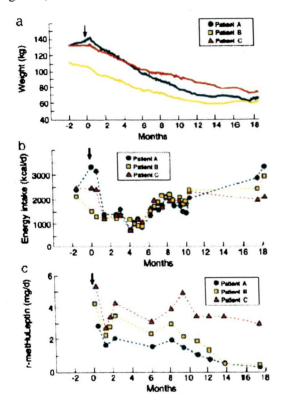

methuLeptin at physiological doses. During the course of therapy, the patient reported improvement in muscle strength, sense of well-being, and energy. Additionally, during the course of leptin replacement, there was increased facial hair, onset of facial acne, development of pubic and axillary hair, growth of penis and testicles, and normal ejaculatory patterns.

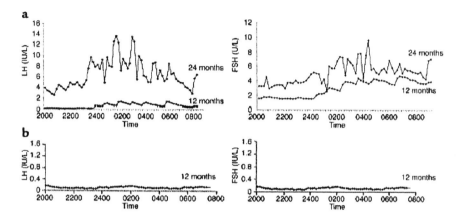

Figure 3: Frequent sampling of LH and FSH levels at 12 months and 24 months of r-metHuleptin in Child C showing age appropriate pubertal changes. (b) Frequent sampling values at 12 months of r-metHuleptin in prepubertal children showing no evidence of inappropriate puberty. Reproduced with permission [46].

The first three patients reported by Farooqi did not have clinically altered thyroid function or abnormalities in the HPA axes. The fourth child reported[51] had evidence for mild primary autoimmune hypothyrodism and this resolved after replacement therapy with leptin. Licino and colleagues had reported abnormalities in 24 hour secretion patterns of TSH in the adult patients. There was no follow-up of TSH secretion during leptin therapy in their subsequent paper. The same authors studied cortisol secretion over 24 hours and reported that cortisol dynamics are characterized by a higher number of smaller peaks, with smaller morning rise, increased relative variability, and increased pattern irregularity in the absence of leptin which change to higher 24-h mean concentrations after leptin replacement, with fewer pulses, of greater height, including a greater morning rise. In light of these limited observations, these authors have proposed that leptin has a role in organizing the dynamics of human hypothalamic–pituitary–adrenal (HPA) function.

The data on GH secretion and IGF-1 levels are hard to interpret due to the small numbers of patients. However, it is safe to conclude that there were no profound abnormalities in the observed heights of either the children or the adults at baseline. [39,45,46,49,50]. From the limited data on these patients, it appears that leptin may have some regulatory effects on levels of some IGF-1 binding proteins [50].

Immunologial effects of leptin therapy

The first implication that leptin deficient patients may have an immunological abnormality was made by Ozata in his Turkish kindred with leptin mutations [49] where an increased rate of infant and childhood mortality was described in the kindred compared to expected rates in the same environment. A number of immunological parameters were studied in two children with congenital leptin mutations by Farooqi and colleagues[46]: The most extensively studied child had a normal total lymphocyte number and a normal number of $CD3^+$ T cells, but there was a reduction in $CD4^+$ T cell number and an increase in $CD8^+$ and B cells, causing a marked reduction in the $CD4^+/CD8^+$ ratio. The absolute number of naive ($CD4^+CD45RA^+$) T cells was reduced (193.6 ± 16.3, 17.0% ± 3.0%, vs. 1,789.0 ± 219.0, 80.4% ± 8.7%, in controls) and consistently lower than that of memory ($CD4^+CD45RO^+$) T cells (676.6 ± 31.3, 82.1% ± 8.1%, vs. 366.6 ± 219.4, 17.8% ± 9.0%, in controls), as was the naive/memory T cell ratio (0.28 vs. 4.88 in controls). R-metHuLeptin therapy normalized this suggested immunophenotype. Thus, $CD4^+$ T cell number was increased to a normal level, as was the $CD4^+/CD8^+$ T cell ratio, while the number of $CD8^+$ and $CD19^+$ B cells was reduced. During the period of r-metHuLeptin therapy, the number of naive $CD4^+CD45RA^+$ T cells and the naive/memory T cell ratio were increased (410.6 ± 78.4 and 0.48, respectively). Finally, the proportion of NK cells, as defined by $CD3^-/CD16^+/CD56^+$ expression, was normal and maintained constant before and after leptin treatment.

Lymphocytes from two children with congenital leptin mutations showed reduced proliferative responses and lower production of cytokines to a variety of polyclonal stimuli such as OKT3, PHA, PMA/Iono, and the recall antigen PPD, prior to r-metHuLeptin therapy. The T cell hyporesponsiveness persisted even when further stimuli were added (IL-2, anti-CD28 mAb, allogeneic stimulator cells). Immunoglobulin levels were within the normal age-related range before treatment, with slightly increased IgM (data not shown), which is in agreement with data from *ob/ob* mice[52,53]. Chronic r-metHuLeptin replacement increased the proliferative responses and cytokine production of the patient's lymphocytes in all assays, in some even to a level comparable with lymphocytes from age-matched controls. The most significant and best-maintained increases after treatment were observed in the production of IFN-γ, which was restored to a level similar to that of control cells.

2. EFFECTS OF LEPTIN IN LIPODYSTROPHY: A STATE OF SEVERE LEPTIN DEFICIENCY

Aside from mutations of the leptin gene, leptin deficiency can be caused by the lack (or deficiency) of adipose tissue. This condition is known as lipodystrophy. Lipodystrophy is characterized by partial or complete deficiency of white adipose tissue, [54]. This rare condition is associated with very low leptin levels, [55-57], hyperphagia, diabetes, moderate to severe insulin resistance, hypertriglyceridemia and nonalcoholic hepatic steatosis (NASH). [54,58] A patient with generalized lipodystrophy (NIH-1) is shown in Figure 4 demonstrating the severity of fat loss and skin manifestations of hypertriglyceridemia. Multiple murine models of lipodystrophy have been created using a variety of different strategies. Regardless of the strategy, the animal models display the metabolic features observed in human lipodystrophy syndromes and suggest that the metabolic features are a consequence of fat loss. Even though the planning stage for a clinical study in human lipodystrophy had been in progress since 1998, the human trial gained momentum after the landmark study by Shimomura and colleagues was published in 1999[59]. This seminal paper showed dramatic amelioration of metabolic abnormalities of lipodystrophy in mice after only 3 weeks of leptin replacement, setting the stage for the human studies. Further, these observations were validated in the aZIP over expression animal model of lipodystrophy[60].

The human trial involving lipodystrophic patients with reduced leptin levels has expanded our knowledge on the metabolic and therapeutic effects of r-metHuLeptin in humans. Restoration of blood leptin levels in nine lipodystrophic patients by subcutaneous injections for 4 months resulted in a reduction in HbA1c by 1.9% in the face of significant reductions in underlying diabetes therapy, a decrease in fasting triglyceride levels by 60%, and a significant improvement in insulin resistance [55]. In addition, there was a decrease in liver volume of 28% and improvement in serum liver enzymes (ALT and AST). The response of NIH 1 is demonstrated in Figure 5. The decrease in daily caloric intake and resting metabolic rate has raised the question whether the observed metabolic changes could be attributable to altered nutrient intake. To address this, we suspended r-metHuLeptin replacement in one subject while clamping her caloric intake. After cessation of r-metHuLeptin, an increase in fasting insulin and triglyceride levels were noted on day 2 and 4, respectively.

Reinitiating r-metHuLeptin treatment reversed these elevations. This study demonstrated the important role of leptin as a therapeutic agent to improve deranged carbohydrate and lipid metabolism in this group of patients with lipodystrophy [55].

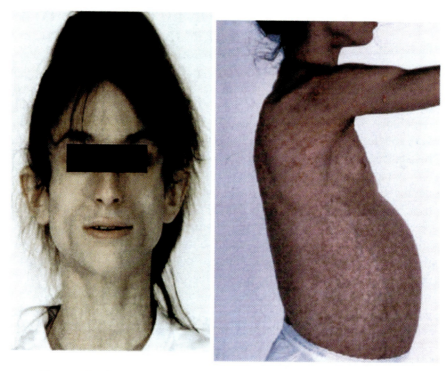

Figure 4: Patient NIH-1, a 17-year old patient with acquired generalized lipodystrophy. Severe hepatomegaly and diffuse multiple cutenous xanthomata. The severity of her symptoms during her clinical presentation to the NIH in 1998 was one of the driving forces that led to the launching of the leptin replacement trial in human lipodystrophy. . Reproduced with permission [55].

Effects of r-metHuLeptin on liver and muscle

Marked hepatic steatosis in lipodystrophic mice has been shown to be reversed by leptin administration [59,60] or by transgenic expression of leptin [60]. A similar effect has been demonstrated in lipodystrophic humans. An 80% decrease in liver lipid content [56,61] and 28% reduction in liver volume [55,62] in response to r-metHuLeptin treatment has been seen in patients with lipodystrophy. This dramatic reduction in hepatic triglyceride content was associated with a marked increase in hepatic and peripheral insulin sensitivity [56].

More recently, Javor et al reported improvement of liver histopathology with significant reductions in the semi-quantitative scores of nonalcoholic steatohepatitis associated with lipodystrophy on biopsy specimens of patients before and after a short-period of r-metHuLeptin therapy[63]. These remarkable observations suggest that nonalcoholic hepatic steatosis (NASH) pathology can be reversed in the setting of a metabolic disease either in

Clinical applications of leptin

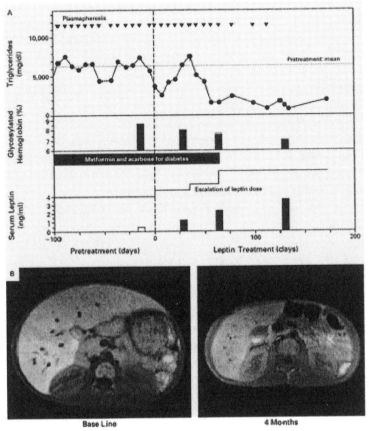

Figure 5: A. Clinical course of patient NIH-1 before and after r-metHuleptin therapy. Effects on triglyceride levels, HbA1c level and circulating leptin levels with the daily dose of leptin therapy are shown. Before r-methumleptin, patient was receiving fenofibrate and lipitor, in addition to at least weekly plasmapharesis, for lipid control. Diabetes was inadequately controlled with metformin and acarbose combination therapy. r-methumleptin allowed for discontinuation of lipid and glucose lowering therapies including weekly plasmapharesis. These effects have been sustained after 5 years of therapy. B. T1-weighted magnetic resonance images of the abdomen using 1.5 Tessla magnet from patient NIH-1 at baseline of study and after 4 months demonstrating a remarkable decrease in liver volume. Reproduced with permission [55].

association with amelioration of the metabolic conditions or through direct actions of leptin on liver.

There is a strong relationship between insulin resistance and the lipid content of the liver [64-66] and muscle tissue [56,66-77]. Studies in these lipodystrophic patients showed that leptin treatment decreased the lipid content not only in the liver but in muscle tissue as well [56,61]. A mean reduction of 42% in intramyocellular lipid content was achieved by chronic leptin administration [61]. Similarly, Petersen and colleagues demonstrated a 33% reduction in intramyocellular triglyceride content which was accompanied by a 30% decrease in muscle total fatty acyl CoA concentration [56], suggesting increased fatty acid oxidation. These changes were accompanied by an increase in insulin sensitivity [56,61]. It has been proposed that reduction in intramyocellular lipid content of the skeletal muscle contributes to the reversal of insulin resistance by improving insulin signaling and glucose consumption [78,79].

These clinical observations are supported by animal studies investigating the molecular mechanisms of leptin action. Leptin has been shown to stimulate fatty acid oxidation in the muscle [80,81], possibly by activating 5'-AMP-activated protein kinase [80]. Increased lipid stores in nonadipose tissues lead to insulin resistance [82]. Leptin-induced increase in fatty acid oxidation may be the mechanism accounting for the decrease in intramyocellular lipid and improvement in insulin resistance [61]. It has been proposed that intracellular accumulation of fatty acid-derived metabolites, such as fatty acyl CoA, can trigger a cascade of events leading to diminished activation of glucose transporter-4 translocation in skeletal muscle which would culminate in decreased sensitivity to insulin action [56,73,74]. Leptin may break this chain of events. An increase in fatty acid overproduction may also be one of the mechanisms responsible for lipid accumulation in the liver as seen in leptin deficient subjects [83]. A possible mechanism of leptin's anti-steatotic action may be due the enhancement of fatty acid oxidation in the liver [84].

More detailed look at energy balance

A subset of the lipodystrophic patients included in the original report were studied in an effort to more objectively determine effects of r-metHuLeptin replacement on satiety and satiation[85]. Satiation and satiety were determined before and again during leptin treatment. Satiation was measured as the time to voluntary cessation of eating from a standardized food array after a 12-h fast. Satiety was determined as the time to hunger sufficient to consume a full meal after consumption of a standardized preload. During leptin treatment, satiation time decreased (41.2 ± 18.2 to 19.5 ± 10.6 min; $P = 0.01$), satiety time increased (62.9 ± 64.8 to 137.8 ± 91.6 min; $P = 0.04$), energy consumed to produce satiation decreased (2034 ± 405 to 1135 ± 432 kcal or 8.5 ± 1.7 to 4.7 ± 1.8 MJ; $P < 0.01$), and the amount of food desired in the postabsorptive state decreased ($P < 0.02$). Ghrelin concentrations also decreased during leptin administration (284.3 ± 127.9 to 140.6 ± 104.5 pmol/liter; $P < 0.002$). Based on these data, we concluded that r-metHuLeptin administration results in reduced caloric, shorter, more satiating meals and longer-lived satiety. These data support the hypothesis that leptin plays an important, permissive role in human appetite regulation.

Effects on neuroendocrine regulation

As seen in patients with congenital leptin deficiency, patients with lipodystrophy exhibited reproductive dysfunction. This is particularly evident in reproductive age female patients. Seven of the original nine cases were included in a more detailed report assessing hypothalamic-pituitary and endocrine axes. Five of the seven patients were in reproductive age range and only one of these patients was cycling regularly. Four of these patients had either primary or secondary amenorrhea. It was interesting to note that these patients also had hyperandrogenism even if their baseline LH and FSH levels were low and their response to LHRH was prepubertal. R-metHuLeptin replacement corrected their LHRH response, improved their estradiol levels and ameliorated levels of testosterone. These biochemical improvements were associated with gain of regular or near-regular menstrual cycles.

There were no clinically evident abnormalities in thyroid or adrenal function in patients with lipodystrophy. The ability to respond to TRH by pituitary TSH secretion was slightly altered after r-metHuLeptin therapy; but this did not translate into a clinically significant change in circulating free thyroid hormones. The ACTH and cortisol response to CRH administration were comparable before and after r-metHuLeptin replacement. It is important to note that the circadian rhythms of secretion in the various axes were not assessed in the lipodystrophic patients.

Circulating IGF-1 levels were significantly lower than the lower limit of normal in the lipodystrophic patients before r-metHuLeptin replacement therapy (E.A. Oral, unpublished observations). These levels significantly increased after 4 to 8 months of leptin replacement. We have proposed these changes might be a direct effect of leptin on the GH axis as well as IGF-1 binding protein abnormalities possibly associated with the severe state of insulin resistance at baseline. We have not assessed the levels of these binding proteins yet.

Effects on bone mineral density and function

Body composition and bone mineral density were studied in fourteen lipodystrophic patients at baseline, 4 months and 1 year of leptin therapy[62]. Dual energy x-ray absorptiometry (DEXA) demonstrated modest, but statistically significant decreases in fat mass (5.4 +/- 0.8 kg to 5.0 +/- 0.8 kg; P =.003) and lean body mass (51.2 +/- 3.2 kg to 48.3 +/- 3.4 kg; P =.003) at 4 months on therapy. The potential confounding changes in tissue lipid were not completely addressed in these measurements. There was no impact of leptin therapy on bone mineral content or bone mineral density in this small cohort.

Simha and colleagues reported bone mineral density and studies of bone metabolism in 2 female patients who were studied at baseline and during 18 months of therapy[86]. At baseline, the bone mineral density for both patients, measured at the lumbar spine and total hip, was within 1 SD of the peak bone mass. There was no significant change in bone mineral density in both patients after 16-18 months of leptin therapy. Similarly, concentrations of serum osteocalcin and bone-specific alkaline phosphatase or urinary excretion of deoxypyridinoline and N-telopeptides remained unchanged after 6-8 months of leptin therapy, suggesting no dramatic effects of leptin on osteoblastic or osteoclastic activity in these two subjects.

Effects on immune function

We assessed immunological status of 10 of the lipodystrophic patients at baseline, and during the first 8 months of r-metHuLeptin therapy[87]. In contrast to the patients with congenital deficiency, there was no evidence to suggest clinical immunodeficiency such as recurrent infections or unexplained fevers. First, we studied lymphocyte subsets at baseline and then at 4 and 8 months of therapy. Leptin therapy caused a significant increase in the absolute number of T-cells. This occurred in both alpha/beta and gamma/delta lineages. The number of CD4 and CD8 cells increased concurrently, allowing the CD4/CD8 ratio to remain similar to baseline. The baseline numbers of CD4 cells were in the normal range, though on the low side of normal at baseline. Leptin therapy also caused a number of significant changes in T-lymphocyte subset distribution resulting in significant increments in cytotoxic T-cells and NK cells. The changes noted at 4 months were sustained at 8 months.. The leptin deficient lipodystrophy patients had relatively higher B-lymphocytes (CD20+ cells, 21.2±1.6%, normal: 4.8-15.9%). The absolute number of B-cells was also higher than the upper limit of the normal range 434±376 (normal: 88-330). There were no changes in the absolute number of B-cells with therapy (433±369). This led to the near-normalization of the high B-cell percentage observed at baseline (4 months: 16.6±7.7%, normal: 4.8 to 15.9%).

In addition, in vitro peripheral blood mononuclear cells were studied functionally for cytokine release and proliferation following stimulation with lipopolysaccharide (LPS), LPS + interferon-gamma, phytohemagglutin (PHA) and PHA+ interleukin 12 at baseline and 4-months. TNF-α secretion (a T-lymphocyte dependent cytokine) measured from PBMC of these patients was remarkably increased after 4-months of leptin therapy as compared to baseline state. In addition, patients' baseline state was significantly lower than healthy control state. Maximum stimulation post-therapy slightly exceeded normal range. In contrast, interferon-γ secretion at rest slightly decreased (p=0.06) after r-metHuLeptin therapy. This effect was not apparent with stimulated levels. None of these levels were outside normal range. The proliferation responses from patients at baseline state were not different after therapy under rest or stimulated conditions. These values were comparable to normal control responses. We concluded that our data supported the growing body of evidence that leptin had immunomodulatory actions in humans; however, there were slight differences between the details observed from patients with congenital leptin deficiency and our lipodystrophic patients.

Long-term effects

Most recent data analyses on the NIH lipodystrophy trial with 20 patients reported and data from 15 completing one year have been summarized[88]. The following synopsis of metabolic improvements were taken from this report: Reductions were seen in serum fasting glucose (from 205 ± 19 to 126 ± 11 mg/dl; $P < 0.001$), HbA$_{1c}$ (from 9 ± 0.4 to $7.1 \pm 0.5\%$; $P < 0.001$), triglycerides (from $1,380 \pm 500$ to 516 ± 236 mg/dl; $P < 0.001$), LDL (from 139 ± 16 to 85 ± 7 mg/dl; $P < 0.01$), and total cholesterol (from 284 ± 40 to 167 ± 21 mg/dl; $P < 0.01$). HDL was unchanged (from 31 ± 3 to 29 ± 2 mg/dl; $P = 0.9$). Liver volumes were significantly reduced (from $3,663 \pm 326$ to $2,190 \pm 159$ cm^3; $P < 0.001$), representing loss of steatosis. Decreases were seen in total body weight (from 61.8 ± 3.6 to 57.4 ± 3.4 kg; $P = 0.02$) and resting energy expenditure (from $1,929 \pm 86$ to $1,611 \pm 101$ kcal/24 h; $P < 0.001$). The conclusion was that r-metHuLeptin led to significant and sustained improvements in glycemia, dyslipidemia, and hepatic steatosis. The first lipodystrophic patient included in this trial has completed 5 years of therapy with persistence of her metabolic and neuroendocrine improvements. The long-term metabolic efficacy of r-metHuLeptin therapy was independently validated in 2 Japanese patients receiving the same therapy using a similar protocol [89]. The beneficial effects of r-metHuLeptin therapy on the reproductive function of female patients were also sustained with long-term therapy[90].

3. ANOTHER RARE FORM OF LEPTIN DEFICIENCY: RABSON MENDENHALL SYNDROME

The effect of leptin was studied in the Rabson-Mendenhall syndrome [91], a condition characterized by severe insulin resistance usually caused by compound heterozygous mutations in the insulin receptor gene [92,93]. The clinical findings in these children include marked insulin resistance, hyperinsulinemia, acanthosis nigricans and growth retardation. In contrast to lipodystrophic patients, the two siblings with Rabson-Mendenhall syndrome in this study had no hypertriglyceridemia nor hepatic steatosis [91]. Treatment with r-metHuLeptin for ten months resulted in a significant decrease in fasting glucose, insulin levels and HbA1c, indicating a substantial improvement in insulin resistance. Three months after withdrawal of the treatment, the improvement was lost and the fasting glucose and insulin levels returned to the high pretreatment levels. It should be mentioned that, although pretreatment leptin levels were low, these patients had considerably higher baseline leptin levels than lipodystrophic patients, and yet, they exhibited a marked improvement in insulin resistance in response to leptin replacement. It is of interest to note that the period on r-metHuLeptin therapy for these two children marked their greatest height velocity observed to that point.

4. A COMMON FORM OF LEPTIN DEFICIENCY: HYPOTHALAMIC AMENORRHEA

It has been known for a long time that energy deficits may cause a disruption of hypothalamic–gonadal and other endocrine axes. After the discovery of leptin and its potential regulatory role in neuroendocrine regulation, low levels of leptin were implicated in the mediation of hypothalamic amenorrhea in response to energy deficits. In a case-control study, Welt and colleagues hypothesized that exogenous r-metHuLeptin replacement would improve reproductive and neuroendocrine function in women with hypothalamic amenorrhea[94]. Eight women with hypothalamic amenorrhea, and a relatively low leptin level compared with weight matched controls, were initially monitored for one month before receiving r-metHuLeptin for up to three months. Six control subjects with hypothalamic amenorrhea received no treatment and were studied for a mean (±SD) of 8.5±8.1 months. Luteinizing hormone (LH) pulsatility (demonstrated in Figure 6), body weight, ovarian imaging, and gonadal hormone levels were monitored in both groups. The control subjects showed no significant

Clinical applications of leptin

change in these parameters. The women in the study group revealed no evidence of ovulation during the one-month run in period before r-metHuLeptin therapy. In contrast, r-metHuLeptin treatment not only increased mean LH levels and LH pulse frequency, maximal follicular diameter, the number of dominant follicles, ovarian volume, but it appeared to recapitulate a normal pattern of gonadal regulation after only two weeks (Figure 6).

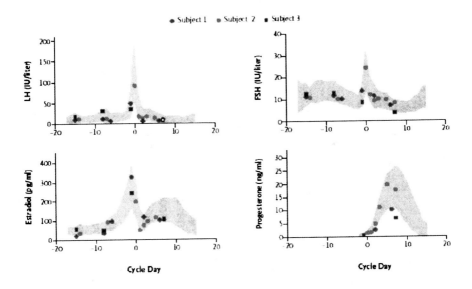

Figure 6: Levels of LH, FSH, Estradiol, and Progesterone in three subjects with hypothalamic amenorrhea who ovulated while on r-metHuLeptin therapy show a normal pattern. Used with permission [94].

Also, r-metHuLeptin significantly increased levels of free triiodothyronine, free thyroxine, insulin-like growth factor 1, insulin-like growth factor–binding protein 3, bone alkaline phosphatase, and osteocalcin but not cortisol, corticotropin, or urinary N-telopeptide. There were neither significant adverse events nor intolerances to the treatment. The authors concluded that r-metHuLeptin administration for the relative leptin deficiency in women with hypothalamic amenorrhea appears to improve reproductive, thyroid, and growth hormone axes and markers of bone formation, suggesting that leptin, a peripheral signal reflecting the adequacy of energy stores, is required for normal reproductive and neuroendocrine function. While this study has important physiological implications, the potential clinical applications in this population will require further study of the role of leptin in modulating pubertal development, bone mass accretion, gonadal function, fertility, as well as the relevance of the other pituitary hormones that appear to be modulated. The potential for an effect on weight was also assessed within this study. At physiological replacement doses weight remained stable, while at pharmacological doses, there was a modest weight loss. This will need to be considered in any clinical application in this population.

5. LEPTIN IN THE TREATMENT OF OBESITY (WEIGHT LOSS AND WEIGHT MAINTENANCE)

The weight loss promoting effects of leptin in animal studies initially raised the expectation that leptin could be a novel therapeutic agent in the treatment of human obesity. It is notable that this effect of leptin in rodents was most evident in the ob/ob mouse and substantially less in the diet-induced obesity model. The weight loss effect of r-metHuLeptin in the Ob human was comparable to the effects in the Ob/Ob mouse. The effects of leptin in diet induced obesity have been studied with two analogues and in different paradigms.

The first study involved a complex design to assess the weight loss of r-metHuLeptin or placebo given twice per day for 6 months. Subjects were given a 500 Cal deficit diet with minimal behavioral intervention, so as to assess the effect of the intervention. The mean weight loss in obese cohorts was proportional to the dose of leptin and is shown in Figure 7. At the highest dose (0.3 mg/kg achieving a maximum serum leptin concentration of 480 ng/ml), the cohort lost 7.1 kg from baseline as compared with 1.3 kg in the placebo group. The only associated adverse event was injection site reactions, which appeared also to be dose dependent. This study demonstrated that obese patients, with high baseline leptin levels, were only moderately responsive to higher doses of exogenous r-metHuLeptin[95]. There appeared to be a wide range of response to r-metHuLeptin. Some individuals lost greater than 15 kg in 24 weeks, while no individual in placebo group lost greater than 10 kg over this same time frame (Figure 8). The factors that might determine a better response to r-metHuLeptin could not be effectively evaluated determined in the context of the small trial published thus far.

In contrast to the Heymsfeld paper, Hukshorn et al [96] using weekly administration of pegylated recombinant human leptin for 12 weeks showed no significant difference in weight loss between placebo and treatment groups, although there were reductions in appetite scores and triglycerides. It is important to note that the serum leptin concentration achieved with treatment (from a baseline of 21.9 ng/ml to 25.7 ng/ml) in this study was much lower than that reported by Heymsfield (480 ng/ml) [95]. Further, Hukshorn et al. did not observe a differential weight loss between placebo

Clinical applications of leptin 345

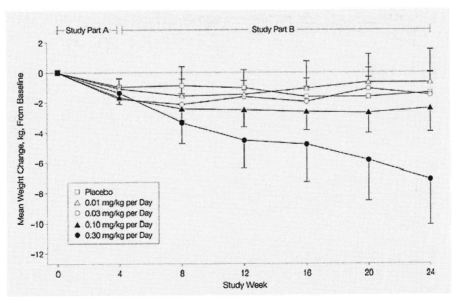

Figure 7: Pattern of weight change from baseline to week 24 in obese subjects who received r-metHuLeptin. Error bars indicate SEM. The number of subjects changes over the course of the study. Reproduced with permission [95].

and treatment groups in a small pilot study utilizing 60 mg/week dose of pegylated leptin, which increased the serum leptin concentration to 2542 ng/ml by the eighth week [97]. Overall, these studies support the premise that leptin is not a robust anti-obesity target in an unselected population as monotherapy.

Of note, a significantly greater weight loss (Figure 9) was observed in pegylated leptin-treated obese individuals, compared to placebo, when the subjects were concomitantly put on a very low energy diet [98]. In this study, pegylated leptin administration resulted in a tremendous increase in serum leptin concentration, which was accompanied by a diminished appetite. The placebo individuals, on the contrary, exhibited an increase in appetite, which was associated with a substantial decline in serum leptin level. The authors concluded that the physiologic function of leptin is as a signal of starvation at times of caloric restriction rather than a signal to suppress energy intake when there is abundance of energy storage [98]. The opportunity to create a leptin responsive state, through the induction of significant weight loss (Very Low Caloric Diet or gastric surgery), and to utilize a leptin analogue to either improve weight loss or assist in the maintenance of weight lost remains to be fully studied.

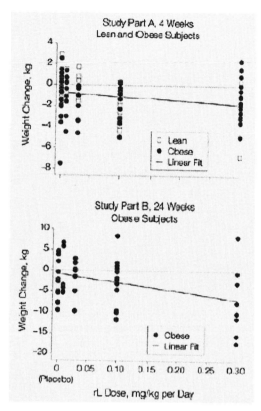

Figure 8: Relationship between r-metHuLeptin (rL) Dose and Body Weight as Measured by Calibrated Scales. Study Part A (4 weeks exposure of lean and obese subjects $P = .02$) and Study Part B (24 weeks exposure of only obese subjects $P = .01$). Reproduced with permission [95].

There is also evidence that leptin may play a therapeutic role in the maintenance of reduced body weight. There is a reduction in serum leptin concentration, energy expenditure and circulating thyroid hormone concentrations associated with maintenance of reduced weight [99,100]. These changes can be responsible for regaining the lost weight [99,101,102]. Restoration of leptin concentration to pre-weight loss levels with r-metHuLeptin was demonstrated to reverse the decline in T3 and T4 levels, and an increase in non-resting and total energy expenditure [103]. These changes were associated with a loss of fat mass during leptin treatment [103].

The clinical response to leptin analogues in leptin replete obese subjects is profoundly reduced as compared with that observed in genetically leptin-deficient patients as already shown in the individual studies and reviewed previously by other authors [104]. The mechanisms responsible for this difference are not clear and research is currently under way to illuminate the possible reasons. One avenue of study is the sexual dimorphism of leptin

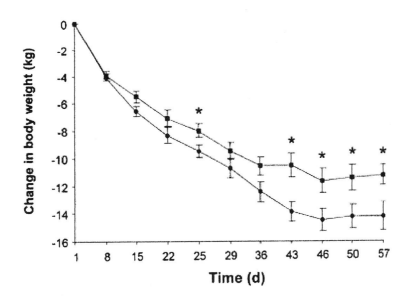

Figure 9: Effect of 80 mg pegylated human recombinant leptin [polyethylene glycol–OB protein (PEG-OB)] (•; n = 12) or matching placebo (■; n = 10) administered weekly in conjucntin with severe energy restriction (2.1 MJ/d) on mean (± SEM) weight loss from the start of the treatment (day 1), through the diet period (day 46), to the end of the 2-wk follow-up period (day 57). *Significantly different from the PEG-OB group, $P < 0.05$ (interaction of time and treatment; two-factor repeated-measures ANOVA with Scheffe's F procedure). Used with permission [98].

production and or clearance, the fasting-induced decline in leptin production is blunted in women with upper body obesity [105] and the clearance in obese women appears to be increased with prolonged fasting [106]. Some have posited that obese individuals with high circulating leptin levels are resistant to the appetite reducing effects of endogenous and exogenously administered leptin [16,107]. Several mechanisms have been postulated to be responsible for the relative insensitivity of obese individuals to leptin [108]. One hypothesis is that there is impaired transport of leptin through the blood brain [109,110]. This is supported by the finding that leptin concentrations in the cerebrospinal fluid (CSF) were much lower than the serum concentrations in the obese [109,111] and comparable to that in lean subjects despite obese individuals had much higher levels of circulating leptin [107]. Although exogenous r-metHuLeptin seems to be able to get into the CSF, as demonstrated by Fujioka, although the ratio of peripheral increase to central increase before and after dosing is reduced[112]. Other mechanisms that might explain a leptin resistance involve impaired leptin-signaling in leptin-responsive neurons in the hypothalamus[33], and post-receptor effects of leptin on hypothalamic neuronal network that regulate energy homeostasis [113].

The potential for the clinical application of leptin in more common forms of insulin resistance and diabetes mellitus remain to be seen. Recently, encouraging results of leptin's efficacy in a lean and leptin responsive animal model of Type 2 diabetes were reported[114]. There has been only a limited description of two clinical trials evaluating efficacy in r-metHuLeptin treatment of obese subjects with Type 2 Diabetes Mellitus (A.M. DePaoli, Oral Presentation, NAASO 2000). One study in drug naïve and one in sulphonylurea treated subjects. The data from the monotherapy study revealed a reduction in HbA1c from placebo of 0.4% at 4 months with a small weight loss of less than 2 kg compared with placebo. The glucose lowering effects were found to be independent of the weight loss. The study in sulphonylurea treated subjects showed a 0.25% reduction in HbA1c compared to placebo after 4 months. There was no weight loss in this second study. Based on the profound effect of r-metHuLeptin on insulin resistance and hyperglycemia in the lipodystrophic studies, it is intriguing to consider the potential investigation of r-metHuLeptin in subjects with type 2 diabetes mellitus with relatively normal or low leptin, potentially a 'leptin responsive' population.

6. SAFETY AND TOLERABILITY OF LEPTIN THERAPY

Studies of physiological replacement doses of leptin in humans with any cause of leptin deficiency utilized 0.02 mg/kg/day to 0.10 mg/kg/day. The leptin levels reported in both the lipodystrophic patients and the patients with congenital leptin deficiency were comparable (5 to 12 ng/mL) early in the course of therapy. In some of these patients, non-neutralizing antibodies were detected beyond one month of therapy, which were not associated with any efficacy or safety parameter alterations. The development of binding antibodies was associated with higher serum leptin concentrations and a delay in the peak concentration after leptin administration. No neutralizing antibodies were observed in any subject with endogenous leptin. There were two subjects with congenital leptin deficiency (who lack circulating leptin, and thus administration of a leptin molecule would be foreign to them), that had a transient loss of biological efficacy associated with evidence of a transient neutralizing antibody, increasing the dose recaptured efficacy.

R-metHuLeptin was generally well tolerated. Neither the patients with congenital leptin deficiency nor the patients with lipodystrophy had significant adverse events that can be attributed definitely to leptin. There were two subjects with lipodystrophy that had a significant progression of their underlying renal disease while on replacement therapy [115]. Importantly, there were no significant injection site reactions in any of the studies utilizing the lower dose range.

The obesity trials utilized higher doses of leptin. Antibody status (positive or negative for the presence of anti-leptin antibodies) had no statistically significant independent effect on weight loss at 4 weeks ($P = .77$) or at 24 weeks ($P = .12$) after accounting for the effects of treatment and dose cohort on weight loss. At 4 weeks, there was no association of the occurrence of adverse events ($P = .11$) with antibody status. By 24 weeks, all subjects had experienced at least 1 adverse event; thus, an association between the overall incidence of adverse events and antibody status could not be determined.

Injection site reactions mild (86%) to moderate (14%) in severity were the most common adverse events are reported in the obesity trials. Injection site reactions were generally well tolerated by most subjects; and withdrawals due to these were rare. The next most common adverse event was headache, which occurred in 38% and 44% of the placebo- and recombinant leptin-treated subjects, respectively. None of the subjects taking recombinant leptin experienced clinically significant adverse effects on major organ systems (central nervous system, cardiovascular, hepatic, renal, gastrointestinal, hematological) as evidenced by adverse event incidence, physical examinations, laboratory values, electrocardiograms, and vital signs.

The data on the safety and tolerability of pegylated-leptin are also encouraging. Overall, the only side effects to note were local injection site reactions which were reported as mild[96-98]. Also, the papers mentioned above note a statistical drop in total protein levels with no change in urinary proteins. Overall, leptin analogues have been well tolerated with no significant attributable adverse events.

Some experimental studies and epidemiological correlative studies of human circulating leptin levels have implicated leptin to be an adverse mediator of hypertension[116], atherogenesis[117-119], hypercoagulopathy[120], hepatic fibrosis[121], bone marrow transformation[122], diabetic retinopathy[123] and other microvascular complications of diabetes[124]. To date, we have not observed any adverse consequences of r-metHuLeptin therapy in the humans receiving long-term therapy to suggest a role for leptin in any of these disease processes. Likewise, we did not observe any adverse effects on bone mass as suggested by some rodent models [125]. Longer follow-up will help to further define these issues.

7. OTHER POTENTIAL APPLICATIONS AND ONGOING STUDIES

While the therapeutic efficacy of r-metHuLeptin in human lipodystrophy syndromes is remarkable, the rarity of these syndromes may be an obstacle in their study. More recently, lipodystrophy has been characterized as part of the HIV syndrome. This is not an uncommon condition and shares features similar to the lipodystrophy syndromes in which the efficacy of r-metHuLeptin therapy is now established. There are ongoing trials assessing the safety and efficacy of r-metHuLeptin therapy in HIV-related lipodystrophy. The results of these studies should become available soon.

Another interesting observation from the lipodystrophy trials was the remarkable anti-steatotic effect of leptin in muscle and liver. Whether these effects of leptin can be translated into therapeutic indications in common lipotoxicity that we observe in human obesity and Type 2 diabetes mellitus remain to be seen. We have begun a pilot study testing the efficacy of leptin therapy in individuals with biopsy proven nonalcoholic steatohepatitis and other metabolic derangements.

Further studies in hypothaloamic amenorrhea will also provide greater insight into the actions of r-metHuLeptin in common states of leptin deficiency. The important implications for women's health need to be further clarified. For example, some experimental studies are suggestive that pharmacological use of leptin may have a role in ovulation induction[126]

As preclinical and clinical leptin research continues to unravel this biology, it wild not be surprising to see therapeutic roles of leptin in unexpected applications, such as wound healing [20,21], Likewise, there is a body of literature supporting a therapeutic role for leptin in sleep disorders such as narcolepsy [127] and sleep apnea[128,129] or even in primary immunodeficiency syndromes.

8. CONCLUSIONS

It is quite clear that leptin has a wide spectrum of physiological actions. It is also noteworthy that a "leptin deficiency syndrome" is characterized by increased appetite, perturbed neuroendocrine (particularly reproductive) function, and immunologic changes. Many features of the leptin deficiency syndrome resemble those seen in the state of profound caloric deprivation. Taken together, the data suggest a threshold leptin level for its regulatory functions. Below this threshold level, leptin deficiency syndrome manifests. Thus, it is not surprising to see the biggest impact of leptin therapy when leptin deficiency syndrome is present.

It is important to distinguish between physiological replacement and pharmacological applications of an agent such as leptin. The spectrum of clinical utility is likely wider than the correction of leptin deficiency. The challenge lies in understanding the mechanisms of leptin responsiveness.

The study of both animal and human states of leptin deficiency has been very fruitful in furthering our understanding of the physiological importance of this hormone in humans. The future therapeutic applications of leptin will be based on further understanding of the regulation and physiological actions of this hormone. Exploration of the therapeutic benefits beyond physiological replacement will require open minds, creative approaches, and more human studies.

While leptin trials in human obesity did not produce the expected weight loss in leptin replete obese humans, these studies suggest that at least a subset of the patients may be responsive to the weight loss effects of leptin. Understanding the heterogeneity underlying obesity and other disorders of adiposity and embracing the possibility of long-term combination therapy may increase our likelihood of success in dealing with these clinical conditions. As is so often the case of a novel therapeutic, the future clinical applications of leptin will likely touch upon areas that were not originally foreseen.

ACKNOWLEDGEMENTS

We wish to thank Drs. Simeon Taylor, Abhimanyu Garg and Phil Gorden for their leadership roles in the lipodystrophy studies. Similarly, Drs. Sadaf Farooqi, Steven O'Rahilly, and Julio Licinio pioneered our understanding of leptin deficient humans. Dr. Chris Mantzoros has spearheaded many important aspects of leptin biology in humans. Equally importantly, we wish to express our gratitude to the subjects who participated in all of the clinical trials. As described in the body of the Chapter, the clinical presentation of patient NIH-1 was one of the driving forces that made the lipodystrophy trial possible; her courage to endure difficulties and trust in science were inspiring. Also, the monumental efforts of all physicians and clinical staff taking part in these studies need to be acknowledged. We especially would like to mention the efforts of Elaine Cochran, R.N whose dedication has been instrumental in the continuation of the lipodystrophy trial into long-term follow-up phase. Dr. Oral has been supported by the NIH-funded Michigan Diabetes and Research Center as well as Michigan Peptide Research Center. Finally, Daphne Scace and Roberta Wilcox provided excellent secretarial and administrative support to the authors.

REFERENCES

1. P. E. Scherer, S. Williams, M. Fogliano, G. Baldini, H. F. Lodish. A novel serum protein similar to C1q, produced exclusively in adipocytes. *J Biol Chem*. 1995;270:26746-9.
2. C. M. Steppan, S. T. Bailey, S. Bhat, E. J. Brown, R. R. Banerjee, C. M. Wright, H. R. Patel, R. S. Ahima, M. A. Lazar. The hormone resistin links obesity to diabetes. *Nature*. 2001;409:307-12.
3. G. S. Hotamisligil, N. S. Shargill, B. M. Spiegelman. Adipose expression of tumor necrosis factor-alpha: direct role in obesity-linked insulin resistance. *Science*. 1993;259:87-91.
4. R. S. Ahima, J. S. Flier. Adipose tissue as an endocrine organ. *Trends Endocrinol Metab*. 2000;11:327-32.
5. R. S. Ahima, J. S. Flier. Leptin. *Annu Rev Physiol*. 2000;62:413-37.
6. A. Fukuhara, M. Matsuda, M. Nishizawa, K. Segawa, M. Tanaka, K. Kishimoto, Y. Matsuki, M. Murakami, T. Ichisaka, H. Murakami, E. Watanabe, T. Takagi, M. Akiyoshi, T. Ohtsubo, S. Kihara, S. Yamashita, M. Makishima, T. Funahashi, S. Yamanaka, R. Hiramatsu, Y. Matsuzawa, I. Shimomura. Visfatin: a protein secreted by visceral fat that mimics the effects of insulin. *Science*. 2005;307:426-30.
7. C. Hug, H. F. Lodish. Medicine. Visfatin: a new adipokine. *Science*. 2005;307:366-7.
8. S. Kralisch, J. Klein, M. Bluher, R. Paschke, M. Stumvoll, M. Fasshauer. Therapeutic perspectives of adipocytokines. *Expert Opin Pharmacother*. 2005;6:863-72.
9. D. Modan-Moses, G. Paret. Leptin and transplantation: pieces are still missing in the puzzle. *Isr Med Assoc J*. 2002;4:207-8.
10. J. Kratzsch, M. Hockel, W. Kiess. Leptin and pregnancy outcome. *Curr Opin Obstet Gynecol*. 2000;12:501-5.
11. W. G. Haynes, D. A. Morgan, S. A. Walsh, A. L. Mark, W. I. Sivitz. Receptor-mediated regional sympathetic nerve activation by leptin. *J Clin Invest*. 1997;100:270-8.
12. J. C. Dunbar, Y. Hu, H. Lu. Intracerebroventricular leptin increases lumbar and renal sympathetic nerve activity and blood pressure in normal rats. *Diabetes*. 1997;46:2040-3.
13. G. Maor, M. Rochwerger, Y. Segev, M. Phillip. Leptin acts as a growth factor on the chondrocytes of skeletal growth centers. *J Bone Miner Res*. 2002;17:1034-43.
14. H. Masuzaki, Y. Ogawa, N. Sagawa, K. Hosoda, T. Matsumoto, H. Mise, H. Nishimura, Y. Yoshimasa, I. Tanaka, T. Mori, K. Nakao. Nonadipose tissue production of leptin: leptin as a novel placenta-derived hormone in humans. *Nat Med*. 1997;3:1029-33.
15. A. A. Mikhail, E. X. Beck, A. Shafer, B. Barut, J. S. Gbur, T. J. Zupancic, A. C. Schweitzer, J. A. Cioffi, G. Lacaud, B. Ouyang, G. Keller, H. R. Snodgrass. Leptin stimulates fetal and adult erythroid and myeloid development. *Blood*. 1997;89:1507-12.
16. J. M. Friedman, J. L. Halaas. Leptin and the regulation of body weight in mammals. *Nature*. 1998;395:763-70.
17. J. S. Flier. Clinical review 94: What's in a name? In search of leptin's physiologic role. *J Clin Endocrinol Metab*. 1998;83:1407-13.

18. N. Hoggard, L. Hunter, J. S. Duncan, L. M. Williams, P. Trayhurn, J. G. Mercer. Leptin and leptin receptor mRNA and protein expression in the murine fetus and placenta. *Proc Natl Acad Sci U S A*. 1997;94:11073-8.
19. T. Gainsford, T. A. Willson, D. Metcalf, E. Handman, C. McFarlane, A. Ng, N. A. Nicola, W. S. Alexander, D. J. Hilton. Leptin can induce proliferation, differentiation, and functional activation of hemopoietic cells. *Proc Natl Acad Sci U S A*. 1996;93:14564-8.
20. S. Frank, B. Stallmeyer, H. Kampfer, N. Kolb, J. Pfeilschifter. Leptin enhances wound re-epithelialization and constitutes a direct function of leptin in skin repair. *J Clin Invest*. 2000;106:501-9.
21. B. D. Ring, S. Scully, C. R. Davis, M. B. Baker, M. J. Cullen, M. A. Pelleymounter, D. M. Danilenko. Systemically and topically administered leptin both accelerate wound healing in diabetic ob/ob mice. *Endocrinology*. 2000;141:446-9.
22. T. Madej, M. S. Boguski, S. H. Bryant. Threading analysis suggests that the obese gene product may be a helical cytokine. *FEBS Lett*. 1995;373:13-8.
23. F. Zhang, M. B. Basinski, J. M. Beals, S. L. Briggs, L. M. Churgay, D. K. Clawson, R. D. DiMarchi, T. C. Furman, J. E. Hale, H. M. Hsiung, B. E. Schoner, D. P. Smith, X. Y. Zhang, J. P. Wery, R. W. Schevitz. Crystal structure of the obese protein leptin-E100. *Nature*. 1997;387:206-9.
24. Y. Zhang, R. Proenca, M. Maffei, M. Barone, L. Leopold, J. M. Friedman. Positional cloning of the mouse obese gene and its human homologue. *Nature*. 1994;372:425-32.
25. N. Isse, Y. Ogawa, N. Tamura, H. Masuzaki, K. Mori, T. Okazaki, N. Satoh, M. Shigemoto, Y. Yoshimasa, S. Nishi, et al. Structural organization and chromosomal assignment of the human obese gene. *J Biol Chem*. 1995;270:27728-33.
26. M. Maffei, J. Halaas, E. Ravussin, R. E. Pratley, G. H. Lee, Y. Zhang, H. Fei, S. Kim, R. Lallone, S. Ranganathan, et al. Leptin levels in human and rodent: measurement of plasma leptin and ob RNA in obese and weight-reduced subjects. *Nat Med*. 1995;1:1155-61.
27. R. V. Considine, M. K. Sinha, M. L. Heiman, A. Kriauciunas, T. W. Stephens, M. R. Nyce, J. P. Ohannesian, C. C. Marco, L. J. McKee, T. L. Bauer, et al. Serum immunoreactive-leptin concentrations in normal-weight and obese humans. *N Engl J Med*. 1996;334:292-5.
28. G. Brabant, H. Nave, B. Mayr, M. Behrend, V. van Harmelen, P. Arner. Secretion of free and protein-bound leptin from subcutaneous adipose tissue of lean and obese women. *J Clin Endocrinol Metab*. 2002;87:3966-70.
29. E. Jequier, L. Tappy. Regulation of body weight in humans. *Physiol Rev*. 1999;79:451-80.
30. J. S. Flier. Leptin expression and action: new experimental paradigms. *Proc Natl Acad Sci U S A*. 1997;94:4242-5.
31. M. Maffei, H. Fei, G. H. Lee, C. Dani, P. Leroy, Y. Zhang, R. Proenca, R. Negrel, G. Ailhaud, J. M. Friedman. Increased expression in adipocytes of ob RNA in mice with lesions of the hypothalamus and with mutations at the db locus. *Proc Natl Acad Sci U S A*. 1995;92:6957-60.
32. T. W. Stephens, M. Basinski, P. K. Bristow, J. M. Bue-Valleskey, S. G. Burgett, L. Craft, J. Hale, J. Hoffmann, H. M. Hsiung, A. Kriauciunas, et al. The role of neuropeptide Y in the antiobesity action of the obese gene product. *Nature*. 1995;377:530-2.
33. C. Vaisse, J. L. Halaas, C. M. Horvath, J. E. Darnell, Jr., M. Stoffel, J. M. Friedman. Leptin activation of Stat3 in the hypothalamus of wild-type and ob/ob mice but not db/db mice. *Nat Genet*. 1996;14:95-7.
34. K. L. Houseknecht, C. A. Baile, R. L. Matteri, M. E. Spurlock. The biology of leptin: a review. *J Anim Sci*. 1998;76:1405-20.

35. J. L. Halaas, K. S. Gajiwala, M. Maffei, S. L. Cohen, B. T. Chait, D. Rabinowitz, R. L. Lallone, S. K. Burley, J. M. Friedman. Weight-reducing effects of the plasma protein encoded by the obese gene. *Science.* 1995;269:543-6.
36. L. A. Campfield, F. J. Smith, Y. Guisez, R. Devos, P. Burn. Recombinant mouse OB protein: evidence for a peripheral signal linking adiposity and central neural networks. *Science.* 1995;269:546-9.
37. M. A. Pelleymounter, M. J. Cullen, M. B. Baker, R. Hecht, D. Winters, T. Boone, F. Collins. Effects of the obese gene product on body weight regulation in ob/ob mice. *Science.* 1995;269:540-3.
38. I. S. Farooqi, J. M. Keogh, S. Kamath, S. Jones, W. T. Gibson, R. Trussell, S. A. Jebb, G. Y. Lip, S. O'Rahilly. Partial leptin deficiency and human adiposity. *Nature.* 2001;414:34-5.
39. C. T. Montague, I. S. Farooqi, J. P. Whitehead, M. A. Soos, H. Rau, N. J. Wareham, C. P. Sewter, J. E. Digby, S. N. Mohammed, J. A. Hurst, C. H. Cheetham, A. R. Earley, A. H. Barnett, J. B. Prins, S. O'Rahilly. Congenital leptin deficiency is associated with severe early-onset obesity in humans. *Nature.* 1997;387:903-8.
40. A. Strobel, T. Issad, L. Camoin, M. Ozata, A. D. Strosberg. A leptin missense mutation associated with hypogonadism and morbid obesity. *Nat Genet.* 1998;18:213-5.
41. K. Clement, C. Vaisse, N. Lahlou, S. Cabrol, V. Pelloux, D. Cassuto, M. Gourmelen, C. Dina, J. Chambaz, J. M. Lacorte, A. Basdevant, P. Bougneres, Y. Lebouc, P. Froguel, B. Guy-Grand. A mutation in the human leptin receptor gene causes obesity and pituitary dysfunction. *Nature.* 1998;392:398-401.
42. H. Rau, B. J. Reaves, S. O'Rahilly, J. P. Whitehead. Truncated human leptin (delta133) associated with extreme obesity undergoes proteasomal degradation after defective intracellular transport. *Endocrinology.* 1999;140:1718-23.
43. J. A. Edwardson, C. A. Hough. The pituitary-adrenal system of the genetically obese (ob/ob) mouse. *J Endocrinol.* 1975;65:99-107.
44. P. U. Dubuc. The development of obesity, hyperinsulinemia, and hyperglycemia in ob/ob mice. *Metabolism.* 1976;25:1567-74.
45. I. S. Farooqi, S. A. Jebb, G. Langmack, E. Lawrence, C. H. Cheetham, A. M. Prentice, I. A. Hughes, M. A. McCamish, S. O'Rahilly. Effects of recombinant leptin therapy in a child with congenital leptin deficiency. *N Engl J Med.* 1999;341:879-84.
46. I. S. Farooqi, G. Matarese, G. M. Lord, J. M. Keogh, E. Lawrence, C. Agwu, V. Sanna, S. A. Jebb, F. Perna, S. Fontana, R. I. Lechler, A. M. DePaoli, S. O'Rahilly. Beneficial effects of leptin on obesity, T cell hyporesponsiveness, and neuroendocrine/metabolic dysfunction of human congenital leptin deficiency. *J Clin Invest.* 2002;110:1093-103.
47. I. A. Barash, C. C. Cheung, D. S. Weigle, H. Ren, E. B. Kabigting, J. L. Kuijper, D. K. Clifton, R. A. Steiner. Leptin is a metabolic signal to the reproductive system. *Endocrinology.* 1996;137:3144-7.
48. J. A. Cioffi, A. W. Shafer, T. J. Zupancic, J. Smith-Gbur, A. Mikhail, D. Platika, H. R. Snodgrass. Novel B219/OB receptor isoforms: possible role of leptin in hematopoiesis and reproduction. *Nat Med.* 1996;2:585-9.
49. M. Ozata, I. C. Ozdemir, J. Licinio. Human leptin deficiency caused by a missense mutation: multiple endocrine defects, decreased sympathetic tone, and immune system dysfunction indicate new targets for leptin action, greater central than peripheral resistance to the effects of leptin, and spontaneous correction of leptin-mediated defects. *J Clin Endocrinol Metab.* 1999;84:3686-95.
50. J. Licinio, S. Caglayan, M. Ozata, B. O. Yildiz, P. B. de Miranda, F. O'Kirwan, R. Whitby, L. Liang, P. Cohen, S. Bhasin, R. M. Krauss, J. D. Veldhuis, A. J. Wagner, A. M. DePaoli, S. M. McCann, M. L. Wong. Phenotypic effects of leptin

replacement on morbid obesity, diabetes mellitus, hypogonadism, and behavior in leptin-deficient adults. *Proc Natl Acad Sci U S A*. 2004;101:4531-6.
51. W. T. Gibson, I. S. Farooqi, M. Moreau, A. M. DePaoli, E. Lawrence, S. O'Rahilly, R. A. Trussell. Congenital leptin deficiency due to homozygosity for the Delta133G mutation: report of another case and evaluation of response to four years of leptin therapy. *J Clin Endocrinol Metab*. 2004;89:4821-6.
52. G. Fantuzzi. Adipose tissue, adipokines, and inflammation. *J Allergy Clin Immunol*. 2005;115:911-9; quiz 920.
53. J. M. Montez, A. Soukas, E. Asilmaz, G. Fayzikhodjaeva, G. Fantuzzi, J. M. Friedman. Acute leptin deficiency, leptin resistance, and the physiologic response to leptin withdrawal. *Proc Natl Acad Sci U S A*. 2005;102:2537-42.
54. M. L. Reitman, E. Arioglu, O. Gavrilova, S. I. Taylor. Lipoatrophy revisited. *Trends Endocrinol Metab*. 2000;11:410-6.
55. E. A. Oral, V. Simha, E. Ruiz, A. Andewelt, A. Premkumar, P. Snell, A. J. Wagner, A. M. DePaoli, M. L. Reitman, S. I. Taylor, P. Gorden, A. Garg. Leptin-replacement therapy for lipodystrophy. *N Engl J Med*. 2002;346:570-8.
56. K. F. Petersen, E. A. Oral, S. Dufour, D. Befroy, C. Ariyan, C. Yu, G. W. Cline, A. M. DePaoli, S. I. Taylor, P. Gorden, G. I. Shulman. Leptin reverses insulin resistance and hepatic steatosis in patients with severe lipodystrophy. *J Clin Invest*. 2002;109:1345-50.
57. V. C. Pardini, I. M. Victoria, S. M. Rocha, D. G. Andrade, A. M. Rocha, F. B. Pieroni, G. Milagres, S. Purisch, G. Velho. Leptin levels, beta-cell function, and insulin sensitivity in families with congenital and acquired generalized lipoatropic diabetes. *J Clin Endocrinol Metab*. 1998;83:503-8.
58. E. A. Oral. Lipoatrophic diabetes and other related syndromes. *Rev Endocr Metab Disord*. 2003;4:61-77.
59. I. Shimomura, R. E. Hammer, S. Ikemoto, M. S. Brown, J. L. Goldstein. Leptin reverses insulin resistance and diabetes mellitus in mice with congenital lipodystrophy. *Nature*. 1999;401:73-6.
60. K. Ebihara, Y. Ogawa, H. Masuzaki, M. Shintani, F. Miyanaga, M. Aizawa-Abe, T. Hayashi, K. Hosoda, G. Inoue, Y. Yoshimasa, O. Gavrilova, M. L. Reitman, K. Nakao. Transgenic overexpression of leptin rescues insulin resistance and diabetes in a mouse model of lipoatrophic diabetes. *Diabetes*. 2001;50:1440-8.
61. V. Simha, L. S. Szczepaniak, A. J. Wagner, A. M. DePaoli, A. Garg. Effect of leptin replacement on intrahepatic and intramyocellular lipid content in patients with generalized lipodystrophy. *Diabetes Care*. 2003;26:30-5.
62. S. A. Moran, N. Patten, J. R. Young, E. Cochran, N. Sebring, J. Reynolds, A. Premkumar, A. M. Depaoli, M. C. Skarulis, E. A. Oral, P. Gorden. Changes in body composition in patients with severe lipodystrophy after leptin replacement therapy. *Metabolism*. 2004;53:513-9.
63. E. D. Javor, M. G. Ghany, E. K. Cochran, E. A. Oral, A. M. DePaoli, A. Premkumar, D. E. Kleiner, P. Gorden. Leptin reverses nonalcoholic steatohepatitis in patients with severe lipodystrophy. *Hepatology*. 2005;41:753-60.
64. G. Marchesini, M. Brizi, A. M. Morselli-Labate, G. Bianchi, E. Bugianesi, A. J. McCullough, G. Forlani, N. Melchionda. Association of nonalcoholic fatty liver disease with insulin resistance. *Am J Med*. 1999;107:450-5.
65. G. Marchesini, M. Brizi, G. Bianchi, S. Tomassetti, E. Bugianesi, M. Lenzi, A. J. McCullough, S. Natale, G. Forlani, N. Melchionda. Nonalcoholic fatty liver disease: a feature of the metabolic syndrome. *Diabetes*. 2001;50:1844-50.
66. L. Ryysy, A. M. Hakkinen, T. Goto, S. Vehkavaara, J. Westerbacka, J. Halavaara, H. Yki-Jarvinen. Hepatic fat content and insulin action on free fatty acids and glucose metabolism rather than insulin absorption are associated with insulin

requirements during insulin therapy in type 2 diabetic patients. *Diabetes.* 2000;49:749-58.
67. M. Krssak, K. Falk Petersen, A. Dresner, L. DiPietro, S. M. Vogel, D. L. Rothman, M. Roden, G. I. Shulman. Intramyocellular lipid concentrations are correlated with insulin sensitivity in humans: a 1H NMR spectroscopy study. *Diabetologia.* 1999;42:113-6.
68. S. Jacob, J. Machann, K. Rett, K. Brechtel, A. Volk, W. Renn, E. Maerker, S. Matthaei, F. Schick, C. D. Claussen, H. U. Haring. Association of increased intramyocellular lipid content with insulin resistance in lean nondiabetic offspring of type 2 diabetic subjects. *Diabetes.* 1999;48:1113-9.
69. N. G. Forouhi, G. Jenkinson, E. L. Thomas, S. Mullick, S. Mierisova, U. Bhonsle, P. M. McKeigue, J. D. Bell. Relation of triglyceride stores in skeletal muscle cells to central obesity and insulin sensitivity in European and South Asian men. *Diabetologia.* 1999;42:932-5.
70. A. Virkamaki, E. Korsheninnikova, A. Seppala-Lindroos, S. Vehkavaara, T. Goto, J. Halavaara, A. M. Hakkinen, H. Yki-Jarvinen. Intramyocellular lipid is associated with resistance to in vivo insulin actions on glucose uptake, antilipolysis, and early insulin signaling pathways in human skeletal muscle. *Diabetes.* 2001;50:2337-43.
71. L. S. Szczepaniak, E. E. Babcock, F. Schick, R. L. Dobbins, A. Garg, D. K. Burns, J. D. McGarry, D. T. Stein. Measurement of intracellular triglyceride stores by H spectroscopy: validation in vivo. *Am J Physiol.* 1999;276:E977-89.
72. A. B. Mayerson, R. S. Hundal, S. Dufour, V. Lebon, D. Befroy, G. W. Cline, S. Enocksson, S. E. Inzucchi, G. I. Shulman, K. F. Petersen. The effects of rosiglitazone on insulin sensitivity, lipolysis, and hepatic and skeletal muscle triglyceride content in patients with type 2 diabetes. *Diabetes.* 2002;51:797-802.
73. A. Dresner, D. Laurent, M. Marcucci, M. E. Griffin, S. Dufour, G. W. Cline, L. A. Slezak, D. K. Andersen, R. S. Hundal, D. L. Rothman, K. F. Petersen, G. I. Shulman. Effects of free fatty acids on glucose transport and IRS-1-associated phosphatidylinositol 3-kinase activity. *J Clin Invest.* 1999;103:253-9.
74. M. E. Griffin, M. J. Marcucci, G. W. Cline, K. Bell, N. Barucci, D. Lee, L. J. Goodyear, E. W. Kraegen, M. F. White, G. I. Shulman. Free fatty acid-induced insulin resistance is associated with activation of protein kinase C theta and alterations in the insulin signaling cascade. *Diabetes.* 1999;48:1270-4.
75. J. K. Kim, O. Gavrilova, Y. Chen, M. L. Reitman, G. I. Shulman. Mechanism of insulin resistance in A-ZIP/F-1 fatless mice. *J Biol Chem.* 2000;275:8456-60.
76. J. K. Kim, J. J. Fillmore, Y. Chen, C. Yu, I. K. Moore, M. Pypaert, E. P. Lutz, Y. Kako, W. Velez-Carrasco, I. J. Goldberg, J. L. Breslow, G. I. Shulman. Tissue-specific overexpression of lipoprotein lipase causes tissue-specific insulin resistance. *Proc Natl Acad Sci U S A.* 2001;98:7522-7.
77. G. Perseghin, P. Scifo, F. De Cobelli, E. Pagliato, A. Battezzati, C. Arcelloni, A. Vanzulli, G. Testolin, G. Pozza, A. Del Maschio, L. Luzi. Intramyocellular triglyceride content is a determinant of in vivo insulin resistance in humans: a 1H-13C nuclear magnetic resonance spectroscopy assessment in offspring of type 2 diabetic parents. *Diabetes.* 1999;48:1600-6.
78. K. F. Petersen, G. I. Shulman. Pathogenesis of skeletal muscle insulin resistance in type 2 diabetes mellitus. *Am J Cardiol.* 2002;90:11G-18G.
79. A. V. Greco, G. Mingrone, A. Giancaterini, M. Manco, M. Morroni, S. Cinti, M. Granzotto, R. Vettor, S. Camastra, E. Ferrannini. Insulin resistance in morbid obesity: reversal with intramyocellular fat depletion. *Diabetes.* 2002;51:144-51.
80. Y. Minokoshi, Y. B. Kim, O. D. Peroni, L. G. Fryer, C. Muller, D. Carling, B. B. Kahn. Leptin stimulates fatty-acid oxidation by activating AMP-activated protein kinase. *Nature.* 2002;415:339-43.

81. D. M. Muoio, G. L. Dohm, F. T. Fiedorek, Jr., E. B. Tapscott, R. A. Coleman, G. L. Dohn. Leptin directly alters lipid partitioning in skeletal muscle. *Diabetes.* 1997;46:1360-3.
82. N. B. Ruderman, A. K. Saha, D. Vavvas, L. A. Witters. Malonyl-CoA, fuel sensing, and insulin resistance. *Am J Physiol.* 1999;276:E1-E18.
83. A. W. Ferrante, Jr., M. Thearle, T. Liao, R. L. Leibel. Effects of leptin deficiency and short-term repletion on hepatic gene expression in genetically obese mice. *Diabetes.* 2001;50:2268-78.
84. Y. Lee, M. Y. Wang, T. Kakuma, Z. W. Wang, E. Babcock, K. McCorkle, M. Higa, Y. T. Zhou, R. H. Unger. Liporegulation in diet-induced obesity. The antisteatotic role of hyperleptinemia. *J Biol Chem.* 2001;276:5629-35.
85. J. R. McDuffie, P. A. Riggs, K. A. Calis, R. J. Freedman, E. A. Oral, A. M. DePaoli, J. A. Yanovski. Effects of exogenous leptin on satiety and satiation in patients with lipodystrophy and leptin insufficiency. *J Clin Endocrinol Metab.* 2004;89:4258-63.
86. V. Simha, J. E. Zerwekh, K. Sakhaee, A. Garg. Effect of subcutaneous leptin replacement therapy on bone metabolism in patients with generalized lipodystrophy. *J Clin Endocrinol Metab.* 2002;87:4942-5.
87. E. A. Oral, E. Javor, L. Ding, Uzel G., E. K. Cochran, J. R. Young, A. DePaoli, S. M. Holland, P. Gorden. Leptin replacement therapy modulates circulating lymphocyte subsets and T-cell responsiveness in severe lipodystrophy. *J Clin Endocrin and Metabolism.* 2005.
88. E. D. Javor, E. K. Cochran, C. Musso, J. R. Young, A. M. Depaoli, P. Gorden. Long-term efficacy of leptin replacement in patients with generalized lipodystrophy. *Diabetes.* 2005;54:1994-2002.
89. K. Ebihara, H. Masuzaki, K. Nakao. Long-term leptin-replacement therapy for lipoatrophic diabetes. *N Engl J Med.* 2004;351:615-6.
90. C. Musso, E. Cochran, E. Javor, J. Young, A. M. Depaoli, P. Gorden. The long-term effect of recombinant methionyl human leptin therapy on hyperandrogenism and menstrual function in female and pituitary function in male and female hypoleptinemic lipodystrophic patients. *Metabolism.* 2005;54:255-63.
91. E. Cochran, J. R. Young, N. Sebring, A. DePaoli, E. A. Oral, P. Gorden. Efficacy of recombinant methionyl human leptin therapy for the extreme insulin resistance of the Rabson-Mendenhall syndrome. *J Clin Endocrinol Metab.* 2004;89:1548-54.
92. Y. Takahashi, H. Kadowaki, A. Ando, J. D. Quin, A. C. MacCuish, Y. Yazaki, Y. Akanuma, T. Kadowaki. Two aberrant splicings caused by mutations in the insulin receptor gene in cultured lymphocytes from a patient with Rabson-Mendenhall's syndrome. *J Clin Invest.* 1998;101:588-94.
93. P. Roach, Y. Zick, P. Formisano, D. Accili, S. I. Taylor, P. Gorden. A novel human insulin receptor gene mutation uniquely inhibits insulin binding without impairing posttranslational processing. *Diabetes.* 1994;43:1096-102.
94. C. K. Welt, J. L. Chan, J. Bullen, R. Murphy, P. Smith, A. M. DePaoli, A. Karalis, C. S. Mantzoros. Recombinant human leptin in women with hypothalamic amenorrhea. *N Engl J Med.* 2004;351:987-97.
95. S. B. Heymsfield, A. S. Greenberg, K. Fujioka, R. M. Dixon, R. Kushner, T. Hunt, J. A. Lubina, J. Patane, B. Self, P. Hunt, M. McCamish. Recombinant leptin for weight loss in obese and lean adults: a randomized, controlled, dose-escalation trial. *Jama.* 1999;282:1568-75.
96. C. J. Hukshorn, W. H. Saris, M. S. Westerterp-Plantenga, A. R. Farid, F. J. Smith, L. A. Campfield. Weekly subcutaneous pegylated recombinant native human leptin (PEG-OB) administration in obese men. *J Clin Endocrinol Metab.* 2000;85:4003-9.
97. C. J. Hukshorn, F. M. van Dielen, W. A. Buurman, M. S. Westerterp-Plantenga, L. A. Campfield, W. H. Saris. The effect of pegylated recombinant human leptin

(PEG-OB) on weight loss and inflammatory status in obese subjects. *Int J Obes Relat Metab Disord.* 2002;26:504-9.
98. C. J. Hukshorn, M. S. Westerterp-Plantenga, W. H. Saris. Pegylated human recombinant leptin (PEG-OB) causes additional weight loss in severely energy-restricted, overweight men. *Am J Clin Nutr.* 2003;77:771-6.
99. R. L. Leibel, M. Rosenbaum, J. Hirsch. Changes in energy expenditure resulting from altered body weight. *N Engl J Med.* 1995;332:621-8.
100. M. Rosenbaum, J. Hirsch, E. Murphy, R. L. Leibel. Effects of changes in body weight on carbohydrate metabolism, catecholamine excretion, and thyroid function. *Am J Clin Nutr.* 2000;71:1421-32.
101. R. S. Ahima, D. Prabakaran, C. Mantzoros, D. Qu, B. Lowell, E. Maratos-Flier, J. S. Flier. Role of leptin in the neuroendocrine response to fasting. *Nature.* 1996;382:250-2.
102. M. Rosenbaum, M. Nicolson, J. Hirsch, E. Murphy, F. Chu, R. L. Leibel. Effects of weight change on plasma leptin concentrations and energy expenditure. *J Clin Endocrinol Metab.* 1997;82:3647-54.
103. M. Rosenbaum, E. M. Murphy, S. B. Heymsfield, D. E. Matthews, R. L. Leibel. Low dose leptin administration reverses effects of sustained weight-reduction on energy expenditure and circulating concentrations of thyroid hormones. *J Clin Endocrinol Metab.* 2002;87:2391-4.
104. D. W. Lee, M. C. Leinung, M. Rozhavskaya-Arena, P. Grasso. Leptin and the treatment of obesity: its current status. *Eur J Pharmacol.* 2002;440:129-39.
105. S. Klein, J. F. Horowitz, M. Landt, S. J. Goodrick, V. Mohamed-Ali, S. W. Coppack. Leptin production during early starvation in lean and obese women. *Am J Physiol Endocrinol Metab.* 2000;278:E280-4.
106. S. L. Wong, A. M. DePaoli, J. H. Lee, C. S. Mantzoros. Leptin hormonal kinetics in the fed state: effects of adiposity, age, and gender on endogenous leptin production and clearance rates. *J Clin Endocrinol Metab.* 2004;89:2672-7.
107. L. A. Campfield, F. J. Smith. Overview: neurobiology of OB protein (leptin). *Proc Nutr Soc.* 1998;57:429-40.
108. K. El-Haschimi, H. Lehnert. Leptin resistance - or why leptin fails to work in obesity. *Exp Clin Endocrinol Diabetes.* 2003;111:2-7.
109. J. F. Caro, J. W. Kolaczynski, M. R. Nyce, J. P. Ohannesian, I. Opentanova, W. H. Goldman, R. B. Lynn, P. L. Zhang, M. K. Sinha, R. V. Considine. Decreased cerebrospinal-fluid/serum leptin ratio in obesity: a possible mechanism for leptin resistance. *Lancet.* 1996;348:159-61.
110. M. W. Schwartz, E. Peskind, M. Raskind, E. J. Boyko, D. Porte, Jr. Cerebrospinal fluid leptin levels: relationship to plasma levels and to adiposity in humans. *Nat Med.* 1996;2:589-93.
111. S. Y. Nam, J. Kratzsch, K. W. Kim, K. R. Kim, S. K. Lim, C. Marcus. Cerebrospinal fluid and plasma concentrations of leptin, NPY, and alpha-MSH in obese women and their relationship to negative energy balance. *J Clin Endocrinol Metab.* 2001;86:4849-53.
112. K. Fujioka, J. Patane, J. Lubina, D. Lau. CSF leptin levels after exogenous administration of recombinant methionyl human leptin. *Jama.* 1999;282:1517-8.
113. C. M. Kotz, J. E. Briggs, M. K. Grace, A. S. Levine, C. J. Billington. Divergence of the feeding and thermogenic pathways influenced by NPY in the hypothalamic PVN of the rat. *Am J Physiol.* 1998;275:R471-7.
114. Y. Toyoshima, O. Gavrilova, S. Yakar, W. Jou, S. Pack, Z. Asghar, M. B. Wheeler, D. LeRoith. Leptin improves insulin resistance and hyperglycemia in a mouse model of type 2 diabetes. *Endocrinology.* 2005;146:4024-35.
115. E. D. Javor, S. A. Moran, J. R. Young, E. K. Cochran, A. M. DePaoli, E. A. Oral, M. A. Turman, P. R. Blackett, D. B. Savage, S. O'Rahilly, J. E. Balow, P. Gorden.

Proteinuric nephropathy in acquired and congenital generalized lipodystrophy: baseline characteristics and course during recombinant leptin therapy. *J Clin Endocrinol Metab.* 2004;89:3199-207.

116. R. Schutte, H. W. Huisman, A. E. Schutte, N. T. Malan. Leptin is independently associated with systolic blood pressure, pulse pressure and arterial compliance in hypertensive African women with increased adiposity: the POWIRS study. *J Hum Hypertens.* 2005;19:535-41.

117. P. F. Bodary, S. Gu, Y. Shen, A. H. Hasty, J. M. Buckler, D. T. Eitzman. Recombinant Leptin Promotes Atherosclerosis and Thrombosis in Apolipoprotein E-Deficient Mice. *Arterioscler Thromb Vasc Biol.* 2005;25:1634.

118. P. F. Bodary, S. Gu, Y. Shen, A. H. Hasty, J. M. Buckler, D. T. Eitzman. Recombinant leptin promotes atherosclerosis and thrombosis in apolipoprotein E-deficient mice. *Arterioscler Thromb Vasc Biol.* 2005;25:e119-22.

119. P. F. Bodary, R. J. Westrick, K. J. Wickenheiser, Y. Shen, D. T. Eitzman. Effect of leptin on arterial thrombosis following vascular injury in mice. *Jama.* 2002;287:1706-9.

120. M. T. Guagnano, M. Romano, A. Falco, M. Nutini, M. Marinopiccoli, M. R. Manigrasso, S. Basili, G. Davi. Leptin increase is associated with markers of the hemostatic system in obese healthy women. *J Thromb Haemost.* 2003;1:2330-4.

121. K. Ikejima, H. Honda, M. Yoshikawa, M. Hirose, T. Kitamura, Y. Takei, N. Sato. Leptin augments inflammatory and profibrogenic responses in the murine liver induced by hepatotoxic chemicals. *Hepatology.* 2001;34:288-97.

122. M. Hino, T. Nakao, T. Yamane, K. Ohta, T. Takubo, N. Tatsumi. Leptin receptor and leukemia. *Leuk Lymphoma.* 2000;36:457-61.

123. E. Suganami, H. Takagi, H. Ohashi, K. Suzuma, I. Suzuma, H. Oh, D. Watanabe, T. Ojima, T. Suganami, Y. Fujio, K. Nakao, Y. Ogawa, N. Yoshimura. Leptin stimulates ischemia-induced retinal neovascularization: possible role of vascular endothelial growth factor expressed in retinal endothelial cells. *Diabetes.* 2004;53:2443-8.

124. G. Wolf, S. Chen, D. C. Han, F. N. Ziyadeh. Leptin and renal disease. *Am J Kidney Dis.* 2002;39:1-11.

125. P. Ducy, M. Amling, S. Takeda, M. Priemel, A. F. Schilling, F. T. Beil, J. Shen, C. Vinson, J. M. Rueger, G. Karsenty. Leptin inhibits bone formation through a hypothalamic relay: a central control of bone mass. *Cell.* 2000;100:197-207.

126. D. Barkan, V. Hurgin, N. Dekel, A. Amsterdam, M. Rubinstein. Leptin induces ovulation in GnRH-deficient mice. *Faseb J.* 2005;19:133-5.

127. S. W. Kok, F. Roelfsema, S. Overeem, G. J. Lammers, M. Frolich, A. E. Meinders, H. Pijl. Altered setting of the pituitary-thyroid ensemble in hypocretin-deficient narcoleptic men. *Am J Physiol Endocrinol Metab.* 2005;288:E892-9.

128. P. O'Donnell C, C. D. Schaub, A. S. Haines, D. E. Berkowitz, C. G. Tankersley, A. R. Schwartz, P. L. Smith. Leptin prevents respiratory depression in obesity. *Am J Respir Crit Care Med.* 1999;159:1477-84.

129. K. Tatsumi, Y. Kasahara, K. Kurosu, N. Tanabe, Y. Takiguchi, T. Kuriyama. Sleep oxygen desaturation and circulating leptin in obstructive sleep apnea-hypopnea syndrome. *Chest.* 2005;127:716-21.

INDEX

Abdominal adipocytes, 94
Acetylcholine, 85
Acquired generalized lipodystrophy, 223
Acquired murine lipodystrophy, 226
Acquired partial lipodystrophy, 222
Activated protein kinase, 229
Activity levels, 85
Acute fast, 280
Acute phase response, 128
Acute lymphoblastic leukemia, 204
Acute promyelocytic leukemia, 203
Acute sepsis, 39
Acute starvation, 135
ACTH, 110-111, 255, 337
Activity levels, 6
Acyl CoA synthetase, 262
Adenoviral gene therapy, 85
Adhesion molecules, 128
Adrb-2 deficient mice, 142
Adipocytes, 39, 43, 110, 114-115, 151, 162, 232 262, 273-274, 326
Adipocyte hypertrophy, 132
Adipocyte-insular axis, 97
Adipocyte size, 38
Adipogenesis, 90
Adiponectin, 115, 197, 225-226, 230, 232, 330
Adipo-insular axis, 87, 90
Adipose tissue, 37, 39-40, 42-43, 115-116, 153, 230, 275
Adipose tissue deposits, 34
Adipose tissue unilocularity, 276
Adipostatic theory, 305
Adjacent mucosa, 201
Adrenal, 17, 42, 106, 180, 337
Adrenal function, 110, 112
Adrenalectomy, 164, 275
Adrenocorticotropic hormone (ACTH), 278
Adult male mice, 167
Aggregation of platelets, 186
Aggressive behaviour, 312
Agouti-related disease, 181, 306

Agouti-related peptide, 18, 56, 229
Agouti yellow mice, 141, 182
Agouti obese mouse, 176, 179
Agouti-related protein (AgRP), 57, 60-61, 67, 108, 116, 278
Alpha adrenergic, 182
Alternative splicing, 277
Aminopeptidases (A&B), 271
AML, 204, 206
Amnion, 160, 164
Amniotic fluid leptin levels, 164
Amphetamine-regulated transcript, 56
Anandamide, 194
Androgens, 151
Androgen receptor, 167
Angiogenic properties, 268
Angiogenesis, 125, 133, 162, 176, 195, 271, 326
Angiostatin, 131
Animals, 105
Animal leptin assays, 318-321
Anorectic, 55
Anorectic peptides, 61
Anorexia nervosa, 194
Anterior pituitary, 106, 152, 278
Antibodies, 134
Antiestrogen therapy, 205
Anti-diabetogenic protein, 79
Anti-inflammatory mediators, 132
Anti-leptin antibodies, 270, 309, 347
Antiretroviral drug-induced lipodystrophy, 226
Antiosteogenic action of leptin, 142
Approximate entropy (ApEn), 255
ARC, 60-61, 63, 65-66
Arcuate nucleus, 40, 55, 116, 151-152, 278, 309
ARKO mice, 167
Arterial baroreceptors, 180
Arterial pressure, 176, 182
Arthritis, 134
Apoptosis, 129
Appetite regulation, 5
ATF4-RANKL, 143
Atherogenesis, 348

Atherothrombosis, 42
Autoimmune hypothyroidism, 321
Autoimmunity, 127, 129-131, 135
Autonomic nervous system, 176

Baboon, 17, 160-163
Backfat thickness, 21
Baroreflex activation, 177
Barraquer-Simons syndrome, 223
Basal FSH & LH concentrations, 330
Basal temperature, 312
Bat, 17
B cells, 128
Benign prostatic hyperplasia, 199
Berardinelli-Seip congenital
  lipodystophy 2 (BSCL2) gene, 219
Beta-endorphin, 278
BeWo choriocarcinoma cells, 165
Binding protein for leptin, 20
Bioactive leptin, 160
Blastocyst endometrial dialogue, 161
Blood brain barrier, 19-20, 40, 56, 160, 261
Blood brain transport, 66
Blood flow, 261
Blood glucose levels, 80
Blood mononuclear cells, 270
Blood pressure, 42, 176, 181, 185, 326
Body fat, 151, 257
Body mass index (BMI), 151
Body temperature, 5-6, 85, 265
Body weight regulation, 55
Bone alkaline phosphatase, 342
Bone and cartilage, 267
Bone formation, 139, 268
Bone marrow adipocytes, 140
Bone marrow human, 195
Bone marrow transformation, 348
Bone marrow transplant, 186
Bone mass, 69, 139, 142-144, 162, 267
Bone metabolic markers, 143
Bone mineral density, 21, 338
Bone remodeling, 269
Bone resorption, 139, 142-143, 162
Bone specific alkaline phosphatase, 338
Bovine, 274, 283
Bovine mammary gland, 263
Brain, 17
Brain-derived neurotrophic factor (BDNF), 59
BRCA1, 197
Breast cancer, 133, 195-198, 205
Brown adipose tissue, 84, 177, 180-181
Brush border, 271
B-lymphocytes, 339

Calcium dependent, 264
Caloric deprivation, 116
Caloric restriction, 105
cAMP, 64, 93
Cancer, 18
Cancer cachexia, 201

Cancer and leptin, 193
Capacitated sperm, 167
Carcinogenesis, 196, 206
Cardiomyocyte hypertrophy, 185
Cardiomyopathy, 184, 219
Cardiovascular disease, 115, 175-176, 229
Cardiovascular homeostasis, 176
Carnitine palmitoyltransferase I, 263, 265
CART, 61, 143
Cartilage and bone, 267
Caspase 8, 226
Catecholamines, 56, 112, 141, 177-178, 253
Cattle adipose tissue, 266
Caudal brain stem nuclei, 61
Caudal dorsomedial nucleus, 152
CC-chemokine ligand, 130
CD3 T cell, 332
CD4 T cell, 126, 129, 332, 338
CD8 T cell, 126, 128-129, 332, 338
Cell mediated immunity, 128
Central administration of leptin, 278
Central hypothyroidism, 309
Central injection of leptin, 55
Central nervous system, 154, 248
Cerebrospinal fluid, 19, 40, 66, 346
Cerebrospinal fluid leptin levels, 40
C/EBP, 96
C/EBPα protein, 274
c-fos, 58, 61, 127
c-jun, 127
C-reactive protein, 201
Chemical symapathectomy, 183
Chemokines, 130
Chemotactic response, 268
Chemotaxis, 127
Chemotherapy, 196
Chicken, 21, 261, 267
Chief cells, 272
Cholecystokinin (CCK), 60-61, 69, 85, 200, 272
Chondrocyte, 140
Chondrocyte differentiation, 268
Chorion, 160-161
Chronic heart failure, 184
Chronic myeloid leukemia, 204
Circadian clock, 253
Circadian rhythm, 108, 248
Circulating human leptin, 255
Circulating norepinephrine levels, 178
Citrate lyase, 266
Class I cytokine receptor, 12, 127, 269, 277-278
Clinical medicine, 143
Clomiphene citrate (CC) medication, 157
CNS melanocortin system, 58
Coagulation, 326
Cocaine and amphetamine-regulated transcript 56,
  116, 180, 229, 278
Collagen-Iα, 268
Colonic epithelial cells, 195
Colonic tumor resections, 201
Colon cancer, 201-202, 206

Colorectal cancer, 133
Combination antiretroviral therapy, 222
Complete caloric restriction, 38
Competitive immunoassays for leptin, 318
Concanavalin A (ConA), 130
Congenital leptin deficiency, 109, 306, 347
Congenital leptin mutations, 332
Congenital generalized lipoatrophy (CGL), 218-219
Congenital murine lipoatrophy (CGL), 223
Conjoined twins, 3
Controlled ovarian hyperstimulation (COH), 157-159
Coronary heart disease, 165, 176
Corpus luteu, 160
Corticosteroids, 253
Corticosterone, 110, 307, 311
Corticotropes, 106, 342
Corticotropin-releasing hormone (CRH), 56, 111, 117, 180
Cortisol, 39, 93, 112, 153, 248, 255, 275, 307, 312, 331, 337, 342
Cow, 278, 282-283
CRH, 59-61, 69, 111, 337
Critical body weight, 281
Cultured cytotrophoblast cells, 161
Cultured omental adipose tissue, 110
Cytokines, 39, 115, 130, 161, 269, 339
Cytokine signaling (SOCS), 40, 108
Cytostolic calcium concentration, 81
Cytotrophoblast cells, 160
C-terminal leptin fragment, 320

Dairy cattle, 21
Day length, 283
db/db, 128, 140, 179-181, 270
db/db mice, 43, 54, 85, 115, 179-180, 185-186 202, 229, 265, 306
Decidual tissue, 160-161, 163-164
Deoxypyridinoline, 338
Dephosphorylation of IRS-1, 262
Depressor effects of leptin, 182
Dermal fibroblasts, 270
Development of pubic and axillary hair, 331
Dexamethasone, 112, 164, 273
Diabetes, 79, 95, 115-116, 229
Diabetes (*db*) genes, 3
Diabetes mellitus, 165
Diabetic (*db/db*) mouse, 3-7, 12, 18-19
Diabetic retinopathy, 131-132, 348
Diacylglycerol acyltransferase, 262
Diet-induced mice, 42, 182
Diet-induced obesity, 40, 63, 66, 87, 89, 179, 229, 342
Digestive mucosa, 201
DIO, 67, 230
Distal pulmonary epithelial cells, 162
Diurnal leptin rhythms, 247-248
Diurnal oscillations, 249
Diurnal pattern, 36
Diurnal secretion of TSH, 108
DMN, 60-61, 63, 65

DNA synthesis, 110
Dog, 176
Domain structure of leptin receptor, 12
Dominant follicles, 159, 341
Dsylipidemia, 176
Dual energy x-ray absorptiometry, 338
Ductal breast tumors, 196
DU 145, 199
Dunnigan variety, 220

E_2 levels, 159
Early onset obesity, 306
Embryo development, 131, 161
Embryonic chick muscel cell cultures, 264
Endochondral ossification, 162
Endocrine organ, 115
Endocrine system, 103
Endogenous leptin secretion, 253
Endometriosis, 21
Endometrial, 164, 195, 198
Endostatin, 131
Endothelial cells, 183
Endotoxemia, 269
Energy balance, 150, 336
Energy expenditure, 40, 54, 265
Energy homeostasis, 55, 69
Energy intake, 40
Environmental, 54
Enzyme linked immunosorbent assay (ELISA) 319
Epididymal fat pads, 267
Epinephrine, 177
erB2, 15
ERK, 15
ERK2 phosphorylation, 200
Erythroid development, 203
Esophageal cancer, 203
Esophagus, 195
Estradiol benzoate, 166
Estradiol benzoate-treated ovariectomized female rats, 152-153
Estrogen, 35, 151, 154, 277, 280
Estrogen deficiency, 269
Estrogen independent tumors, 197
Estrogen induced leptin mRNA expression, 282
Estrogen receptor, 196, 205
Euglycemic clamp, 94
Ewe, 277-278, 280-283
Exercise induced hypothalamic amenorrhoea, 194
Exogenous leptin administration, 255
Experimental autoimmune encephalomyelitis (EAE), 12, 129
Experimentally induced colitis (EIC), 130
Experimentally induced glomerulonephritis, 130
Experimentally induced hepatitis (EIH), 129

fa/fa rats, 43, 94, 115
Facial hair, 331
Familial partial lipodystrophy, 220-221
Fasting, 61, 153, 322
Fasting plasma leptin, 257

Fat, 17
Fat cell volume, 38, 151, 275-276
Fat distribution, 34
Fatty acid esterification, 262
Fatty acid oxidation, 336
Fatty acid synthetase (FAS), 96, 263, 266
Fatty acid translocase, 263
Fetectomy, 163-164
Feed efficiency, 21
Feed intake regulation, 265
Feedback regulator-appetite suppression, 5
Feeding behavior, 261, 278
Female rhesus monkeys, 111
Fertility, 68, 150, 277, 342
Fetal adipose tissue, 159, 164, 275-276
 adrenal gland, 163
 circulation, 164
 cortisol, 164
 development, 162
 HPA, 164-165
 leptin levels, 257
 lungs, 162
 pigs, 275-276
 placental units, 159
 programming paradigm, 165
 sheep, 266, 275-277
Fever, 269
Fibrinolysis, 186
Fibroblast growth factor (FGF), 131
First menarche, 281
Fish, 261
Follicle stimulating hormones (FSH), 194
Follicular development, 284
 diameter, 341
 fluid, 158
 phase, 156
Forebrain, 60
Food intake, 55
Free fatty acids, 261
Free leptin, 37, 155, 320
Free thyroxine, 308, 342
Free triiodothyronine, 342
FSH, 107, 152, 158

Galanin, 56, 152
Galanin hypothalamic neurons, 278
Galanin-like peptide (GALP), 59, 152
GALP neurons, 59, 63
Gamma-aminobutyric acid(GABA), 278
Ganglionic blockade, 182-183
Gastric cancer, 200-202, 205
Gastric cells, 200
 leptin infusion, 271-272
 mucosal biopsies, 200
Gastrin, 200
Gastrointestinal, 195, 200
Gastrointestinal tract, 271
Gel electrophoresis, 323
Gemfibrozil, 226
Gender, 34, 151

Gender differences, 165-166
Genetic, 54
 disorders, 305
 models of obesity, 176
Gestational diabetes, 165
Gestational steroids, 162
Ghrelin, 59, 69, 194, 201, 337
Gilt, 277, 281-282
Glomerular filtration, 183-184
Glomerular pathology associated obesity, 184
Glucagon-like peptide (GLP-1), 80-82, 91
Glucocorticoids, 38-39, 129, 164, 253, 255, 273, 279
Glucokinase (GK), 83
Gluconeogenesis, 264
Glucose, 36, 253
Glucose-6-phosphatase (Glc-6-pase), 83
Glucose-dependent insulinotropic polypeptide, 85
Glucose homeostasis, 56, 84
Glucose stimulated insulin secretion, 81
Glucose transporter 4, 336
Glucostatic theory, 5
Glumerosclerosis, 184
Glutamine:fructose amidotransferase, 36
GLUT4, 83
Glycerol phosphate acyltransferase, 262
Glycogen synthesis, 264
Glycosylated hemoglobin, 227
GnRH neurons, 278
GnRH release, 152
gp130 receptor family, 12
Gonadal, 106, 341
 estrogen production, 166
 hormone levels, 341
 steroidogenesis, 166, 280
Gonadectomy-induced bone loss, 142
Gonadotropes, 106-107
Gonadotropin, 151, 158, 161
Gonadotropin-releasing hormone (GnRH), 117, 156
Gonadotropin secretion, 278
Granulocyte-macrophage colony stimulating factor (GM-CSF), 204
Granulosa, 283-284
Grb2, 16, 194
Green fluorescence protein (GFP), 60
Growth hormone (GH), 69, 105, 107, 113-114, 117, 274, 279, 312, 331
Growth hormone releasing hormone (GHRH), 117
Growth plate chondrocytes, 268
Growth of penis and testicles, 331
Growth spurt, 330
Gut, 200, 261

Half-life of leptin, 37
hCG secretion, 161
hCG stimulated testosterone production, 166
Heart, 17, 84
Heart rate, 182-183
Head circumference, 162
Heifer, 277, 281-282

Helicobacter pylori, 201
Hematopoiesis, 126, 203, 326
Hen, 154
Hepatic fibrosis, 348
Hepatic glucose production, 83-84
Hepatic insulin resistance, 326
Hepatic steatosis, 326, 334
Hepatocyte cultures, 264
Heterophilic interference, 323
Heterozygous relatives of our leptin deficient subjects, 311
Hexosamine (UPD-GlcNAc) biosynthesis, 36, 38
High carbohydrate meals, 248
High fat diet, 40, 176, 184, 248
Hindbrain, 60-61
Histochemical staining of testes, 167
HIV lipodystrophy, 222, 232, 349
HIV-1 infection, 133
Homeopoiesis, 269
Homozygous frame shift mutation, 327
Hormonal regulation leptin gene expression, 274
Hormone secretion, 261
HPA axis, 111, 331
HPLC, 320, 323
Humans, 38, 81, 87, 94, 105, 116, 132, 143-144, 160-161, 200, 262, 281-283, 306-307, 349
    adipocytes, 112
    anti-mouse antibodies, 323
    cytotrophoblast cells, 153, 162
    female, 281
    islets, 91
    lipodystrophy, 218, 227, 333
    monocytes, 126
    osteoblast proliferation, 268
    pituitary adenomas, 106, 205
    placental explants, 161
    recombinant leptin, 270
    umbilical endothelial cells, 271
huOb-ra, huOb-rb, 199
Hydrocortisone, 275-276
Hypercorticisterosenemia, 326
Hyperandrogenic, 157
Hypercoagulopathy, 348
Hyperglycemia, 86, 89, 95, 326
Hyperglycemic clamp, 94
Hyperinsulinemia, 84-87, 89, 97, 195-196
Hyperinsulinemic-euglycemic clamps, 36, 86
Hyperinsulinemic glucose clamps, 83
Hyperleptinemia, 84, 165, 185, 196, 229
Hyperphagic, 7, 68, 228, 307
Hyperplasia, 132
Hypertension, 42, 164, 182, 348
Hypertensive men, 185
Hyperthyroid subjects, 109
Hypoglycemia, 68, 80, 261
Hypogonadism, 143, 228, 306
Hypogonadotropic hypogonadism, 306, 330
Hypoinsulinemia, 68, 80
Hypoleptinemic, 90
Hypophysectomized, 275

Hypothalamic, 61, 151, 194, 252
Hypothalamic amenorrhea, 159, 194, 340-342, 349
Hypothalamic arcuate nucleus, 178
Hypothalamic ARC, 68
Hypothalamic hypothyroidism, 312
Hypothalamic lesions, 4, 305
Hypothalamic LHRH pulse generator, 252
Hypothalamic neurons, 110, 180
Hypothalamic NPY neurons, 278
Hypothalamic pituitary function, 38, 111
Hypothalamic pituitary adrenal axis (HPA), 248, 251, 280, 331
Hypothalamic pituitary gonadal (HPG), 251
Hypothalamic pituitary thyroid axis, 38, 68, 106, 108, 309
Hypothalamic SOCS-3 expression, 41
Hypothalamic ventromedial (VMH), 54
Hypothalamus, 54-56, 59-61, 64-65, 67, 69, 97, 105, 111, 152, 156, 278, 346
Hypothermia, 177
Hypothyroid subjects, 109
Hypoxia, 162

ICV, 84
IFNβ, 129
IFNγ, 332, 339
IGF-I, 199, 201, 268, 274-275, 282, 312, 331, 337
IgG2a, 128
IL-2, 128
IL-4, 129
IL-6, 268-269, 277
IL-11, 269
IL-12, 269
Ileum, 271
Immune functions 68, 125-127, 203, 269, 326, 338
Immune homeostasis, 135
Immune suppression, 105, 127-128
Immunity, 229
Immunocompromised hosts, 133
Immunodeficiency, 228, 309
Immunoelectron microscopy, 106
Immunological abnormalities, 326-327, 332
Immunoradiometric Assay (IRMA), 319
Immunoreconstitution, 133
Implantation, 159, 164
Increased arterial pressure, 181
Increased energy expenditure, 6
Infant length, 162
Infertile male patients, 167
Infertility, 20, 157, 167
Inflammation, 125-126, 128, 195
Inflammatory bowel disease (IBD), 131
Inherited lipodystrophy, 218
Initiation of labor, 164
Inner zone of medulla, 184
Insulin, 36, 59, 61, 65, 69, 80, 93, 96, 114, 201, 253, 262, 275
Insulin biosynthesis, 97
Insulin clamp, 83
Insulin-like growth factor-I (IGF-I) 83,195, 279, 342

Insulin mediated neoplasia, 195
Insulin regulation leptin gene expression, 275
Insulin release, 80
Insulin resistance, 7, 79-80, 85, 87, 89, 97, 115, 167, 195, 229, 333
Insulin secretion, 80, 82, 84, 97
Insulin sensitivity, 262, 336
Insulin stimulated glucose uptake, 83
Insulin treatment, 274
Insulinoma, 96
Intense hyperphagia, 306
Intensive 24-h sampling paradigm, 249
Interleukin-6, 182, 199, 259
Intestinal growth, 272
Intracerebral CRH, 181
Intracerebroventricular leptin, 84, 111, 113, 141
Intrafollicular fluid leptin levels, 158
Intraperitoneal leptin in *ob/ob* mice, 85
Intrauterine growth restriction (IUGR), 162, 164
Intravenous infusion of leptin, 181
In vitro fertilization, 157
IRS1, 15
Isoproterenol, 142
IVF patients, 158

Jackson Laboratories, 2-3
JAK/STAT, 14-16, 127, 150, 200
JAK/STAT signal transduction pathway, 40-42
JAK2/STAT3, 15, 62-64, 67
JAK2 activation, 15-16
JAK2 phosphorylation, 63
JAK2 tyrosine kinase, 127
Janus-activated kinases (JAK), 127, 278
Janus kinase/signal transducer, 14, 92, 104
Japanese men, 21
Jejunum, 271

K-ATP channels, 59, 81
Keratinocytes in epidermis, 270
Ketogenesis, 264
Kidney, 42, 181, 195
Koletsky rats, 19, 60, 68

Lactase, 271
Lactating cows, 282-284
Lactating ruminants, 285
Lactotrophs, 107
Large adipocytes, 38
Late embryonic testes, 166
Lateral hypothalamus (LH), 54, 84, 152-153, 159
Leptin, 84, 106-107, 110, 143, 151, 153, 167, 176 227, 257, 274, 281-282
  administration, 183, 260
  adipocyte axis, 126
  analogue, 261
  antibody, 161
  antiserum, 113
  binding proteins, 36, 155, 273
  clearance, 20
  concentration, 322

Leptin concentration:BMI ratio, 158
Leptin deficiency, 182, 307, 311, 330, 349
Leptin deficient children, 307
Leptin dependent increases in NO, 185
Leptin discovery, 149
Leptin gene expression, 273, 275-276
Leptin induced STAT3, 42, 65
Leptin induced sympathoactivation, 177, 180
Leptin pulse amplitude, 258, 273
Leptin pulsatility, 249-252, 273
Leptin radioimmunoassay, 151
Leptin receptors, 11-12, 15-16, 54-55, 61, 81, 104, 164, 176, 261, 263, 270, 277, 283, 312
Leptin receptor deficiency, 312
Leptin receptor expression, 18, 81, 161
Leptin receptor gene, 20
Leptin receptor isoforms, 17, 104
Leptin receptor signaling, 67, 80
Leptin regulation, 115, 162
Leptin resistance, 39-43, 56, 65-66, 70, 80, 87, 90-91, 151, 160, 185, 195, 204, 230, 310, 346
Leptin secretion, 93, 279
Leptin signal transduction, 61
Leptin signaling in hypothalamus, 66, 70
Leptin synthesis, 38, 112
Leptin to insulin, 79
Leptin testes relationship, 168
Leptin transport, 56
Leptin treatment, 7, 144, 330
LEP mRNA, 159, 163, 261
LEP^{ob} neonates, 162
LEPR$_L$, 160, 162
LEPR$_S$, 160, 162
LepR1138 mouse, 18-19
Lesions in hypothalamus, 55
Lesions in VMH, 54
Leukemia, 195, 203
Leukemic promyelocytes, 204
Leydig cells, 167
LH, 60, 63, 65, 107, 156, 282-283
LH pulse frequency, 282
LH secretion, 280
LHRH, 69
Linear bone growth, 268
Linear growth, 114, 326
Lipid metabolism, 261
Lipids, 42
Lipodystrophy, 217-218, 221, 227, 232, 333, 347
Lipodystrophic mice, 7
Lipolysis, 262
Lipostat, 5, 260
Lipostatis theory, 33, 105, 151
Lipotoxicity, 42-43
Litter size, 21
Liver damage, 130
Liver histopathology, 336
Locomotor activity, 18
Long day length, 283
Loss of leptin pattern, 258
Lungs, 17

Lung cancer, 133, 205
Luteal phase, 156-157, 280
Luteal steroidogenesis, 157
Luteinizing, 194, 340
Lymph nodes, 17, 129
Lymphocytes, 131, 332
Lymphoid cells, 127
Lymphoid organs homeostatis, 126
Lymphopoiesis, 203
Lysosomal, 264

Macrophages, 129
Male physiology, 165
Malignant cells, 196
Malnourished humans, 128
Mammary glands, 196, 206
Mandibuloacral dysplasia, 221
MAP-kinase ERK1/2, 271
Mares, 283
Mass spectrometry, 323
Maternal adiposity, 160, 162
Maternal hyperleptinemia, 159
Maternal hypertension, 164
Maternal nutrition, 276-277
Maternal serum leptin, 162
Matrix metalloproteinases, 161
MC4, 58, 108, 143
Meal consumption timing, 248
Median eminence, 40, 152
Medullary cells, 112
Melanin concentrating hormone (MCH), 56, 61, 69, 278, 306
Melanocortin pathway, 141, 180, 182
Melanocortin 3 receptor, 58
Melanocortin 4 receptor, 141, 306
Melanocortin system, 278
Melatonin, 283
Men, 167
Menarche, 330
Menstrual cycle, 156-157
Metabolic complications in obesity, 41, 176
Metabolic mass, 281
Metabolic rate, 6, 85
Metabolic syndrome, 155
Metabolite concentrations, 261
Metastasis, 196
MEK/ERK pathway, 16
Mice, 17, 66, 70, 81, 106, 110, 115, 128, 150, 161, 270, 278, 281
Microvascular complications of diabetes, 348
Milk leptin concentrations, 285
Mitochondrial β-oxidation, 265
Mitrogen activated protein kinase (MAPK),115, 128, 150, 197-198
Monkeys, 153
Monoamines, 180
Monochorionic twin pregnancies, 162
Monocytes/macrophages, 128, 203
Monogenic disorders, 306, 312
Monosodium glutamate, 108

Morbid obesity, 20, 38, 327-329
Motility of duodenum, 272
Motility of jejunum, 272
Mouse islet, 80
Mouse placenta, 160-161
Mouse soleus muscle, 265
MPOA, 68
mRNA, 92, 106, 108, 115, 152, 159, 261, 274
Multi species RIA, 321
Multiple sclerosis, 129
Murine leptin deficiency, 307
Murine models of lipodystrophy, 333
Murine C_2C_{12} myogenic cell cultures, 264
Murine lipodystrophy, 218, 223
Myeloid development, 203
Myocardial hypertrophy, 185
Myocardium, 185
Myocyte hypertrophy, 185

Narcolepsy, 349
Natural killer (NK) cells, 127-128, 332
Neonatal pigs, 267
Neonatal sheep, 266
Neonatal samples, 166
Neonatal skeletal growth, 261
Neuroendocrine functions of leptin, 68
Neuroendocrine regulation, 200, 337
Neuroendocrine response fasting, 106
Neuroendocrinology, 55
Neurotensin, 56
Neuropeptide Y, 18, 56, 116, 151, 180, 194, 253
Neutrophils, 127-128
New Zealand obese mouse model, 19
Nitric oxide (NO), 183, 229
Nonalcoholic hepatic steatosis (NASH), 336, 349
Nonconservative mis-sense leptin gene mutation, 328
Nonhodgkins lymphoma, 21, 132-133
Nonhuman, 152, 155, 160
Nonhuman primates, 178
Norepinephrine, 177, 182
Normal biosynthesis, 309
Normal ejaculatory patterns, 331
Normal fetal pituitary, 106
NOS, 152
NPY, 58, 60-61, 63, 67, 194, 229, 253, 278
NT, 60, 67
Nucleus tractus solitarius (NTS), 60
N-telopeptides, 338
N-terminal leptin fragment, 320

Ob protein, 6
Obese agouti mice, 42
Obese (*ob*) genes, 3
  cloning and sequencing, 5
Obese humans, 41, 66, 87, 89, 113, 311, 349
Obese (*ob/ob*) mouse 1, 2, 4-6, 11, 18, 54, 56, 60 68, 80-81, 85, 91, 114, 130, 150, 154, 182, 185 186,265, 268, 271, 277,278, 306,307, 332, 342

ob/ob, 128, 140, 270
ob/ob mouse islets, 91
Obese men, 167
Obese subjects, 38, 158, 342, 346
Obesity, 4, 20, 34, 54, 79, 86, 116, 132, 158, 165 196, 201, 203, 205, 228, 252
Obesity hormone, 5
Obesity hypertension, 176, 182
ObR, 14, 20, 61, 63
- a, b, c, d, e, f, l, 14-20, 42-43, 55, 92, 104
Obesity induced renal damage, 184
ObRb knockout mouse, 18-19
ObRb mRNA, 105, 195
Ocytocin antagonist, 61
Oestradiol, 131
Onset of puberty, 281
Orexigenic, 55-56, 61
Orexin, 56, 58, 63, 278
Osteoblasts, 139, 142, 162, 195, 268, 338
Osteocalcin, 268-269, 338, 342
Osteoclasts, 142, 162, 338
Osteoporosis, 139, 142-143
Osteoprotegerin, 268
Otsuka Long-Evans Tokushima Fatty (OLETF) rat, 86
Ovarian, 159, 195, 198, 261, 341
Ovarian cancer cell lines, 198
Ovarian dysfunction, 158
Ovarian function, 261
Ovarian steroids, 157
Ovarian surface epithelium, 198
Ovarian volume, 341
Ovariectomized prepubertal gilt, 280
Ovariectomized rats, 269
Ovariectomy, 153, 157
Ovariectomy-induced bone loss, 140
Ovary, 277
Overexpressing leptin, 182
Overfeeding, 323
Ovine pregnancy, 164
Ovulation in female mice, 106
Ovulation induction, 153, 157, 349
Oxidative enzymes, 263
Oxidative stress, 42, 182
Oxygen consumption, 265
Oxygen radicals, 127
Oxytocin, 60-61

P cells, 272
Pancreastatin release, HP75 cells, 107
Pancreatic β–cell, 80-81, 87, 89-91, 97
Pancreatic islets, 80, 229
Parabiosis, 3, 4, 33, 54, 305
Paraventricular nuclei (PVN), 54, 108, 309
PC-3, 199
Passive immunization against leptin, 284
Pegylated recombinant leptin, 41, 343, 345
Peripheral metabolism, 260
Peroxisome proliferator activated receptor (PPAR), 262
Pepsinogen, 200
Perfused rat pancreas, 80
Perfused rodent liver, 264
Peripheral blood mononuclear cells, 327
Peripubertal male rhesus monkey, 153
Perirenal adipose tissue, 275
PFH, 65
Phagocytosis, 128
Phenotypes associated leptin deficiency, 310
Phosphatase SHP2, 16
Phosphatidylinositol-3 kinase (PI3K)-phosphodiesterase 3B (PDE3B)-cAMP pathway, 64, 67, 70, 104
Phosphoenolpyruvate carboxykinase (*PEPCK*) 83
Phosphoinositol-3 kinase, 104
Phosphorylated leptin receptor, 15
Phosphorylation of JAK2, 63
Physiological breast cells, 196
Pig studies, 277
Pigs, 21, 154, 272, 274, 278, 280-281
Pimi Indians, 20
Pituitary, 151, 154, 156
Pituitary adrenal function, 249
Pituitary gland, 277
Pituitary TSH secretion, 337
Placenta, 17, 150, 154, 159-160, 162-164
Placental estrogens, 162
Placental leptin mRNA, 162
Plasma concentration, 177
Plasma cortisol, 111
Plasma glucose, 83
Plasma IGF-1, 114
Plasma insulin, 311-312
Plasma leptin, 66, 249, 258
Plasminogen activator inhibitor-1 activity, 186
Platelet aggregation, 42
Polycystic ovarian syndrome (PCOS), 157-158
Polymorphisms, 20
Polymorphonuclear neutrophils (PMN), 203
Polyps, 201
POMC gene, 278
POMC neurons, 58-59, 61, 63, 65, 67
Porcine, 152, 164, 263-264, 283
Porcine adipocyte culture, 264
Porcine aortic smooth muscle cells, 271
Porcine hepatocytes, 264
Postmenopausal, 142, 196
Potassium excretion, 184
Poultry, 270
PPAR, 96, 262
PPARα, 262
PPARγ, 221, 262
Preadipocytes, 273-274-5
Preclampsia, 164-165
Pregnancy, 20-21, 150, 154, 158-159
Pregnancy associated diabetes, 165
Premature pubarche, 155
Preovulatory follicle, 158-159
Preproinsulin gene expression, 97

Prepubertal gilt, 280
Prepubertal Leydig cells, 166
Pressor effects of leptin, 182-183
Primary culture, 94
Primary immunodeficiency syndrome, 349
Primate, 278
Primate pregnancy, 161
Primate trophoblast, 153
Progesterone, 153, 157
Proinflammatory cytokines, 182, 203
Proinflammatory mediators, 128, 132
Proinsulin mRNA, 81, 90-91
Prolactin, 69, 131, 152, 263
Prolactin-releasing peptide (PrRP), 59
Prolactin secretion, 283
Proopiomelanocortin, 18, 116, 180, 229
Proopiomelanocortin neurons (POMC), 56, 60, 278
Propranolol, 141
Prostaglandins, 161
Prostate cancer human, 195, 198-200, 206
Protein synthesis, 263
Protein tyrosine phosphatase PTP1B, 41, 63
Proteinuria, 184
Proteolytic systems, 264
Psuedomonas aeruginosa exotoxin A, 130
Pubertal development, 308, 330, 342
Puberty in humans, 68, 150, 155
Puberty in mice, 68, 154
Pulsatile, 111, 247-248
Pulsatile leptin secretion, 322
Pulse amplitude, 273
Pulse frequency, 273
Pulses of secretion, 248
PVN, 60-61
PI3K, 65, 67, 128, 180
P38 MAPK, 198

Q223R mutation, 20-21

Rabbit, 176, 261, 265
Rabbit chondrocytes, 267
Rabson Mendenhall syndrome, 340
Radical prostatectomy, 199
Radiotherapy, 196
Ram, 282
RANKL, 142-143
Rat, 17, 66, 70, 81, 83, 95-96, 150, 154, 164, 178, 181, 263, 272, 278, 283
Rat chondrocytes, 267
Rat epididymal adipocytes, 110
Rat models, 4
Rat pregnancy, 160
Rat testes, 166
Reactive oxygen species, 182
Receptor coupled inhibitory G protein, 262
Receptor isoforms, 12, 14
Recombinant murine leptin, 84, 106, 109, 111
Recombinant methionyl-human leptin, 227, 327, 335, 337, 339, 342, 346-349
Recombinant ovine leptin, 262

Recombinant rhesus leptin, 153
Rectal cancer, 202
Reduced food intake, 6, 141
Relative hypoleptinemia, 311
Renal cancer, 205
Renal effects of leptin, 184
Renal sympathetic outflow, 180
Reproduction, 19, 105, 149, 158, 194, 228, 277, 326
Reprductive dysfunction, 337
Reproductive function, 277
Reproductive hormone, 38
Reproductive neuroendocrinology, 68
Resistance to leptin, 179
Resistant tuberculosis, 133
Resting metabolic rate, 312
Restored T3, T4, 109
Rhesus monkey, 155
Rhesus pubertal development, 156
Rheumatoid factors, 323
rho/rac, 15
Ritonavir, 226
Rodent adipocytes, 38, 43, 112
Rodent leptin assays, 321
Rodent models of obesity, 41
Rodent pituitary, 107
Rodent pregnancy, 160
Rodents, 38, 94, 105, 110, 116, 165, 200, 257, 262-263, 278, 281, 306
Rommey Marsh sheep, 283
Rosiglitazone, 226
Ruminants, 261

Salivary glands, 200
Sandwich ELISA for canine leptin, 321
Satiety, 150, 337
Satiety factor, 4-5
Satiety signal, 34
Seasonal reproduction, 282
Secretin, 272
Selective leptin resistance, 41, 179, 182
Semen leptin concentrations, 167
Seminal plasma, 167
Seminiferous tubules, 167
Sepsis, 258
Serine kinase ERK, 15
Serotonins, 56
Serum, 285
Serum corticosterone, 111
Serum insulin, 282
Serum leptin, 36
Serum leptin levels, 37, 111
Serum leptin binding protein, 36
Serum osteocalcin, 338
Serum testosterone, 168
Severe burns, 259
Sex differences, 255, 257
Sex steroid concentrations, 330
Sexual dimorphism, 131, 257
Sexually immature rats, 166

SF-1, 166
Sheep, 130, 154, 261, 270, 283
Short day lengths, 283
Short-term fasting, 37, 105
Siberian hamster, 283
Signaling pathways, 15
Signal transducer/activator of transcription (STAT) 3, 57, 104, 127
Simivistatin, 21
Skeletal maturation, 114
Skeletal muscle, 84, 263-266
Skin, 84
Sleep apnea, 21, 349
Sleep duration, 259
Small adipocytes, 38
Small intestine, 271
Soay rams, 283
Solid tumor, 196
Soluable binding-protein, 13
Soluable circulating leptin receptor (solLEPR), 150, 160-161
Soluable leptin receptor, 21, 163, 320
Somatropes, 106-107
Somatostatin (SS), 113, 117, 200
SOCS, 92
SOCS3, 15, 18, 43, 58, 63, 66, 92, 127
SOCS3-expression, 40
SOCS3 protein, 63
Spleen, 17, 84
Splenic T cells, 130
Spine ossification, 21
Starved animals, 128
Starvation, 105, 107, 110, 116
STAT1, 15
STAT3, 15, 18-19, 43, 57, 63, 66, 104, 115, 270-271
STAT5, 15
STAT6, 16
STAT signaling, 180
Steroid hormones, 153, 156
Steroid synthesis, 284
Steroidogenesis in bovine granulose, 284
Steroidogenic acute regulatory protein (StAR), 166, 284
Steroidogenic pathway, 166
Stomach, 200, 272
Streptozotocin, 95
Streptozotocin (STZ)-induced diabetic rats, 86
Stromal cells, 195
Subclinical hypothyroidism, 308
Subcutaneous adipose tissue, 34, 163, 262, 275
Subcutaneous fat, 163
Subcutaneous injections of leptin, 307
Subcutaneous insulin implants, 95
Surfactant synthesis, 162
Suppressor of cytokine signaling-3 (SOCS3), 58
Swine, 261-263, 267, 269-270, 273
Sympathetic nervous system, 42, 139, 143, 176-178
Sympathoactivation, 177, 179
Syncytiotrophoblast, 163

T cells, 127, 270, 307
T lymphocytes, 195, 203
Temperature, 282
Testes, 166-167
Testicular *Lepr* mRNA, 166
Testosterone, 35, 38, 106, 151, 155, 166-167
TGFβ, 268, 274
Th1 differentiation, 129
Th1- and Th2-type cytokines, 129, 309
Theca cells, 283
Thermogenic brown adipose tissue, 42
Thermogenesis, 105, 265
Thermoregulation, 18, 261, 311
Thiazolidinediones, 93
Thrombi formation, 186
Thrombosis, 42
Thrombosis and leptin, 186
Thrombospondin-1, 132
Thymic atrophy, 127, 203
Thymic maturation, 129
Thymic size, 129
Thymic T cells, 128
Thymocytes, 129
Thyroid, 106, 109-110
Thyroid function, 18, 38, 107, 331
Thyroid hormone, 105, 110
Thyroid-releasing hormone (TRH) 59, 69, 108, 117
Thyroid thermogenesis, 228
Thyroglobulin mRNA expression, 110
Thyroxine (T4), 275-276
Timing of sample collection, 322
Tissue distribution, 16
Tissue plasminogen activator activity, 186
TNFά, 38, 115, 134, 339
Total leptin, 323
Transgenic mouse models, 7, 63, 182
Transplantation of adipose tissue, 7, 230
TRH biosynthesis, 309
TRH secretion, 309
Triglyceride fatty acid cycling, 265
Triglycerides, 40, 227, 265
Trophoblast, 159, 165
Trophoblast-derived BeWo cells, 165
TSH induced iodide uptake, 110
TSH levels, 308
TSH positive cells, 107
TSH pulsatility, 108
TSH rhythm, 109
T lymphocyte function, 126
Tumor growth and progression, 132
Tumor necrosis factor (TNF), 128-130, 182, 259
Turkey, 21
Twin pregnancies, 160
Two-site sandwich immunoassays, 319
Type 1 CGL, 219
Type 2 CGL, 219
Type 1 cytokine, 125
Type 2 diabetes, 80, 87, 89, 97, 167, 329, 346, 349

Tyrosine kinase receptor, 15
T3 and T4 levels, 346

Ubiquitin Ub-ATP dependent, 264
UCP, 267
Ultradian oscillations, 248-249
Umbilical cord blood, 162
Umbilical vasculature, 160
Uncoupling protein, 266
Urine free cortisol, 111
Uterine endometrium, 161

Vagal stimulation, 272
Vascular endothelial cells, 268, 271
Vascular endothelial growth factor (VEGF), 131, 162, 195
Ventromedial hypothalamus (VMH), 84, 278
Ventromedial nucleus (VMN), 55, 61, 63
Viable blastocyst, 161
Villous tissue, 160, 163
Visceral adipose tissue mass, 34

Weight gain, 37, 176
Weight loss, 37
White adipose tissue, 84, 93
Women, 165
Wortmannin, 180
Wounds healing, 131, 270-271, 326, 349

Zucker rat, 176, 184

α-melanocyte stimulating hormone, 56, 58, 229, 278
β-agonists, 93
β-cell, 81-82
γ-aminobutyric acid (GABA), 58
γ-MSH, 278
2-deoxyglucose, 265
3rd ventricle, 61
3T3-L1 cells, 112
11β-hydroxysteroid dehydrogenase, 39, 112
50 kDa, 161
P450scc, 166